Eating Disorders

Eating Disorders

Editor: Lewis Humphries

FOSTER ACADEMICS
www.fosteracademics.com

www.fosteracademics.com

FOSTER ACADEMICS

Cataloging-in-Publication Data

Eating disorders / edited by Lewis Humphries.
p. cm.
Includes bibliographical references and index.
ISBN 978-1-63242-502-7
1. Eating disorders. 2. Eating disorders--Treatment. 3. Eating disorders in adolescence.
4. Eating disorders in children. I. Humphries, Lewis.
RC552.E18 E28 2017
616.852 6--dc23

Foster Academics,
118-35 Queens Blvd., Suite 400,
Forest Hills, NY 11375, USA

ISBN 978-1-63242-502-7 (Hardback)

Printed and bound in China.

Contents

Preface

This book has been a concerted effort by a group of academicians, researchers and scientists, who have contributed their research works for the realization of the book. This book has materialized in the wake of emerging advancements and innovations in this field. Therefore, the need of the hour was to compile all the required researches and disseminate the knowledge to a broad spectrum of people comprising of students, researchers and specialists of the field.

This book on eating disorders discusses the environmental, psychosocial and physiological factors that cause eating disorders. Symptoms of the various disorders that comprise this condition include milder physical complaints to more serious physiological problems. This book includes some of the vital pieces of work being conducted across the world, on various topics related to eating disorders. This book provides significant information of this discipline to help develop a good understanding of eating disorders and related fields. A number of latest researches have been included to keep the readers up-to-date with the global concepts in this area of study. It will serve as a valuable source of reference for graduate and post graduate students.

At the end of the preface, I would like to thank the authors for their brilliant chapters and the publisher for guiding us all-through the making of the book till its final stage. Also, I would like to thank my family for providing the support and encouragement throughout my academic career and research projects.

Editor

Stigmatizing attitudes towards individuals with anorexia nervosa: an investigation of attribution theory

Kristy Zwickert* and Elizabeth Rieger

Abstract

Background: Guided by Attribution Theory, this study assessed stigmatizing attitudes towards an individual with anorexia nervosa (AN) compared to obesity and skin cancer, and examined the extent to which manipulating a target individual's level of blameworthiness affects levels of stigmatizing attitudes. One hundred and thirty-five female undergraduate students were randomly assigned to one of three conditions. Before and after receiving blameworthy or non-blameworthy information relating to the target's condition, participants completed a series of self-report inventories measuring their emotional reactions, desire for social distance, and causal attributions regarding the target.

Results: Participants reported a significantly greater desire for social distance from the target with AN compared to targets with obesity or skin cancer, and yet (contrary to Attribution Theory) attributed less blame to the target with AN. There were significant increases in stigmatization towards targets described as blameworthy relative to targets described as non-blameworthy.

Conclusion: The findings provide insight into the elevated levels of stigmatizing attitudes held towards individuals with AN, and the role of Attribution Theory in partially accounting for this stigma.

Keywords: Stigmatization, Attribution theory, Blameworthy, Anorexia nervosa, Eating disorders

Background

Research investigating attitudes towards mental illness indicates that stigmatization is widespread [1-3]. Until recently, mental illness stigma research has focused primarily on conditions such as schizophrenia and depression, to the neglect of other psychological disorders [1]. In particular, stigma towards individuals with anorexia nervosa (AN) has received little empirical attention.

Anorexia nervosa is primarily characterized by a relentless pursuit of thinness resulting in weight loss substantially below a normal body weight [4] that predominantly affects young women [5], with a lifetime prevalence rate of approximately 1.9% and an additional 2.4% who partially meet the criteria for the disorder [6]. The disorder is often associated with a poor outcome, including a significantly elevated mortality rate, with a recent meta-analysis providing an estimate of 5.10 deaths per 1000 person-years [7]. Investigating the prevalence, characteristics, and triggers of stigmatizing attitudes towards AN is therefore an important area of research as stigma may impact on outcome. For instance, stigma has been shown to act as a barrier to accessing treatment in individuals with other forms of eating disorder psychopathology (e.g., bulimia nervosa, binge eating disorder, and eating disorder not otherwise specified) [8,9] and may also prolong the recovery process and increase the chance of relapse [10].

Attribution Theory [11] has been widely investigated in an attempt to understand the bases of stigmatizing attitudes held towards those with a mental illness. This theory asserts that when an individual's illness is attributed to forces within his/her control,

* Correspondence: Kristy.Zwickert@anu.edu.au
Research School of Psychology (Building 39), Australian National University, Canberra, ACT 0200, Australia

the person is likely to be held responsible for their condition, and subsequently stigmatized [12]. A number of studies informed by Attribution Theory have documented the existence of a lay perception that mental illnesses are more personally controllable than medical conditions [13] and hence may attract higher levels of stigmatizing attitudes. Medical conditions (e.g., cancer) are more likely to be perceived as onset-uncontrollable, and elicit pity and a willingness to help, whereas psychological disorders are often perceived as onset-controllable, and elicit anger and neglect [11].

Despite the scarcity of research in the area, preliminary evidence suggests that stigmatization of individuals with AN does exist [14,15]. These stigmatizing attitudes have been found to be prevalent among the general public [16], medical and nursing staff [17], and university students [18]. In accordance with Attribution Theory, individuals with AN are often perceived as being responsible for the onset of their illness and as having a significant amount of control over their eating disordered behaviours [19,20]. Such attributions of controllability have been identified in two college-aged samples. In the first, approximately two-thirds of female respondents agreed that individuals with AN only have themselves to blame for their condition [21]. In the second mixed-gender sample, attributing greater levels of responsibility for the development of AN was associated with higher stigmatizing attitudes towards the individual with the condition [22]. It has also been suggested that individuals exposed to sociocultural versus medical causal accounts are more likely to hold individuals with AN responsible for their condition [23] and demonstrate less willingness to provide assistance to individuals with AN [24]. However, research to date on Attribution Theory and stigma in the context of AN is limited by the preponderance of correlational methodologies, with experimental paradigms needed to provide more definitive support for the role of blame-based accounts in causing stigmatizing attitudes.

In contrast to the paucity of research on AN, stigma towards another weight condition – namely, obesity – has received a significant amount of research attention [25]. Obesity stigmatization has been described as extremely pervasive to the extent that, "negative attitudes towards obese people constitute one of the last socially acceptable forms of discrimination" [26]. The rising prevalence of obesity does not appear to have attenuated stigmatizing attitudes towards obese individuals. In fact, these attitudes may be on the increase [27].

Preliminary research suggests that levels of stigma may be equivalent towards individuals with AN and obesity. Specifically, an early study found that participants of high school and university age demonstrated comparable levels of rejection towards individuals with AN and obese individuals (although no significance testing was undertaken) [15]. As such, the obesity literature may be useful in advancing understandings of AN stigma. Stigmatization towards obese individuals draws further parallels with AN stigma in that negative attitudes occur in the context of beliefs about controllability and personal responsibility (i.e., for excess body weight) [25]. For instance, among a sample of respondents from six nations, attributions of controllability (together with holding a negative view of fatness) predicted stigmatizing attitudes towards obese people [28]. Given that perceptions of blameworthiness and personal control appear to be common towards both obesity and AN, it seems appropriate to draw on the expansive body of obesity stigma literature to more clearly define the levels and potential causes of stigmatizing attitudes held towards individuals with AN.

The present study aimed to investigate (i) the relative level of stigma towards individuals with AN and (ii) primarily through the use of an experimental design, the factors that may account for the existence of stigmatizing attitudes. Obesity was selected as a point of comparison as it is a weight condition with a substantial research base of documented negative attitudes and behaviours towards obese individuals. Skin cancer was selected as a control group against which to identify elevated levels of stigma towards individuals with AN given that medical conditions have been found to be associated with lower levels of stigma compared to psychological disorders. For example, participants in one community-based study reported a greater willingness to interact with an individual described as having skin cancer compared to an individual described as having schizophrenia or major depression [29]. Skin cancer also lends itself to a blame-based manipulation given that behavioural factors (such as sun exposure) are implicated in the etiology of the condition.

In line with Attribution Theory, it was hypothesized that AN (a mental illness) would be associated with significantly higher levels of blame and stigmatizing attitudes compared to skin cancer (a medical condition) and comparable levels to that of obesity (a highly stigmatized weight condition). Additionally, and also in accordance with Attribution Theory, it was hypothesized that, after reading a causal explanation of the condition, participants exposed to blame-based accounts would report greater increases in levels of stigma compared to participants exposed to non-blame-based causal accounts irrespective of the type of condition (i.e., AN, obesity or skin cancer).

Methods

Participants

One hundred and fifty-two female undergraduate students from the Australian National University (ANU) were recruited through flyers posted on campus. AN predominantly affects young women between 16 and 24 years of age [5]. Thus, the inclusion criteria required participants to be 24 years or younger as the attitudes held by peers of individuals with AN were the primary focus of this study. Seventeen participants were excluded for incomplete responses or exceeding the age criterion. The final sample consisted of 135 participants, with a mean age of 19.78 years (*SD* = 1.27; Range = 18–23). Participants self-identified as Caucasian (58.6%) or Asian (41.4%). These figures approximate the composition of the Australian population, in that the two largest ethnic groups are represented [30]. The study received ethical approval from the ANU's Human Research Ethics Committee and informed consent was obtained from all participants.

Design

The study employed a 3 (AN, obesity, or skin cancer) × 2 (blameworthy versus non-blameworthy) × 2 (time 1 versus time 2) factorial design. The dependent variables consisted of stigmatizing attitudes (i.e., emotional reactions and desire for social distance) in regards to the target individual and causal attributions regarding the target's condition.

Measures

Participants completed the Affective Reaction Scale (ARS) [31] to assess their emotional reactions towards the target individual. The ARS consists of 10 bipolar items (e.g., apprehensive versus comfortable), with higher scores indicating more positive emotional reactions. Cronbach's alpha for the ARS in the present sample was .82.

Social Distance Scales (SDS) are commonly used in stigma research as a proxy measure of behavioural stigmatization towards individuals with a mental illness [32]. Participants completed the SDS [31] to assess their willingness to have social contact (e.g., live in a share house) with the target individual. An additional item was included to measure participants' willingness to engage in more intimate social interactions with the target (i.e., have as a close personal friend). Each of the eight items was presented on a four-point Likert scale (where 0 = 'definitely unwilling' and 3 = 'definitely willing'), with higher scores indicating a greater willingness to have social contact with the target individual. Cronbach's alpha for the SDS in the present study was .92.

To assess causal attributions, four items relating to genetic factors, social influences, parental influences, and personal choice [33] were each presented on a seven-point Likert scale (ranging from 1 = 'did not contribute at all' to 7 = 'was the main causal factor'). Participants were asked to "rate the extent to which you think the following factors contributed to the development of (the condition) in Kelly". A fifth item (also presented on a seven-point Likert scale) measured the extent to which participants perceived the target to be blameworthy for her condition.

Materials

Two vignettes (A and B) were developed for the AN, obesity, and skin cancer conditions. The information contained in each vignette is outlined in the Appendix. Vignette A outlined the target individual's medical, cognitive, social, and emotional problems. These problems were selected so as to be veridical representations of each condition while also being comparable across conditions. Vignette B either described the target as being responsible for her condition (blameworthy group) or the target's condition as being largely due to genetic influences (non-blameworthy group). For example, the blameworthy AN vignette depicted the target as deliberately choosing to restrict her food intake and exercise excessively, ignoring support from friends and family, and disregarding advice from her doctor and dietitian. In contrast, the non-blameworthy AN vignette described the target as feeling compelled to restrict her eating, having a strong family history of the illness, actively engaging in psychotherapy, and attempting to consume larger portions of food despite intense feelings of anxiety. The vignettes were approximately 150 words in length and were designed to be comparable in their descriptions of symptom severity regardless of whether they were describing a target with AN, obesity or skin cancer.

A series of pilot studies were conducted in which the vignettes were sequentially modified based on feedback from pilot participants. Data from the final pilot study indicated that, as desired, all three versions of Vignette A were equivalent in terms of perceived severity of the condition (i.e., on a 7-point scale of severity, a score of 6.5 for the AN, 6.5 for the obesity, and 6.3 for the skin cancer vignettes). In addition, the blameworthy versions of Vignette B elicited stronger attributions of blame (i.e., on a 7-point scale of blameworthiness, a score of 4.6 for the AN, 5 for the obesity, and 6 for the skin cancer vignettes) compared to the non-blameworthy versions of Vignette B (i.e., on a 7-point scale of blameworthiness, a score of 2 for the AN, 3.5 for the obesity, and 3.9 for the skin cancer vignettes).

Procedure

Participants were randomly assigned to one of six experimental groups: AN blameworthy; AN non-blameworthy; obesity blameworthy; obesity non-blameworthy; skin cancer blameworthy; or skin cancer non-blameworthy. Participants began by reading Vignette A that described the target's ("Kelly's") symptoms (relating to AN, obesity or skin cancer). Participants then completed a series of self-report inventories assessing their attitudes towards the target in terms of levels of stigma (i.e., the Affective Reaction Scale and the Social Distance Scale) and causal attributions (i.e., genetic factors, social influences, parental influences, personal choice, and overall levels of blameworthiness). The participants were then asked to read Vignette B in which the target was described as either blameworthy or non-blameworthy for her condition. The measures assessing stigmatizing attitudes and levels of blameworthiness were then re-administered. Finally, participants provided demographic information including age, ethnicity, and country of birth. Height and weight were also collected to calculate Body Mass Index (BMI = kg/m^2).

Statistical analysis

Differences in age and BMI across conditions were assessed using one-way between-groups analysis of variance (ANOVA). A series of planned contrasts were undertaken to determine whether there were significant differences in stigmatizing attitudes (i.e., the ARS and SDS) and causal attributions between the AN and obesity conditions, and between the AN and skin cancer conditions after reading Vignette A. Difference scores were calculated by subtracting Time 1 scores (after reading Vignette A) from Time 2 scores (after reading Vignette B) for both the ARS and the SDS. Positive difference scores indicated that participants showed an increase in positive emotional and behavioural reactions towards the target from Time 1 to Time 2. A series of planned contrasts were then conducted to investigate the hypotheses that: (i) participants in the blameworthy groups would report significantly greater increases in stigmatizing attitudes from Time 1 (after reading Vignette A) to Time 2 (after reading Vignette B) than the non-blameworthy groups as indexed by mean difference scores on the ARS and SDS; and (ii) there would be no significant interactions between type of condition and level of blameworthiness on ARS and SDS mean difference scores. Confidence intervals were calculated for all analyses and the significance level (two-tailed) was set at $p < 0.05$.

Results

Sample characteristics

A one-way between-groups ANOVA revealed no significant differences between the six groups in terms of mean age (M = 19.78, SD = 1.27), $t_{(132)}$ = 1.727, p = .182, and BMI (M = 21.9, SD = 4.75), $t_{(132)}$ = 1.068, p = .347. As such, age and BMI were not controlled for in subsequent analyses.

Time 1 levels of stigmatizing attitudes across conditions

Planned contrasts were used to compare Time 1 scores on the ARS and SDS across conditions. Consistent with the hypotheses, there was no significant difference in mean scores on the ARS in the AN compared to the obesity condition, $t_{(132)}$ = −1.304, p = .194, 95% CI [−6.31, 1.19]. Yet participants reported significantly lower mean scores on the SDS in the AN compared to the obesity condition, $t_{(132)}$ = −2.981, p = .003, 95% CI [−5.43, -1.01], indicating a greater desire for social distance from the target with AN compared to the obese target. Contrary to hypotheses, there was no significant difference in mean scores on the ARS in the AN compared to the skin cancer condition, $t_{(132)}$ = −1.885, p = .062, 95% CI [−7.63, .33]. As expected, participants reported a significantly lower mean score on the SDS in the AN as compared to the skin cancer condition, $t_{(132)}$ = −2.925, p = .004, 95% CI [−5.23, -.97], indicating a greater desire for social distance in the former relative to the latter. Table 1 outlines the mean scores on the ARS and SDS across the three conditions.

Time 1 levels of causal attributions across conditions

Contrary to expectations, planned contrasts revealed significant differences in levels of blame attributed to the AN versus obese target, with the obese target eliciting significantly higher mean blame scores compared to the AN target, $t_{(132)}$ = −3.811,

Table 1 Mean (SD) scores on causal attribution scales across the three conditions

Dependent variable		Disorder		
		Anorexia nervosa n = 48	Obesity n = 42	Skin cancer n = 45
ARS	*M*	38.96	41.52	42.60
	(*SD*)	(9.31)	(8.48)	(10.02)
SDS	*M*	13.54	16.76	16.64
	(*SD*)	(5.49)	(4.99)	(4.80)
Blame	*M*	3.33	4.48	3.27
	(*SD*)	(1.58)	(1.04)	(1.54)
Genetic influences	*M*	4.08	4.86	4.89
	(*SD*)	(1.40)	(1.20)	(1.30)
Social influences	*M*	6.15	5.48	5.07
	(*SD*)	(.92)	(1.04)	(1.37)
Parental influences	*M*	4.65	5.12	3.51
	(*SD*)	(1.34)	(1.19)	(1.77)
Personal Choice	*M*	5.04	5.64	5.42
	(*SD*)	(1.60)	(1.10)	(1.10)

$p < .001$, 95% CI [−1.72, -.58]. Also unexpectedly, there was no significant difference on mean blame scores in the AN versus the skin cancer condition, $t_{(132)} = .226$, $p = .821$, 95% CI [−.60, .72]. Similar results were obtained for the degree to which the condition was attributed to personal choice. Specifically, the mean personal choice score was significantly higher for obesity as compared to AN, $t_{(132)} = -2.191$, $p = .030$, 95% CI [−1.18, -.02], but not significantly different for the AN and skin cancer targets, $t_{(132)} = -1.413$, $p = .160$, 95% CI [−.96, .20].

Mean scores for the degree to which the condition was attributed to genetic influences were significantly lower for the AN target compared to both the obese and skin cancer targets, $t_{(132)} = -2.804$, $p = .006$, 95% CI [−1.33, -.23] and $t_{(132)} = -2.972$, $p = .004$, 95% CI [−1.38, -.24] respectively. The AN target received significantly higher attributions of social influence than both the obese and skin cancer targets, $t_{(132)} = 2.816$, $p = .006$, 95% CI [.26, 1.08] and $t_{(132)} = 4.620$, $p < .001$, 95% CI [.60, 1.56]. Mean parental influence scores were not significantly different for the AN and obesity targets, $t_{(132)} = -1.536$, $p = .127$, 95% CI [−1.00, .06], but were significantly higher for the AN target compared to the skin cancer target, $t_{(132)} = 3.751$, $p < .001$, 95% CI [.49, 1.79]. Mean scores on the causal attribution scales across the three conditions are shown in Table 1.

Changes (from Time 1 to Time 2) in levels of stigmatizing attitudes following exposure to blame-based attributions

As a manipulation check for the induction of blame-based attributions, mean difference scores for levels of blame were calculated to index the change from Time 1 (after reading Vignette A) to Time 2 (after reading Vignette B). Planned contrasts revealed that Vignette B was effective in altering perceptions of blameworthiness. That is, after reading Vignette B, participants in the blameworthy groups reported significantly greater increases in levels of blame compared to participants in the non-blameworthy groups, $t_{(129)} = -8.635$, $p < .001$, 95% CI [−1.95, -2.11]. There was no significant interaction on blame difference scores between levels of blameworthiness and the AN versus obesity groups, $t_{(129)} = .487$, $p = .627$, 95% CI [−.43, .71], nor between levels of blameworthiness and the AN versus skin cancer groups, $t_{(129)} = .314$, $p = .754$, 95% CI [−.47, .65]. These results suggest that the successful manipulation of blameworthiness in the blameworthy versus non-blameworthy groups was comparable across conditions. Mean blame difference scores across the six experimental groups are presented in Table 2.

Mean difference scores on the ARS and SDS across the six experimental groups are also shown in Table 2. As predicted, planned contrasts revealed significant differences between the blameworthy and non-blameworthy groups on mean ARS and SDS difference scores, $t_{(129)} = 8.788$, $p < .001$, 95% CI [11.74, 13.08] and $t_{(129)} = 9.099$, $p < .001$, 95% CI [5.43, 6.03] respectively. As shown in Figure 1, after reading Vignette B, participants in the blameworthy

Table 2 Mean (SD) difference scores on the blame scale, ARS and SDS across the six experimental groups

Difference scores		Blame					
		Blameworthy			Non-blameworthy		
		AN[1] n = 26	OB[2] n = 22	SC[3] n = 22	AN[1] n = 22	OB[2] n = 20	SC[3] n = 23
Blame Scale	*M*	1.19	1.45	1.18	-.68	-.70	-.87
	(*SD*)	(1.27)	(1.06)	(1.50)	(1.46)	(1.08)	(1.66)
ARS	*M*	−5.50	−10.95	−2.41	6.77	7.85	3.74
	(*SD*)	(7.31)	(10.08)	(8.95)	(7.11)	(6.05)	(8.84)
SDS	*M*	−3.58	−5.91	−2.27	2.50	1.15	1.78
	(*SD*)	(2.55)	(5.18)	(4.03)	(4.61)	(1.63)	(2.64)

Positive scores indicate that participants attributed more blame to the target at Time 2 compared to Time 1.

[1] Anorexia Nervosa.

[2] Obesity.

[3] Skin Cancer.

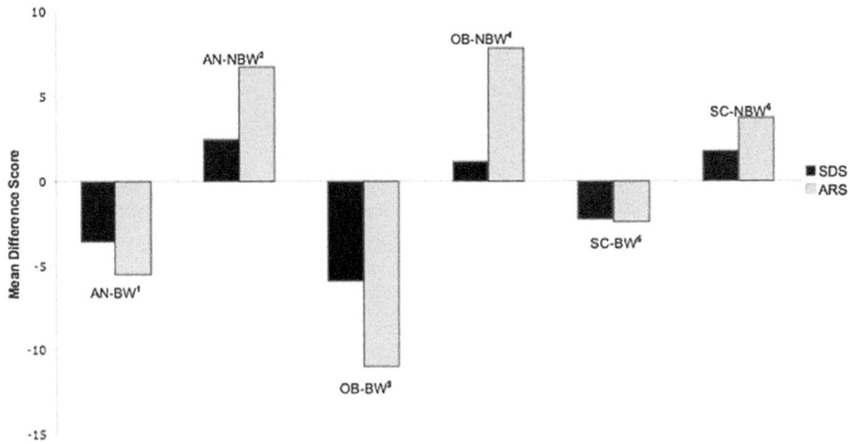

Figure 1 Mean ARS and SDS Difference Scores Across the Six Experimental Groups. AN-BW[1] = anorexia nervosa blameworthy condition; AN-NBW[2] = anorexia nervosa non-blameworthy condition; OB-BW[3] = obesity blameworthy condition; OB-NBW[4] = obesity non-blameworthy condition; SC-BW[5] = skin cancer blameworthy condition; SC-NBW[6] = skin cancer non-blameworthy condition.

groups reported increases in stigmatizing attitudes while participants in the non-blameworthy groups reported decreases in negative attitudes towards the target.

There were no significant interactions between type of condition and level of blame for mean ARS difference scores. Specifically, there was no significant difference between the AN and obesity groups and level of blameworthiness on ARS change scores, $t_{(129)} = -1.886$, $p = .062$, 95% CI [−6.69, 0.16] nor between the AN and skin cancer groups and level of blameworthiness on ARS change scores, $t_{(129)} = 1.001$ $p = .074$, 95% CI [−0.30, 6.42]. Nor were there significant interactions between type of condition and level of blame for mean SDS difference scores. That is, there was no significant difference between the AN and obesity groups and level of blameworthiness on SDS change scores, $t_{(129)} = -.636$, $p = .526$, 95% CI [2.02, 1.04], nor between the AN and skin cancer groups and level of blameworthiness on SDS change scores, $t_{(129)} = 1.333$, $p = .105$, 95% CI [−0.49, 2.51].

Discussion

To our knowledge, this is the first study to document levels of stigmatizing attitudes held towards individuals with AN relative to both obesity (a highly stigmatized weight disorder) and a medical condition (namely, skin cancer). Moreover, in contrast to previous correlational research, the present study's adoption of an experimental methodology allows for the most robust examination of the causes of stigma, specifically, the effect of blame-based accounts in contributing to stigmatizing attitudes.

While it was hypothesized that stigmatizing attitudes would be held towards the target with AN, such attitudes were even stronger than anticipated. That is, participants reported comparable levels of negative affective reactions to the targets with AN and another highly stigmatized condition (i.e., obesity) yet were even more resistant to having social contact with the AN target compared to the obese target. Regarding the latter finding, participants reported that, on average, they were reluctant to associate (even indirectly) with the AN target, yet were 'probably or definitely willing' to have social contact with the obese target. Despite the pervasive nature of obesity stigma, these results provide evidence of even greater levels of stigmatizing attitudes towards people with AN, at least in the domain of social contact with such individuals.

The findings were partially supportive of the hypothesis that psychological conditions are more highly stigmatized than medical conditions, with the AN target attracting a significantly greater desire for social distance compared to the skin cancer target in terms of mean scores on the Social Distance Scale (SDS). Mean SDS scores indicated that while participants were somewhat reluctant to associate (even indirectly) with the AN target, they were 'probably or definitely willing' to have social contact with the skin cancer target. However, the difference between mean Affective Reaction Scale (ARS) scores in the AN and skin cancer groups failed to reach significance, suggesting that willingness to engage in social contact may be a more sensitive index of stigmatizing attitudes than negative emotional reactions.

The second aim of the study was to evaluate the role of blameworthy attributions in the manifestation of stigmatizing attitudes. This aim was initially addressed by investigating the types of causal attributions attributed to target individuals with AN, obesity or skin cancer after reading Vignette A. It was found that participants accorded significantly higher levels of blame and personal control to the obese target relative to the target with AN. The unexpected finding that participants attributed significantly less blame to the AN target and yet reported more stigmatizing attitudes (in terms of a desire for social distance) towards AN compared to obesity appears contrary to Attribution Theory and suggests that factors other than blame-based attributions contribute to stigma. One such factor may be personal contact with a member of a stigmatized group. In the case of the present study, AN and obesity have highly contrasting prevalence rates (approximately 1.9% for AN [6] versus 28.3% for obesity [34]). Given these differences, people are comparatively less likely to have personal contact with an individual diagnosed with AN. Research indicating that individuals who have not had contact with a person with AN are more likely to endorse stigmatizing attitudes compared to those who are familiar with a person who has AN may be one factor that accounts for why AN was more stigmatized in the current study [33]. However, given evidence that the type of contact can impact differentially on attitudes towards individuals with AN (e.g., living with a person with AN being associated with negative attitudes and watching a relevant movie or television show featuring an individual with AN being associated with more positive attitudes), caution is required in selecting contact strategies that are conducive to reducing stigma [21]. A second explanation for the attenuated ratings of blame towards individuals with AN despite elevated stigma is that some symptoms associated with the condition may be perceived as desirable [21]. For example, one study found that despite holding stigmatizing attitudes towards individuals with AN, participants reported admiring their ability to control their eating and exercise [18].

Other findings were consistent with Attribution Theory. For instance, genetic influences were perceived as significantly less relevant to AN than both obesity and skin cancer. The perceived lesser role of this non-blameworthy factor may, according to Attribution Theory, contribute to the observed higher levels of stigmatizing attitudes evident towards those with AN. Although research in the area is in its infancy (particularly in terms of the reliance on family and twin studies and an absence of adoption studies), there is some support for the role of genetic factors in the development of AN [35,36]. A lack of awareness of the possible genetic underpinnings of AN may be one of the reasons that individuals with AN are stigmatized by members of the general public [20]. Furthermore, two recent studies provide support for the dissemination of information relating to the biological underpinnings of AN in that participants exposed to such explanations demonstrated less blaming attitudes compared to participants provided with a sociocultural explanation of the condition [23,24].

In addition to being attributed less to genetic factors, the finding of significantly higher endorsement of social influences for AN can also be interpreted using Attribution Theory. Specifically, individuals with AN may be perceived as having succumbed to social pressures to be thin, with attributions of blame for 'giving in' to social pressures possibly translating into negative responses towards them [24].

The experimental manipulation of blame-based accounts of the three conditions provided the most methodologically robust means for evaluating the causal role of blameworthy attributions in eliciting stigmatizing attitudes. The results of the experimental manipulation were consistent with Attribution Theory's key premise that attributions of blame result in negative affective reactions and social responses towards the target person, with the blameworthy groups experiencing significantly greater deterioration in their negative emotional reactions and desire for social distance from the target than the non-blameworthy groups. As can be seen in Figure 1, across each condition, participants in the blameworthy groups demonstrated an increase in negative emotional reactions and a desire for social distance while participants in the non-blameworthy groups demonstrated a decrease in these negative responses. There was no significant interaction between levels of blameworthiness and type of condition in terms of the desire for social distance suggesting that, irrespective of the type of condition, blame-based accounts resulted in a stronger increase in the desire for social distance from the target than non-blameworthy accounts. However, there was a trend towards significance in terms of a greater change in affective reactions in the obesity versus the AN groups, and in the AN versus skin cancer groups, when exposed to blameworthy versus non-blameworthy accounts. Given that these findings may have become significant with a larger sample, the issue as to whether blameworthy accounts may be of even greater relevance in accounting for stigma in certain conditions relative to others requires further investigation.

Study limitations

Several limitations of the present study must be noted. First, although the sample was generally representative of the broader population in terms of ethnicity, participants were young female undergraduate students, primarily studying psychology. Thus, the current findings may not generalize to more diverse samples with regard to age, gender, and educational background. In particular, the attitudes of mothers warrant investigation as a higher level of maternal criticism has been found to be a strong predictor of poorer treatment response among adolescents with an eating disorder [37]. Moreover, the attitudes of young men may also be worthy of exploration given initial findings that some hold unsympathetic attitudes towards those with an eating disorder [38].

Second, the measures of stigmatizing attitudes used in this study were explicit rather than implicit. However, in addition to concerns about the validity and reliability of implicit measures [39], there are currently no tests available to measure implicit stigmatizing attitudes towards AN, hence the current study's reliance on explicit measures. Additionally, levels of blame were assessed with one item given the absence of psychometrically sound instruments to assess causal attributions in the context of AN. Hence these measures need to be developed as they have been for other conditions (e.g., the Anti-Fat Attitudes Scale for obesity [40]).

Third, the present study investigated anticipated emotional and social reactions towards a fictional character with AN. As such, an important limitation of this study is that *actual* emotional and social reactions towards a person with AN were not examined. Although this is an important first step, more ecologically-valid research is needed to understand the relationship between causal attributions and responses towards stigmatized individuals [1].

Finally, the study may not have had sufficient power to detect significant interactions between level of blameworthiness and type of condition. Post-hoc analyses for the two interaction contrasts (i.e., level of blameworthiness and AN versus obesity on ARS scores, and level of blameworthiness and AN versus skin cancer on ARS scores) revealed a moderate ability to detect a medium effect size (i.e., with power of 65% and 67% respectively at a significance level of .05). Therefore, the notion that blame-based accounts result in comparable increases in stigma irrespective of the type of condition must be considered a preliminary finding given that the findings on the ARS approached significance.

Future directions

Given the lack of research in the area of AN stigma, much remains to be deciphered. Future research should explore additional factors that potentially reduce stigmatizing attitudes towards individuals with AN. Carefully selected contact strategies such as those involving people with personal experience of the disorder may assist with disconfirming faulty beliefs regarding personal blame for the illness [41,42]. In addition, information disseminated to the community could provide nuanced explanations of AN, emphasising that it is a serious psychological condition influenced by a range of biopsychosocial factors, including genetics.

Additionally, it will be important to ascertain the impact of stigma from the perspective of individuals with AN [43] as has been conducted for other mental illnesses such as schizophrenia [44]. It is possible that the perception and experience of stigma in individuals with AN may differ from those with other psychological disorders. For instance, the fact that individuals with AN often experience the condition as egosyntonic may prove protective against the negative attitudes of others towards them [45]. Conversely, given the association between eating disorder symptomatology and rejection sensitivity [46], individuals with an eating disorder may be even more vulnerable to the negative consequences of stigmatizing attitudes.

Conclusions

This study contributes to the small body of research examining stigmatizing attitudes held towards individuals with AN. Elevated levels of stigma towards individuals with AN were found, with some evidence (i.e., in the domain of desired social contact) that these attitudes may be even stronger than those held towards obese individuals. In addition, blame-based accounts were found to increase stigma towards an individual with AN (as well as those with obesity and skin cancer), providing support for the etiological significance of blameworthy attributions for AN stigma. In demonstrating that stigmatizing attitudes in AN can be modified via the manipulation of levels of blameworthiness, the results may help to inform interventions designed to ameliorate such attitudes.

Appendix

Table 3 provides an overview of the information contained in each vignette.

Table 3 Summary of vignettes for the six experimental groups

Anorexia nervosa	Obesity	Skin cancer
Vignette A		
• 19-year-old psychology student who has AN	• 19-year-old psychology student who is obese	• 19-year-old psychology student who has melanoma
• Extremely underweight	• Extremely overweight	• Most dangerous form of skin cancer that required chemotherapy
• Very self-conscious about her body	• Very self-conscious about her body	• Very self-conscious about her hair loss
• Avoids social situations, especially those that require her to eat in public	• Avoids social situations, especially those that require her to eat in public	• Avoids social situations due to embarrassment
• Feels very sad and anxious about her body	• Feels very sad and anxious about her body	• Feels very scared and anxious about her recent health condition
• Experiences irregular heartbeats and is at high risk of heart attack	• Experiences high blood pressure and is therefore at high risk of heart attack	• At risk of the cancer returning and spreading throughout her body
Vignette B – Blameworthy version		
• Deliberately chooses to restrict eating and exercise excessively	• Deliberately chooses to overeat and avoid exercise	• Deliberately spent time in the sun to get a tan
• Not willing to consider other ways to feel good about herself	• Not willing to consider other ways to experience pleasure	• Not willing to consider other ways to feel good about herself
• Chooses to focus solely on continuing to lose weight	• Chooses to focus solely on getting pleasure from eating	• Stuck to usual routine of spending time lying in the sun
• Gets annoyed with friends who provide unwanted advice	• Gets annoyed with friends who provide unwanted advice	• Chose to ignore advice from friends who encouraged her to use sunscreen and wear a hat
• Ignores advice from doctor and dietitian	• Ignores advice from doctor and dietitian	
Vignette B – Non-blameworthy version		
• Driven by illness to restrict eating and exercise excessively	• Driven by strong appetite to engage in overeating	• Illness results in feeling self-conscious about hair-loss
• History of AN within her family	• History of obesity within her family	• History of cancer within her family
• Doctor has explained genetic contributions to the condition	• Doctor has explained genetic contributions to the condition	• Doctor has explained genetic contributions to the condition
• Has made many personal attempts at gaining weight	• Has made many personal attempts at losing weight	• Has made many personal attempts at being cautious in the sun
• Referred to clinical psychologist and actively participating in therapy	• Referred to clinical psychologist and actively participating in therapy	• Referred to cancer specialist and actively monitoring changes in skin
• Trying to eat more even though it makes her anxious	• Trying to walk more even though it is physically uncomfortable	• Trying to keep out of the sun as much as possible

Note. Participants received one copy of Version A corresponding with the condition to which they were assigned (i.e., AN, obesity, or skin cancer) and one copy of Version B (describing the individual as either blameworthy or non-blameworthy).

Competing interests
The authors declare that they have no competing interests.

Authors' contributions
KZ and ER designed the study, conducted the statistical analysis, and drafted the manuscript. KZ carried out the data collection. Both authors read and approved the final manuscript.

References

1. Angermeyer MC, Dietrich S: **Public beliefs about and attitudes towards people with mental illness: a review of population studies.** *Acta Psychiat Scand* 2006, **113**:163–179.
2. Corrigan PW, Watson AC: **The paradox of self-stigma and mental illness.** *Clin Psychol-Sci Pr* 2002, **9**:35–53.
3. Crisp AH, Gelder MG, Rix S, Meltzer HI, Rowlands OJ: **Stigmatisation of people with mental illnesses.** *Brit J Psychiat* 2000, **177**:4–7.
4. American Psychiatric Association: *Diagnostic and statistical manual of mental disorders 4th edition text revision.* Washington, DC: Author; 2000.

5. Wells JE, Oakley Brown MA, Scott KA, McGee MA, Baxter J, Kokaua J: **Prevalence, interference with life and severity of 12 month DSM-IV disorders in Te Rau Hinengaro: the New Zealand mental health survey.** *Aust NZ J Psychiat* 2006, **40:**845–854.
6. Wade TD, Bergin JL, Tiggemann M, Bulik CM, Fairburn CG: **Prevalance and long-term course of lifetime eating disorders in an adult Australian twin cohort.** *Aust NZ J Psychiat* 2006, **40:**121–128.
7. Arcelus A, Mitchell AJ, Wales J, Nielsen S: **Mortality rates in patients with anorexia nervosa and other eating disorders: a meta-analysis of 36 studies.** *Arch Gen Psychiat* 2011, **68**(7):724–731.
8. Evans EJ, Hay PJ, Mond J, Paxton SJ, Quirk F, Rodgers B, Sawoniewska MA: **Barriers to help-seeking in young women with eating disorders: a qualitative exploration in a longitudinal community survey.** *Eat Disord* 2011, **19:**270–285.
9. Hepworth N, Paxton SJ: **Pathways to help-seeking in bulimia nervosa and binge eating problems: a concept mapping approach.** *Int J Eat Disorder* 2007, **40:**493–504.
10. Corrigan PW: **The impact of stigma on severe mental illness.** *Cogn Behav Pract* 1998, **5:**201–222.
11. Weiner B, Perry RP, Magnusson J: **An attributional analysis of reactions to stigma.** *J Pers Soc Psychol* 1988, **55:**738–748.
12. Weiner B: *Judgments of responsibility: A foundation for a theory of social conduct.* New York: Guilford; 1995.
13. Corrigan PW, River L, Lundin RK, Uphoff Wasowski K, Campion J, Mathisen J, Gagnon C: **Stigmatizing attributions about mental illness.** *J Community Psychol* 2000, **28:**91–102.
14. Chiodo J, Stanley M, Harvey JH: **Attributions about anorexia nervosa and bulimia.** *J Soc Clin Psychol* 1984, **2:**280–285.
15. Smith MC, Pruitt JA, McLaughlin Mann L, Thelan MH: **Attitudes and knowledge regarding bulimia and anorexia nervosa.** *Int J Eat Disorder* 1986, **5**(3):545–553.
16. Crisp A: **Stigmatization of and discrimination against people with eating disorders including a report of two nationwide surveys.** *Eur Eat Disord Rev* 2005, **13:**147–152.
17. Fleming J, Szmukler GI: **Attitudes of medical professionals towards patients with eating disorders.** *Aust NZ J Psychiat* 1992, **26:**436–443.
18. Roehrig JP, McLean CP: **A comparison of stigma toward eating disorders versus depression.** *Int J Eat Disorder* 2010, **43:**671–674.
19. Holliday J, Wall E, Treasure J, Weinman J: **Perceptions of illness in individuals with anorexia nervosa: a comparison with lay men and women.** *Int J Eat Disorder* 2005, **37:**50–56.
20. Stewart M, Keel PK, Schiavo RS: **Stigmatisation of anorexia nervosa.** *Int J Eat Disorder* 2006, **39:**320–325.
21. Mond JM, Robertson-Smith G, Vetere A: **Stigma and eating disorders: is there evidence of negative attitudes towards anorexia nervosa among women in the community?** *J Ment Health* 2006, **15**(5):519–532.
22. Ebneter DS, Latner JD, O'Brien KS: **Just world beliefs, causal beliefs, and acquaintance: associations with stigma towards eating disorders and obesity.** *Pers Indiv Differ* 2011, **51:**618–622.
23. Crisafulli MA, Von Holle A, Bulik CM: **Attitudes towards anorexia nervosa: the impact of framing on blame and stigma.** *Int J Eat Disorder* 2008, **41:**333–339.
24. Crisafulli MA, Thompson-Brenner H, Franko DL, Eddy KT, Herzog DB: **Stigmatization of anorexia nervosa: characteristics and response to intervention.** *J Soc Clin Psychol* 2010, **29**(7):756–770.
25. Puhl RM, Heuer CA: **The stigma of obesity: a review and update.** *Obesity* 2009, **19:**941–964.
26. Puhl RM, Brownell KD: **Stigma, discrimination, and obesity.** In *Eating disorders and obesity: a comprehensive handbook.* 2nd edition. Edited by Fairburn CG, Brownell KD. New York: The Guilford Press; 2002:108–112.
27. Puhl RM, Andreyeva T, Brownell KD: **Perceptions of weight discrimination: prevalence and comparison to race and gender discrimination in America.** *Int J Obesity* 2008, **32:**992–1000.
28. Crandall CS, D'Anello S, Sakalli N, Lazarus E, Nejtardt GW, Feather NT: **An attribution-value model of prejudice: anti-fat attitudes in six nations.** *Pers Soc Psychol B* 2001, **27**(1):30–37.
29. Breheny M: **Genetic attribution for schizophrenia, depression, and skin cancer: impact on social distance.** *New Zeal J Psychol* 2007, **36:**154–160.
30. Australian Bureau of Statistics: *Reflecting a nation: Stories from the 2011 census, 2012–2013, catalogue number 2071.0.* Canberra: Author; 2011.
31. Penn DL, Guynan K, Dally T, Spaulding WD, Garbin CP, Sullivan M: **Dispelling the stigma of schizophrenia: what sort of information is best?** *Schizophrenia Bull* 1994, **20:**567–578.
32. Corrigan PW, Penn DL, Edwards AB, Green A, Diwan SL: **Prejudice, social distance, and familiarity with mental illness.** *Schizophrenia Bull* 2001, **27:**219–225.
33. Stewart M, Schiavo RS, Herzog DB, Franko DL: **Stereotypes, prejudice and discrimination of women with anorexia nervosa.** *Eur Eat Disord Rev* 2008, **16:**311–318.
34. Australian Bureau of Statistics: *2011-13 Australian Health Survey, catalogue number 4364.0.55.001.* Canberra: Author; 2012.
35. Kaye WH, Bulik CM, Plotnicov K, Thornton L, Devlin B, Fichter MM, Jones I: **The genetics of anorexia nervosa collaborative study: methods and sample description.** *Int J Eat Disorder* 2009, **41:**289–300.
36. Strober M, Freeman R, Lampert C, Diamond J, Kaye W: **A controlled family study of anorexia nervosa and bulimia nervosa: evidence of shared liability and transmission of partial syndromes.** *Am J Psychiat* 2000, **157:**393–401.
37. Van Furth EF, van Strien DC, Martina LML, van Son MJM, Hendrickx JJP, van Engeland H: **Expressed emotion and the prediction of outcome in adolescent eating disoders.** *Int J Eat Disorder* 1996, **20:**19–31.
38. Mond JM, Arrighi A: **Gender differences in perceptions of the severity and prevalence of eating disorders.** *Early Interv Psychiatry* 2011, **5:**41–49.
39. Brendl CM, Markman AB, Messner C: **How do indirect measures of evaluation work? Evaluating the inference of prejudice in the implicit association test.** *J Pers Soc Psychol* 2001, **81:**760–773.
40. Crandall CS: **Prejudice against fat people: ideology and self-interest.** *J Pers Soc Psychol* 1994, **66:**882–894.
41. Corrigan PW, Penn DL, Green A, Lundin R, Kubiak MA: **Familiarity with and social distance from people who have serious mental illness.** *Psychiatr Serv* 2001, **52:**953–958.
42. Couture SM, Penn DL: **Interpersonal contact and the stigma of mental illness: a review of the literature.** *J Ment Health* 2003, **12:**291–305.
43. Crabtree JW, Haslam SA, Postmes T, Haslam C: **Mental health support groups, stigma, and self-esteem: positive and negative implications of group identification.** *J Soc Issues* 2010, **66:**553–569.
44. Schulze B, Angermeyer MC: **Subjective experiences of stigma: a focus group study of schizophrenic patients, their relatives and mental health professionals.** *Soc Sci Med* 2003, **56:**299–312.
45. Nordbo RHS, Espeset EMS, Guliksen KS, Skarderud F, Geller J, Holte A: **Reluctance to recover in anorexia nervosa.** *Eur Eat Disord Rev* 2011, **20**(1):60–67.
46. Gilbert N, Meyer C: **Fear of negative evaluation and the development of eating psychopathology: a longitudinal study among nonclinical women.** *Int J Eat Disorder* 2005, **37:**307–312.

Preliminary examination of a mentor-based program for eating disorders

Marisol Perez[1*], Ashley Kroon Van Diest[1] and Shannon Cutts[2]

Abstract

Background: There is a current and pressing need for recovery resources for individuals suffering from eating disorders. Mentoring programs have been useful with other psychiatric disorders such as addictions, and may be useful for individuals recovering from an eating disorder. The present study sought to examine a mentoring program for individuals working towards recovery from an eating disorder.

Methods: The study included mentors (i.e., individuals who have recovered from an eating disorder for an extended period of time), and mentees (i.e., individuals who were in the process of recovering from an eating disorder and wanting additional support aside from their treatment team). Participants included 141 participants, consisting of 34 mentors, 58 mentees who matched with a mentor, and 49 mentees searching for a mentor. Participants completed questions assessing eating disorder symptoms, quality of life, motivation towards recovery, and treatment compliance.

Results: Matched mentees reported higher levels of quality of life on 7 out of 12 domains, and missed fewer appointments with treatment providers when compared to unmatched mentees. There were no differences between matched and unmatched mentees on motivation, energy or confidence towards recovery.

Conclusions: Findings suggest a mentor model is beneficial for individuals engaged in the process of recovering from an eating disorder in the areas of quality of life and treatment compliance. Specifically, mentees in a mentoring relationship reported better family and close relationships, future outlook, and psychological, emotional, and physical well-being than unmatched mentees. Mentors reported being positively impacted by the mentoring relationship by strengthening the skills they learned while in recovery, and reminding them of how far they had come in their own recovery. The findings in this study suggest that mentor programs warrant further investigation as ancillary support services for individuals recovering from an eating disorder.

Keywords: Mentor program, Eating disorders, Quality of life, Treatment compliance

Background

A recent article by Kazdin & Blasé [1], argues that psychotherapy and clinical practice need a reboot, with the current model of individual psychotherapy unable to significantly reduce the burden of mental illness. The authors suggest that in order to better reduce the burden of mental illness there needs to be a greater array of services available that maximize technology, such as the internet, and expand opportunities for non-professionals to assist in prevention and support services [1]. Kazdin & Blasé's [1] article accurately reflects the field of eating disorders, where there is a current and pressing need for recovery resources for individuals suffering from eating disorders [2,3]. In a recent study of eating disorder services, both patients and carers mentioned support services as one of the top five essential features of high quality eating disorder services [2], yet report a lack of services available [3]. In addition, 294 individuals recovering from an eating disorder reported support during all stages of the recovery process as important for recovery, the need for additional support outside of psychological treatment, and financial costs being the biggest barrier to services [2,3].

Affordable ancillary support services for individuals wanting to recover from an eating disorder have the potential to ease some of the financial burden and the

* Correspondence: marisol.perez@asu.edu
[1]Department of Psychology, Texas A&M University, 4235 TAMU, College Station, TX 77843-4235, USA
Full list of author information is available at the end of the article

pressing need for support during the recovery process [2,3]. Interviews with individuals recovered from an eating disorder indicate that non-professional contacts such as support groups are important components of the recovery process [4]. Ancillary support services can range from local community support groups for carers and sufferers of eating disorders [5-9], to support groups for co-occurring issues such as Alcoholics Anonymous [10] or Overeaters Anonymous [11], nutritional assistance [12], and online resources [13-15]. However the research on ancillary support services for individual suffering from eating disorders is sparse, with limited information on how these services can assist in the recovery process. For example, there are several studies that have assessed the benefits of support groups, but most have been conducted via interviews from the patient's perspective [5-9] with no objective assessments used to ascertain the success or benefits of the groups. In addition, the literature on online eating disorder support groups has focused on thematic content analysis of the discussions [13,14]. A paucity of studies have examined community support groups for eating disorders with co-occurring issues such as Overeaters Anonymous and found these groups to be beneficial and significantly reduce symptoms [11,16]. Given the limited research on ancillary support services and the pressing need for low-cost services, the current study seeks to improve upon the literature by empirically examining the benefits of an additional ancillary support service, a mentor-based program developed for individuals recovering from an eating disorder that is free. The mentor-based program was designed to provide additional support and accountability in-between sessions for individuals in treatment, or keep individuals active in the recovery process if they were not in treatment [17].

Using a mentor model to facilitate recovery in mental health is not a novel concept. The most recognized mentor-type model is the Twelve Step model used in the fellowship of Alcoholics Anonymous [10]. The mentor-mentee model revolves around the willing presence of a volunteer who has achieved the "goal," working in partnership with a person who is aiming to achieve the goal. Straussner and Byrne [18] undertook a review of the benefits of Alcoholics Anounymous and found several studies demonstrating the efficacy of the mentor-mentee program in reducing the mentee's drinking. In addition there is research from Alcoholics Anonymous programs to demonstrate that the mentorship relationship is also beneficial for the mentor with the mentoring relationship helping the mentor stay recovered [19-21]. These findings collectively suggest that the mentor-mentee model of Alcoholics Anonymous benefits both the mentor and mentee in their recovery from alcohol.

The mentor model is also used in many health/behavioral areas including school programs, business, mental health and infant health [22-24]. A review of the organizational and vocational literature for the past 25 years found a positive impact of mentorship for the mentee, mentor, and the organization [22]. In addition, a recent review of school programs where mentors were adults who met with youth mentees, found that mentor programs increase a youth's connectedness with school, family, and community, and reduces dropout rates and problematic behavior in the classroom [23]. Finally, a recent mentor model was implemented with success to facilitate the detection and introduction of services for infant mental health problems by direct medical providers, where the mentors were mental health professionals who specialized in infant mental health [24].

A review of the empirical literature on eating disorders revealed that there are no studies discussing a mentor-mentee program for individuals recovering from an eating disorder. Given the success of the mentor model for other vocational, education, and mental health areas outside of the eating disorders field, a mentor program for eating disorders may have several potential benefits to patients and the field. Some individuals in outpatient treatment would benefit from regular, sustained contact with additional recovery-based support and accountability resources beyond what professional treatment sessions can offer to them [13,14,17]. Reviews of discussions on electronic support groups has found that individuals suffering from eating disorders seek emotional support, and information and feedback, with members with longer periods of recovery serving as role models [13,14]. A mentor program can also assist patients in coping with triggers or negative life events, and decreases in motivation that occur in between therapy sessions [17]. For those contemplating entering treatment or those individuals who do not have access to treatment, a mentor program can offer some form of recovery-based support and serve as a motivator for finding and maintaining treatment [17]. For the field of eating disorders, a mentor program can provide additional no-cost support services that can reduce the financial burden reported by patients that serves as a barrier to needed care [2,3]. Thus, a mentor program for individuals suffering from eating disorders can have numerous potential benefits to the individual sufferer and the field.

The field of eating disorders has debated the role of the recovered individual in the recovery process of others suffering from an eating disorder [25]. Concerns with having recovered individuals involved in the recovery process of others revolve around countertransference issues, taking over the recovery process for the patient, and risk of relapse [25,26]. On the other hand, reports from treatment providers with a history of an eating disorder [26], recovered individuals who have been symptom free for at least 1 year [4], and research from online support groups [13] and Overeaters Anonymous [11] suggest that there are benefits to having recovered individuals involved in the treatment of others. In addition, mentor models are based on the helper therapy principle, which states that there are intrinsic rewards and benefits to helpers when they assist others, including maintaining treatment outcomes [27]. The current study will contribute to this debate by examining if there are benefits to engaging in a mentor relationship for individuals who are in the process of recovery. In addition, we examine the perspectives of the recovered individual who are serving as mentors.

The current study sought to improve upon the ancillary support services literature in 3 ways: 1.) examine the benefits of a mentor model for individuals recovering from an eating disorder for which there is no previous research; 2.) use common, empirically validated, self-report questionnaires deviating from the existing literature that uses interviews and online discussions with thematic content analysis; and 3.) provide the perspective of the mentor and the needs of the sample which is also limited in the existing literature. It was hypothesized that mentees who were working with a mentor, would have more motivation to recover from an eating disorder, spend more time and energy devoted to recovery work, have a higher reported quality of life particularly in the arena of interpersonal relationships, and perhaps exhibit greater treatment compliance than mentees who were searching for mentors but had not yet found one. The current study also sought to quantify specific topics that mentors and mentees regularly discussed, to describe the most common additional support needs that mentees reported, and to ascertain the impact of mentoring on the volunteer mentors.

Method

Study design & procedures

The data collected from this study was part of a larger program evaluation designed to assess unmet need, service use and satisfaction with MentorCONNECT. This was a cross-sectional, retrospective study with the use of online self-report questionnaires. It is common for mentees that would like a mentor to search for several months for a mentor, with the main reason for not finding a mentor being availability (Shannon Cutts, personal communication, April 2011). During the time of the study, there were more mentees wanting mentor services than there were mentors available, creating a natural control group (i.e., people were not randomized into a control group or intervention group). These wait-listed individuals are labeled unmatched mentees in this study.

Prior to the study, all self-report questionnaires were reviewed by a board of 18 individuals including researchers, licensed professionals, and recovered individuals. Numerous board members were concerned with the self-reported weight item as potentially triggering for participants. Given the overwhelming and strong response to the weight item, it was dropped from the questionnaire. This study was reviewed and approved by the Texas A&M University's Institutional Review Board, and all participants completed online consent forms and agreed to participate in the research study before completing the online survey. The online survey was accessible for a 2-month period, but participants could only participate once.

Recruitment

Participants were recruited through a mass email (approximate $N = 1000$) inviting them to participate in a 20-minute online survey over a 2-month period. All members and new members that joined MentorCONNECT during the 2 month study period were invited to participate. A total of 76.7% of the sample did not respond to the mass email with more details provided in Figure 1. It is unknown why only 23.3% of the targeted sample responded to the study. As an incentive to participate, survey participants who completed the survey were entered into a raffle to win numerous prizes related to recovery. Participation was completely voluntary.

Participants

A total of 141 individuals participated in this study, consisting of 34 mentors, 58 matched mentees, and 49 unmatched mentees, see Figure 1 for more details. The racial composition of the entire sample was 81% White, 1% Black, 4% Hispanic, 2% Asian, and 5% other. A total of 9% of the sample was currently living outside of the United States. Participants ranged in age from 15 to 63, with a mean age of 31 (SD = 10.26). Mentors were on average 34 years old (SD = 12.88), and consisted of 4 mental health professionals with no history of an eating disorder, and 30 recovered individuals who reported being recovered for an average of 8 years (SD = 6.00). Almost all of the mentors (93.8%) were living in the United States at the time of this study and all were women. Mentors were asked what eating disorder they most closely identified with during the course of their illness and were allowed to endorse more than one disorder. Approximately 56% of mentors identified with anorexia nervosa, 38% bulimia nervosa, 15% binge eating disorder, and 38% eating disorder not otherwise specified. Mentees ranged in age from 19 to 59 years old with an average of 31 years old (SD = 8.94), and were predominantly women. Table 1 provides the descriptive information for matched and unmatched mentees.

Mentor program

The mentor-based program was created by *MentorCONNECT*, a nonprofit organization that is a global eating disorders-focused mentoring community. Individuals seeking additional support recovery services from eating disorder can become members of *MentorCONNECT*. All

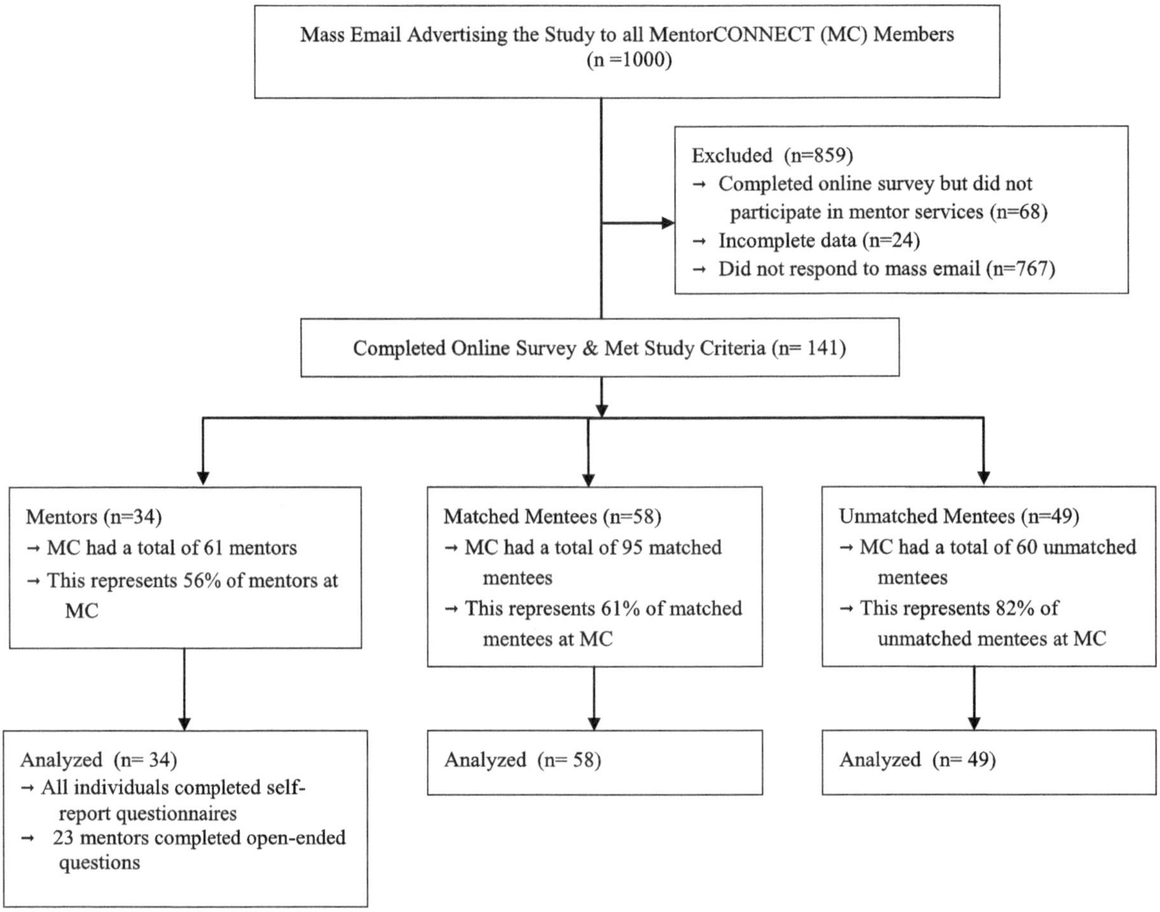

Figure 1 CONSORT diagram.

services are provided for free. Mentors were volunteers who were mental health professionals that specialize in eating disorders, and/or individuals who have personally achieved 12 consecutive months of sustained recovery, defined as "largely free from eating disordered thoughts and coping behaviors". Mentor volunteers were pre-screened by a team of lay and licensed professionals to assess their recovery status before being approved to serve. Mentors receive a package of materials to assist with the mentoring process and are assigned an experienced mentor to assist them. For a review of this mentor model please see Cutts [17]. Each approved volunteer mentor writes a free-form paragraph about their personal recovery history, including why they want to serve as a mentor and what they have to offer, their availability, and preferred method of contact. This information is posted on a password-protected page that mentees can view to request a match with their preferred mentor. A mentor-level volunteer leader serves as the Mentoring Match Coordinator and assists mentees and mentors with finalizing a new match. Once a match is made, the new pair completes an Immediate Action Plan form that outlines their communication preferences and solidifies their commitment to regular communication and to the match itself. Pairs are asked to commit to communicating at least once per week. Mentors are asked to commit a minimum of one hour per week per mentee, up to a maximum number of three mentees per mentor.

The mentoring relationship within this program was modeled after past research from the organizational/vocational literature [28]. The first phase of the mentoring relationship is the initiation phase [28]. In this phase, the mentor and mentee get to know each other, decide if the mentor might be appropriate to meet the mentee's needs, establish the boundaries of the relationship, and establish the mode and frequency of contact. During this phase it is also recommended that mentors review with mentees how both parties can respectfully end the relationship if they need or want to discontinue. During this phase mentors and mentees tend to report feeling both

Table 1 Demographic information on matched and unmatched mentees

	Matched	Unmatched	t or X^2	p
Age (year born)	1982 (8.64)	1980 (9.34)	0.71	.48
International status	19%	20%	0.04	.85
Ethnicity (Caucasian)	90.9%	88.6%	3.38	.64
Self-reported diagnosis				
AN	62%	49%	1.85	.17
BN	29%	37%	0.67	.42
BED	10%	16%	0.84	.36
EDNOS	41%	35%	0.50	.48
EDDS total	1.77 (0.67)	1.50 (0.97)	1.65	.10
Length of time at MC			0.51	.92
Less than 3 months	33%	37%		
3 - 6 months	26%	29%		
7 - 12 months	22%	18%		
More than 1 year	19%	16%		

Note: International status refers to the percentage of the sample born outside the United States. Self-reported diagnosis – participants were asked to endorse the diagnosis they most closely identified with and could choose more than 1 disorder. For age born and EDDS total the Means (Standard Deviations) are reported. MC – *MentorCONNECT*; EDDS – Eating Disorder Diagnostic Scale. Matched mentee group $N = 58$; unmatched mentee group $N = 49$.

excitement and challenge as they start to work together (Shannon Cutts, personal communication, April 2011). The second phase of the mentoring relationship is the cultivation phase [28]. During this phase the mentor and mentee mutually benefit from and develop the relationship further depending on the needs and interest of both parties. The mentoring relationship can change dramatically during this time, particularly if mentees move into or out of inpatient treatment, day hospitalization, and outpatient treatment. The mentoring topics will also gradually shift over time from focusing on what the mentee is doing on a daily basis that is complying with treatment goals and recovery, towards relapse prevention, and increasing quality of life and life satisfaction issues. This phase is usually reported by both parties in a positive light [28]. Over time and through successful treatment and a continuing complementary evolution in the mentoring relationship, the mentee becomes more independent and is less dependent on the mentor, which leads into the third phase, the separation phase. During this phase, the mentor may report feeling not needed, or may feel that there is limited use made of the support they are continuing to offer. Although there may be feelings of sadness as the relationship transitions and often ends, this period is usually celebrated by both parties as a successful conclusion to a mutually productive relationship. It is important to note that the time frame of the mentoring relationship can vary by mentee. Some mentees only need support for a short period of time to help them get through a difficult time, while for others; the mentoring relationship may last several years. After the mentor and mentee decide to end their formal mentoring relationship, they enter into the final phase. In the redefinition phase, the pair can decide to end the relationship and cease communication or change the quality of the relationship to mirror more of a friendship [28].

Measures

Group status

Participants were asked to identify how they used *MentorCONNECT* (i.e. membership level) with the options being, *mentor, matched mentee* (i.e., an individual working with a mentor), and *unmatched mentee* (i.e., an individual searching or waiting for a mentor to come available). Participants' response on this item determined their group status.

Eating Disorder Diagnostic Scale (EDDS)

The EDDS is a brief self-report measure of 22 items designed for diagnosing anorexia nervosa, bulimia nervosa, binge eating disorder, and eating disorder not otherwise specified based on the DSM-IV [29]. The EDDS items can also be standardized and summed for use as a continuous symptom composite scale. The EDDS has good psychometric properties [29,30]. For this study, the internal consistency using the standardized items was 0.95. As mentioned in the Procedure section, the self-reported weight item was removed from this scale. Thus, anorexia nervosa as defined by the DSM-IV could not be computed, instead sub-threshold anorexia nervosa was computed following the EDDS scoring protocol.

Eating Disorder Quality of Life Scale (EDQLS)

The EDQLS assesses functioning or quality of life among adolescents and adults suffering from eating disorders [31]. This measure contains 40 items that assess 12 domains of functioning considered to be important by patients suffering with eating disorders and consistent with the World Health Organization's definition of quality of life: cognitive, education/vocation, family & close relationships, relationships with others, future outlook, appearance, leisure, psychological, emotional, values & beliefs, physical, and eating disorder (i.e., level of impairment in daily functioning directly due to an eating disorder). Items are rated on a 5-point scale ranging from *strongly disagree* to *strongly agree* with higher scores indicating higher levels of functioning. The EDQLS has demonstrated good psychometric properties [31]. Internal consistency of the EDQLS for this study was 0.97 for the total scale, 0.75 for the cognitive domain, 0.80 for education/vocation, 0.58 for family & close relationships, 0.77 for relationships with others, 0.76 for future outlook, 0.85 for appearance, 0.91 for leisure, 0.72

for psychological, 0.76 for emotional, 0.77 for values & beliefs, 0.57 for physical, and 0.89 for eating disorder.

Motivation, energy, & confidence towards recovery

Participants were asked "how motivated are you to recover?," "how much energy do you spend on a daily basis towards recovery?," and "how confident are you that you will recover?," with all three questions using a 5-point scale where higher scores indicate more motivation, energy and confidence towards recovery.

Treatment compliance

Participants were asked, "In the past month, how many appointments with your treatment providers have you missed?" Prior to this question, treatment providers were defined as anyone on the individual's treatment team. Participants entered the number of appointments missed in the past 30 days. Participants only completed this item once.

Length of mentoring relationship

Mentees were asked how long they had been in a mentoring relationship with a mentor from MentorCONNECT, with responses entered in number of months.

Frequency of communication

Both mentors and matched mentees were asked how frequently they communicated, with the options being *daily or almost daily, 2–3 times per week, once a week, twice a month or more*, and *once a month*.

The mentoring process

Mentors and matched mentees were asked what they discussed from a list of 27 topics: dealing with triggers from family and environment; managing or reducing eating disorder thought and behaviors; finding enough quality support services; lack of access to professional treatment; lack of willingness to seek treatment; lack of understanding or support from friends and family; support offered by family and friends isn't what is needed; managing relationships with peers, family, friends, colleagues, society; asking for and accepting help from others; choose who to ask for help; managing relapses; body dissatisfaction and poor body image; setting and working towards recovery goals; dealing with weight stabilization; following a meal plan; grocery shopping/eating out/food-based socializing; learning to name, feel, and deal with emotions; finding time for recovery amidst other obligations; setting and honoring boundaries; choosing recovery; finding reasons to recover; using my voice and expressing needs, wants, desires, and boundaries; staying motivated and committed to doing the hard work of recovery; intimacy and relationship challenges, fears, and issues; finding and expressing preferences, skills, talents, and identity outside of "Ed"; building meaning and quality of life into the recovery process; other co-occurring recovery issues with addiction, trauma, abuse, self-harm, depression, anxiety, etc. Mentors were also given the opportunity to describe topics of communication, or provide more details about any of the topics listed above through open-ended questions.

Impact of program on mentors

Mentors were asked in an open-ended question what the impact of mentoring was on them. They were able to write up to 250 words to describe their experience.

Unmet need

Matched and unmatched mentees were also asked about current needs for which they would like assistance from a mentor.

Results

Descriptive analyses were conducted comparing matched and unmatched mentees and there were no differences in age, international status, ethnicity, eating disorder diagnosis affiliation, and eating disorder symptoms total, see Table 1. There were no differences on income level across the groups with 69% of the matched mentees and 65% of the unmatched mentees earning $100,000 or less, $X^2(6) = 1.61$, $p = .95$.

Quality of life

An independent sample t-test was conducted to compare the matched and unmatched mentees on eating disorder quality of life indices. Details of these results can be viewed in Table 2. A comparison of the matched and unmatched mentees revealed that matched mentees reported significantly higher levels of quality of life in the education/vocation, family and close relationships, future outlook, psychological, emotional, values and beliefs, and physical domains than unmatched mentees. It is important to note that mentors' scores on the EDQLS are consistent with individuals who report low eating disorder symptoms and high levels of functioning [32]. In contrast, both matched and unmatched mentees are reporting quality of life levels consistent with those with high eating disorder symptoms and overall psychiatric symptom severity [32].

Motivation, energy, and confidence towards recovery

Matched and unmatched mentees were compared on motivation to recover, but no differences were found between the groups, $t\ (105) = 0.32$, $p = .75$, with both the matched ($M = 3.98$, $SD = 0.98$) and unmatched ($M = 3.91$, $SD = 1.11$) mentees reporting being "somewhat" to "very" motivated to recover. There were no differences between the groups on amount of energy spent towards recovery on a daily basis, $t\ (105) = 1.14$, $p = .26$, with both the

Table 2 Group comparisons on eating disorder quality of life scale

Quality of life subscales	Mentors	Matched mentees	Unmatched mentees	*t*	*p*
Cognitive	11.21 (4.28)	7.09 (2.72)	6.45 (3.52)	1.06	.29
Education/vocational	11.42 (4.36)	6.60 (3.38)	5.22 (3.33)	2.12	.04
Family & close relations	12.36 (4.27)	9.26 (3.43)	7.41 (4.11)	2.54	.01
Relationship with others	10.36 (4.05)	7.05 (3.06)	5.86 (3.48)	1.89	.06
Future outlook	12.00 (4.39)	9.43 (3.61)	7.20 (4.36)	2.89	.01
Appearance	10.73 (4.38)	6.31 (3.04)	5.39 (3.35)	1.49	.14
Psychological	10.42 (3.87)	7.38 (2.75)	5.76 (3.50)	2.69	.01
Emotional	9.91 (4.10)	6.52 (2.87)	5.27 (3.33)	2.09	.04
Values & beliefs	10.49 (4.06)	6.64 (2.86)	5.06 (3.18)	2.69	.01
Leisure	11.36 (4.13)	8.62 (3.16)	7.59 (4.15)	1.46	.15
Physical	10.12 (3.79)	7.02 (2.87)	5.69 (3.32)	2.21	.03
Eating	25.52 (10.42)	15.29 (6.51)	13.20 (7.68)	1.52	.13
Total score	145.91 (53.54)	97.24 (34.92)	79.78 (43.05)	2.32	.02

Note: Group comparisons are only between matched and unmatched mentees. Information in the mentor, matched, and unmatched mentee columns is reported in Means (Standard Deviations). $N = 107$, and $df = 105$ for all comparisons.

matched ($M = 3.45$, $SD = 0.98$) and unmatched ($M = 3.22$, $SD = 1.05$) mentees reporting spending a considerable amount of energy towards recovery. In addition, there were no differences between the groups on level of confidence that recovery will be achieved, $t\ (105) = 0.63$, $p = .53$, with both the matched ($M = 3.16$, $SD = 1.30$) and unmatched ($M = 3.00$, $SD = 1.22$) reporting being "fairly" confident that they will recover.

Treatment compliance

Participants reported the number of missed sessions over the past month. When comparing the matched and unmatched mentees, matched mentees reported missing fewer treatment appointments than unmatched mentees, $t\ (105) = 4.83$, $p < .001$. Matched mentees reported missing on average 0.98 ($SD = 1.02$) appointments with a range of 0 to 4 sessions and a mode of 1. Unmatched mentees reported missing on average 2.14 ($SD = 1.40$) appointments with a range of 0 to 5 sessions and a mode of 3.

Time and frequency of communication

Frequency of communication between matched mentees and mentors varied greatly from "2-3 times daily" to "once a month", with the average being "2-3 times per week" ($M = 1.74$, $SD = 2.12$). Matched mentees were assessed on the length of time they had been in their mentoring relationship and the frequency of communication with their mentors. Pearson product–moment correlations were computed between length of time and frequency of communication, and those variables that emerged significant in the comparisons reported above. As Table 3 displays, the length of time in a mentoring relationship was not significantly associated with any of the quality of life domains, nor motivation, energy or confidence towards recovery. Frequency of communication with your mentor was positively and significantly associated with higher levels of quality of life in the education/vocation, family and close relationships, future outlook, psychological, emotional, values and beliefs, and physical domains.

The mentoring process

Mentors and matched mentees were asked about what topics were frequently discussed by the pairs. Table 4 lists the top topics endorsed by both mentors and matched mentees. In addition to the topics listed in Table 4, mentors also reported frequently discussing treatment compliance, lack of access to professional treatment, lack of willingness to seek treatment, and dealing with weight stabilization. Both matched and

Table 3 Associations between time, frequency of communication with mentors, and quality of life variables among matched mentees

	Length of time	Freq of communication
Motivation	0.02	0.18
Energy	−0.04	0.08
Confidence	0.02	0.23
Education/Vocation	0.20	0.31*
Family & close Rel.	0.04	0.37**
Future outlook	0.03	0.34**
Psychological	0.11	0.40**
Emotional	0.11	0.31*
Values & beliefs	0.13	0.29*
Physical	0.14	0.26*

Note: Table displays pearson correlation coefficients; *$p < .05$, **$p < .01$; $N = 58$.

Table 4 Top list of topics mentors and matched mentees both report discussing the most

Topic	% Endorsing
1. Managing or reducing eating disorder thoughts and behaviors	21
2. Staying motivated and committed to doing the hard work of recovery	19
3. Managing relapses	17
4. Choosing recovery	17
5. Setting and working towards recovery goals	16
6. Dealing with triggers from family and environment	16

unmatched mentees were also asked about their current needs for support services, and Table 5 displays the percentages of the mentees reporting a need for each topic. Approximately one quarter of the sample reported needing support services for learning to name, feel, and deal with emotions. In addition, the other top most pressing needs were dealing with co-occurring issues such as addiction, trauma, depression, etc., and weight stabilization, following a meal plan, and grocery shopping/eating out/food-based socializing.

Impact of program on mentors

Mentors were asked an open-ended question about the impact of mentoring on them of which 23 out of 34 mentors answered the question. Overall, 91% of mentors believe the mentoring process positively impacted their own recovery process with three main themes emerging from their responses. They were positively impacted by strengthening the skills they learned while in recovery, solidifying the steps required towards recovery, and reminders to them of how far they've come in their own recovery/the unhealthy place they were with the eating disorder.

Discussion

The overall objective of the present study was to examine if a mentoring relationship improved motivation, confidence, and energy towards recovery for individuals suffering from an eating disorder, and quality of life. Compared to unmatched mentees, mentees matched with a mentor reported significant improvement in 7 of the 12 domains of quality of life including family and close relationships, future outlook, psychological, and emotional domains. In addition, the frequency of communication between mentors and mentees was positively correlated with the same 7 domains of quality of life. There were no differences on motivation, energy or confidence toward recovery between the two groups, with both groups reporting being fairly motivated, confident and spending a considerable amount of energy on a daily basis towards recovery. Interestingly, matched mentees reported more treatment compliance than unmatched mentees, with treatment compliance being assessed as number of missed appointments with treatment providers in the past month. In addition, mentors reported believing that the mentoring relationship further facilitated their own recovery process. The results from the current study corroborate previous research suggesting that there is a significant amount of need for ancillary support services for individuals recovering from an eating disorder [2,3]. Indeed, all of the 27 discussion topics

Table 5 The reported need of both matched and unmatched mentees

Topic	% Endorsing need
1. Dealing with triggers from family and environment	17
2. Managing or reducing eating disorder thought and behaviors	14
3. Finding enough quality support services	19
4. Lack of access to professional treatment	14
5. Lack of willingness to seek treatment	11
6. Lack of understanding or support from family and friends	11
7. Support offered by family and friends isn't what is needed	12
8. Managing relationships with peers, family, friends, colleagues, society	17
9. Asking for and accepting help from others	18
10. Choosing who to ask for help	15
11. Managing relapses	18
12. Body dissatisfaction and poor body image	20
13. Setting and working towards recovery goals	18
14. Dealing with weight stabilization	22
15. Following a meal plan	22
16. Grocery shopping/eating out/food-based socializing	22
17. Learning to name, feel, and deal with emotions	24
18. Finding time for recovery amidst other obligations	20
19. Setting and honoring boundaries	13
20. Choosing recovery	14
21. Finding reasons to recover	16
22. Using my voice and expressing needs, wants, desires, and boundaries	16
23. Staying motivated and committed to doing the hard work of recovery	12
24. Intimacy and relationship challenges, fears, and issues	19
25. Finding and expressing preferences, skills, talents, and identity outside of "Ed"	17
26. Building meaning and quality of life into the recovery process	20
27. Other co-occurring recovery issues with addiction, trauma, abuse, self-harm, depression, anxiety, etc.	23

N=107.

offered to mentees were endorsed. The most pressing remaining unmet recovery support needs identified by mentees were support services for managing co-occurring issues such as addiction, depression, anxiety, trauma, abuse, and self-harm.

The findings from this study suggest that a mentor model could be a beneficial ancillary support service to reinforce treatment goals, with matched mentees reporting higher rates of quality of life and treatment compliance. Quality of life is an important outcome in eating disorder treatment and relapse prevention, and is reported as personally important to patients [32-34]. Matched mentees also reported significant improvement on family and close relationships domain, indicating higher levels of perceived social support. Increased social support is important towards treatment outcome because low levels of perceived social support during negative life events can exacerbate eating disorder symptoms [35]. The benefits of the mentor model were further corroborated with more frequent communication between mentors and mentees being positively associated with higher scores in the quality of life domains. In addition, 91% of the mentors that completed the open-ended questions reported that the mentoring relationship positively impacted their own recovery process, supporting the helper therapy principle which states that there are intrinsic rewards and benefits to helpers when they assist others, including maintaining treatment outcomes [27].

There were several programmatic components to implementing a mentor program that warrant discussion. First, we suggest assigning an experienced mentor to a new mentor to answer any questions and facilitate the new mentor's process of learning to become a confident and effective mentor. The mentoring relationship can be a different type of relationship and navigating those boundaries can be facilitated with an experienced mentor as a coach particularly for those mentors who are treatment professionals and can have difficulty defining the boundary between a supportive and a therapeutic relationship. The mentor program was structured as a strictly non-medical, non-clinical source of supplemental peer-based support that can complement but never substitute nor replace the vital work of the treatment professional. Thus, there is a strong emphasis to the mentor program for enhancing recovery and treatment results, but in such a way as to conscientiously refrain from interfering with treatment. Examples of this were evident in the responses from mentors on open-ended questions regarding what they focused on and discussed during their conversations with mentees. For example, under the topic "setting and working toward recovery goals," a frequent theme among mentors with mentees suffering from anorexia nervosa was honesty with treatment providers, with mentors learning that at times their mentees withheld information from their treatment providers and worked with their mentees on being more honest to maximize treatment gains. In sum, a clear definition of a mentor relationship and the boundaries of that relationship are hypothesized to be an important component of the program. However this has not been tested and future research needs to investigate the key components of a mentor model.

Past research has reported that professionals have some reservations about recovered individuals being involved in the recovery process of recovering persons [25]. The findings from this study suggest that a mentor model that includes recovered individuals as mentors is beneficial to individuals in the recovery process of an eating disorder. Aside from the current study, there has been some research, albeit limited, that has investigated the role of recovered individuals in facilitating recovery in others. A couple of studies have found that approximately one-third of treatment providers in the eating disorders field have recovered from an eating disorder [36,37]. Costin and colleagues [25,26,38] have outlined the benefits of having recovered individuals involved in the treatment of others. Specifically, patients and carers consider the experience of a recovered person to be a positive asset in the quality of the relationship and advice given [25]. However, concerns of having recovered individuals involved in the recovery process of others mainly stem around risk of relapse [25,38], and Costin and colleagues highlight that the longer a person is recovered and views themselves as recovered, might reduce risk of relapse [26].

There are several limitations of this study that are worth noting. First, this is a cross-sectional study and a preliminary investigation which limits the findings to correlational associations. It is possible that the higher quality of life functioning and treatment compliance among the matched mentees was due to some confounding variable not measured by this study. It is also unknown if matched and unmatched mentees differed on personality characteristics or some other variables that could have potentially made a mentee more or less likely to find a mentor. Another limitation is the sample, which consisted of matched and unmatched mentees, limiting the generalizability of the findings. Mentees were individuals who self-identified as needing additional support for recovery from an eating disorder and were motivated enough to join and actively search for a mentor. Thus, the entire sample consisted of individuals that had demonstrated a significant level of motivation and action towards recovery, and the findings from this study may not apply to individuals in the contemplation or pre-contemplation phases of treatment. In addition, a significant number of members at MentorCONNECT did not participate in this study, thus raising the possibility that our sample is biased or unrepresentative.

This investigation into a mentor program for eating disorders is preliminary, and needs replication. The beneficial findings of this study will hopefully ignite future research. Indeed the ancillary support services literature for eating disorders is in need of empirical research that examines the benefits of these services and for whom. Future research could address who is most likely to benefit from matching with a mentor, what models of mentorship will yield better results, and what are the essential components of a successful mentor-mentee match.

Conclusion

The findings from this study indicate that a mentor program significantly improves the quality of life and treatment compliance for individuals working towards recovery. The potential benefits of a mentor program in alleviating some of the immediate and pressing needs for additional recovery-based support services and the positive findings in this study suggest that mentor programs warrant further investigation.

Competing interests

Shannon Cutts has a financial and non-financial competing interest in that she founded MentorCONNECT, and as its Executive Director does earn salary from the organization.

Authors' contributions

MP designed the study, carried out the data collection, and drafted the manuscript. AKVD assisted in the writing of the method section, and helped draft the rest of the manuscript. SC conceived of the study, participated in the design and implementation, and edited the manuscript. All authors read and approved the final manuscript.

Authors' information

MP conducted the study and drafted the manuscript while at Texas A&M University but has since moved to Arizona State University.

Author details

[1]Department of Psychology, Texas A&M University, 4235 TAMU, College Station, TX 77843-4235, USA. [2]MentorCONNECT, www.mentorconnect-ed.org, Houston, Texas, USA.

References

1. Kazdin AE, Blasé SL: **Rebooting psychotherapy research and practice to reduce the burden of mental illness.** *Perspect Psychol Sci* 2011, **6:**21–37.
2. Nishiono-Maher A, Escobar-Koch T, Ringwood S, Banker J, van Furth E, Schmidt U: **What are the top five essential features of a high quality eating disorder service? A comparison of the views of US and UK eating disorder sufferers, carers, and health professionals.** *Eur Eat Disord Rev* 2011, **19:**411–416.
3. Escobar-Koch T, Banker JD, Crow S, Cullis J, Ringwood S, Smith G, van Furth E, Westin K, Schmidt U: **Service users' views of eating disorder services: an international comparison.** *Int J Eat Disord* 2010, **43:**549–559.
4. Rorty M, Yager J, Rossotto E: **Why and how do women recover from bulimia nervosa? The subjective appraisals of forty women recovered for a year or more.** *Int J Eat Disord* 1993, **14:**249–260.
5. Franko D: **Anorexia nervosa and bulimia: a self-help group.** *Small Gr Res* 1987, **18:**398–407.
6. Garfinkel P, Garner D: *Anorexia Nervosa: A Multidimensional Perspective.* New York: Brunner/Mazel; 1982.
7. Neuman P, Halvorson P: *Anorexia Nervosa & Bulimia: A Handbook For Counselors And Therapists.* New York: Reinhold; 1983.
8. Rakita-Leon G: *Treating Eating Disorders: Obesity, Anorexia Nervosa, And Bulimia.* Lexington, MA: Lewis; 1983.
9. Deeble EA, Bhat AV: **Women attending a self-help group for anorexia and bulimia: Views on self-help and professional treatment.** *Br Rev Bulim Anorex Nerv* 1991, **5:**23–28.
10. World Services AA: *Alcoholics Anonymous: The Story Of How Many Thousands Of Men And Women Have Recovered From Alcoholism.* 4th edition. New York: Alcoholics Anonymous World Services; 2001.
11. Malenbaum R, Herzog D, Eisenthal S, Wyshak G: **Overeaters anonymous: impact on bulimia.** *Int J Eat Disord* 1998, **7:**139–143.
12. Waisberg JL, Woods MT: **A nutrition and behavior change group for patients with anorexia nervosa.** *Can J Diet Pract Res* 2002, **63:**202–205.
13. Eichhorn KC: **Soliciting and providing social support over the internet: an investigation of online eating disorder support groups.** *J Comput-Mediat Comm* 2008, **14:**67–78.
14. Winzelberg A: **The analysis of an electronic support group for individuals with eating disorders.** *Comput Hum Behav* 1997, **13:**393–407.
15. Gleason NA: **A new approach to disordered eating – using an electronic bulletin board to confront social pressure on body image.** *J of Am College Health* 1995, **44:**78–80.
16. Wasson DH, Jackson M: **An analysis of the role of overeaters anonymous in women's recovery from bulimia nervosa.** *Eat Disord* 2004, **12:**337–356.
17. Cutts S: *Beating ANA: How To Outsmart Your Eating Disorder And Take Your Life Back.* Deerfield Beach, FL: Health Communications Inc.; 2009.
18. Straussner SLA, Byrne H: **Alcoholics Anonymous: key research findings from 2002–2007.** *Alcohol Treat Q* 2009, **27:**349–367.
19. Pagano ME, Friend KB, Tonigan JS, Stout RL: **Helping other alcoholics in Alcoholics Anonymous and drinking outcomes: findings from project MATCH.** *J Stud Alcohol Drugs* 2004, **65:**766–773.
20. Pagano ME, Zemore SE, Onder CC, Stout RL: **Predictors of initial AA-related helping: Findings from project MATCH.** *J Stud Alcohol Drugs* 2009, **70:**117–125.
21. Zemore SE, Kaskutas LA, Ammon LN: **In 12-step groups, helping helps the helper.** *Addiction* 2004, **99:**1015–1023.
22. Kammeyer-Maher JD, Judge TA: **A quantitative review of mentoring research: test of a model.** *J Vocat Behav* 2008, **72:**269–283.
23. Randolph KA, Johnson JL: **School-based mentoring programs: a review of the research.** *Child Sch* 2008, **30:**177–185.
24. Summers SJ, Funk K, Twombly L, Waddell M, Squires J: **The explication of a mentor model, videotaping, and reflective consultation in support of infant mental health.** *Inf Mental Hlth J* 2007, **28:**216–236.
25. Johnston C, Smethurst N, Gowers S: **Should people with a history of an eating disorder work as eating disorder therapists?** *Eur Eat Disord Rev* 2005, **13:**301–310.
26. Costin C, Johnson CL: **Been there, done that: Clinicians' use of personal recovery in the treatment of eating disorders.** *Eat Disord* 2002, **10:**293–303.
27. Riessman F: **The 'helper' therapy principle.** *Soc Work* 1965, **10:**27–32.
28. Russell JEA: **Mentoring.** In *Encyclopedia Of Applied Psychology.* Volume 2nd edition. Edited by Spielberger C. New York: Academic; 2004:609–615.
29. Stice E, Telch CF, Rizvi SL: **Development and validation of the eating disorder diagnostic scale: a brief self-report measure for anorexia, bulimia, and binge eating disorder.** *Psychol Assess* 2000, **12:**123–131.
30. Stice E, Fisher M, Martinez E: **Eating disorder diagnostic scale: additional evidence of reliability and validity.** *Psychol Assess* 2004, **16:**60–71.
31. Adair CE, Marcoux GC, Cram BS, Ewashen CJ, Chafe J, Cassin SE, Brown KE: **Development and multi-site validation of a new condition-specific quality of life measure for eating disorders.** *Health Qual Life Outcomes* 2007, **5:**23. http://www.hqlo.com/content/5/1/23.
32. Adair CE, Marcoux GC: *Eating Disorder Quality Of Life Scale (EDQLS): Administration And Scoring Manual.* Calgary, Alberta, Canada: Adair Marcoux Informetrics; 2008.
33. de la Rie S, Noordenbos G, Donker M, van Furth E: **The patient's view on quality of life and eating disorders.** *Int J Eat Disord* 2006, **39:**1–8.
34. Hay P: **Quality of life and bulimic eating disorder behaviors: findings from a community-based sample.** *Int J Eat Disord* 2003, **33:**434–442.
35. Bodell LP, Smith AR, Holm-Denoma JM, Gordon KH, Joiner TE Jr: **The impact of perceived social support and negative life events on bulimic symptoms.** *Eat Behav* 2011, **12:**44–48.
36. Barbarich NC: **Lifetime prevalence of eating disorders among professionals in the field.** *Eat Disord* 2002, **10:**305–312.

37. Warren CS, Crowley ME, Olivardia R, Schoen A: **Treating patients with eating disorders: an examination of treatment providers' experiences.** *Eat Disord* 2009, **17**:27–45.
38. Costin C, Grabb GS: *8 keys to recovery from an eating disorder: effective strategies from therapeutic practice and personal experience.* New York: W.W. Norton & Company, Inc.; 2012.

3

Psychotropic drug prescribing in an Australian specialist child and adolescent eating disorder service: a retrospective study

Julia K Moore[1,3], Hunna J Watson[1,2,3,4*], Emily Harper[1], Julie McCormack[1] and Thinh Nguyen[5]

Abstract

Background: To describe the rates, indications, and adverse effects of psychotropic drug prescription in a specialist tertiary hospital child and adolescent eating disorder service.

Methods: Retrospective case note study of all active eating disorder patients ($N = 115$) over the period of treatment from referral to time of study ($M = 2$ years), covering patient demographics, clinical characteristics, drug prescriptions, indications, and adverse effects.

Results: Psychotropic drugs were prescribed in 45% of cases, most commonly antidepressants (41%), followed by anxiolytics (29%) and antipsychotics (22%), with 8% initiated before referral to the specialist eating disorder program. Common indications were depressed mood, agitation, anxiety, and insomnia. Patient clinical severity and complexity was associated with prescribing. Adverse effects, mostly minor, were recorded in 23% of antidepressant prescriptions, 39% of antipsychotic prescriptions, and 13% of anxiolytic prescriptions. Second generation antipsychotic prescription was associated with subsequent new onset binge eating, in this preliminary observational study. Self-harm by overdose of psychotropics occurred in 11% of patients prescribed medication.

Conclusions: Psychotropic medications were frequently prescribed to adolescent eating disorder patients to treat distressing symptoms. Prospective randomised controlled trials to clarify efficacy and safety are needed. Given the difficulties of conducting clinical trials in this population, services are encouraged to monitor and audit medication safety and efficacy in everyday practice, and to report their findings.

Keywords: Adolescent, Adverse effects, Binge eating, Child, Drug therapy, Eating disorders, Pharmacology

Background

Eating disorders (EDs) affect up to 15% of women in their lifetime [1] and have their peak incidence in adolescence [2]. The nutritional compromise, particularly in anorexia nervosa (AN), occurs during critical brain development and is associated with brain mass reduction [3] and neuropsychological abnormalities [4]. Adolescent EDs are associated with a mortality of approximately 2.9% over 6 years [5] and profound negative impacts on physical, psychological, and social development [2].

Guidelines for treatment, based on expert consensus and weak to moderate levels of evidence, recommend a specialist multidisciplinary team approach with medical, nutritional, social, and psychological care, including family and/or individual psychotherapy [6-8]. Family-based treatment, a specific treatment modality that directly addresses the ED, has a moderate level of evidence in paediatric AN [2]. There is limited evidence to guide treatment selection among paediatric bulimia nervosa (BN) or EDs not otherwise specified (EDNOS) [6,8]. Medication is not recommended as the sole treatment for any ED [6-9]. Nonetheless, psychotropic drugs are prescribed, often off-label, for comorbidities, distress, agitation, and sometimes in an attempt to treat core ED symptoms. Impact on growth and development is largely unknown, and there is little evidence to guide dosage [10].

Selective serotonin reuptake inhibitors (SSRIs) such as fluoxetine have been prescribed to adolescents with EDs

* Correspondence: Hunna.watson@health.wa.gov.au
[1]Princess Margaret Hospital for Children, Perth, Australia
[2]Centre for Clinical Interventions, Perth, Australia
Full list of author information is available at the end of the article

for comorbid depression, anxiety, and obsessive-compulsive disorder (OCD). In young people without EDs, there is high-quality evidence supporting efficacy of fluoxetine and some other SSRIs for these disorders [11]. However, there is no evidence to support treatment with SSRIs in patients with a low body mass index; the available case reports and studies suggest that SSRIs are ineffective for symptoms of depression, anxiety, or OCD in very underweight patients, which is pertinent to AN [10]. There was no benefit from SSRIs in relapse prevention, core ED symptoms, depressive or obsessive-compulsive symptoms in a retrospective study of partially weight-restored female adolescents with AN [12]. Likewise, fluoxetine did not prevent relapse in weight-restored AN adults receiving cognitive-behavioural therapy [13]. The well-publicised finding of a small but significant increased risk of suicidality in youth after commencement of SSRIs was derived from meta-analyses of trials conducted for depression and anxiety disorders [14]; it is unknown to what extent these findings generalise to EDs. Individuals with EDs have an elevated risk of suicidality and deliberate self-harm [15,16]. Drug overdose is a leading method of suicide particularly among females [17], yet little is known about risk of overdose of prescription drugs in this context.

Second generation antipsychotics (SGAs) such as olanzapine are used as an adjunctive treatment for EDs, for anxiety, agitation, and ruminations on themes of food and body image, and to attempt to promote weight gain in malnourished patients. There has recently been interest in olanzapine treatment for AN, accompanied by increasing caution about potential adverse effects. Studies in adults with AN are mixed, though some trials suggest that SGAs improve core symptoms [18]. Prescribing pharmacotherapy involves weighing up potential benefits and risks. Norris et al. [19] published a retrospective matched-groups comparison of 86 female adolescents with AN, 43 treated with olanzapine, and 43 matched comparators. No conclusions could be drawn regarding efficacy. The most notable finding was of adverse effects in 56% of patients treated with olanzapine, most commonly sedation (40%) and lipid abnormality (29% of those screened), highlighting the need to maintain surveillance of medication safety – most older studies do not report lipid or blood glucose monitoring. Olanzapine, quetiapine, and risperidone can cause weight gain and metabolic adverse effects, such as impaired glucose tolerance and dyslipidaemia in children and adolescents, to a greater extent than in adults [20]. They may have a negative effect on bone density, mediated by hyperprolactinaemia [21]. There is also a potential for cardiac side-effects such as QT_c prolongation associated with SGA usage. The QT_c interval has been shown to be longer in AN than in healthy controls, suggesting particular vulnerability [22]. There is a case report of QT_c prolongation occurring repeatedly in an adolescent with AN treated with olanzapine, then risperidone, in combination with fluoxetine [23]. The cardiac risk is of particular concern for patients with AN due to nutritional deficiencies, impaired calcium and phosphate metabolism, and hypokalaemia in patients with symptoms of purging, which predispose to life-threatening arrhythmias. Hypokalaemia can cause U wave formation and flattened T waves on the ECG, which complicates the measurement of the QT_c interval, and so the QT_c interval needs to be interpreted carefully in such cases [24].

SGAs are known to increase appetite and cause weight gain, and some case reports and series, including one on a child with AN, have linked SGAs to emergence, exacerbation, and recurrence of binge eating [25-30]. McKnight and Park [31] found no published evidence that SGAs contribute to the development of binge eating, but reported their clinical observation that SGAs appear to exacerbate binge eating in patients with pre-existing bulimic symptoms. In a consecutive case series of 74 adolescent and adult psychiatric patients treated with clozapine or olanzapine, emergent binge-eating symptomatology or full-blown EDs were more common among those with a history of EDs than those without [29]. Emergent binge eating in patients with restricting AN is a common event: more than half of a sample of young adult women with restricting AN crossed over to the binge eating/purging subtype or to BN in a 7 year longitudinal study [32]. Given these findings, case reports and clinical impressions are difficult to interpret. Dysregulation of eating behaviours through either restricting or binge eating is distressing and problematic, so it is important to be vigilant regarding binge eating as a potential adverse effect of medication.

Anxiolytic drugs such as benzodiazepines are prescribed to patients with EDs to control insomnia, agitation, and anxiety and to facilitate nutritional resuscitation, but there are currently no randomized controlled trials and little literature of any kind describing their use [18]. In children with anxiety disorders, problems with disinhibition, irritability, and drowsiness have been reported with clonazepam [33]. In adults with anxiety disorders, benzodiazepines may impair memory and learning and in some instances reduce the efficacy of specific psychotherapies [34].

A recent report of psychotropic medication use in American adult women with anorexia nervosa between 1997 and 2009 found that of 539 patients presenting for bone density screening, 53% were currently taking a psychotropic medication, most commonly antidepressants (48%) and antipsychotics (13%) [21]. The use of atypical antipsychotics (most commonly quetiapine) had doubled over the 13 year period of the study. Widespread use of these medications is of concern, given the absence of conclusive evidence of benefit and the potential adverse effects.

Few studies report actual psychotropic prescribing in specialist child and adolescent ED services. In a retrospective case note study of 60 children and adolescents with AN newly referred to an Italian specialist psychiatric unit between 2000 and 2004, 16 (32%) were prescribed psychotropic medication [35]. Seventy-six percent of prescriptions were for antidepressants, most commonly paroxetine and sertraline, prescribed for comorbid depression or OCD. Antipsychotic medications accounted for 21% of prescriptions, most commonly haloperidol and olanzapine, for indications of "anguish" and "thought disorders". Sixteen percent received two or more medications concurrently. Adverse events were reported for 29% of prescriptions. In a retrospective case note study of 308 ED cases seen in seven specialist UK child and adolescent ED services during 2005 to 2006 [36], psychotropic drugs were prescribed for 27% of patients, mainly those with AN. Fluoxetine and olanzapine were the most common prescriptions, and the most common indications were depression, anxiety and "pseudo-psychotic" concerns about weight. Adverse effects were reported for 15% of antidepressant prescriptions and 28% of antipsychotic prescriptions, but 38% of olanzapine prescriptions. No conclusions could be drawn about the effectiveness of medications.

Clinicians treating children and adolescents with EDs currently lack evidence-based guidance about psychopharmacological treatment, including efficacy, appropriate doses, and adverse effects. Little is known about how clinicians apply their experience and expert opinion. This study aimed to report the use of psychotropic drugs in a specialist setting, including medication doses and indications; to identify adverse effects; and to describe characteristics of the patient population including illness severity and comorbidity and to correlate these with prescribing practices. We also aimed to report monitoring for medication safety, including ECG monitoring and QT_c prolongation, and metabolic monitoring; and to document the frequency of significant adverse events such as deliberate overdose, emergent suicidality while prescribed SSRIs, and drug-related hyponatraemia. We hypothesised in general that psychotropic prescription would be associated with greater patient clinical severity and complexity, characterised by more severe eating, depressive, anxiety, and dissociative symptomatology, Axis I comorbidity, onset of deliberate self-harm acts and suicidal ideation, presence of binge eating, and admissions and bed days. Based on clinical observations, we tentatively hypothesised that there would be an association between antipsychotic use and emergent binge eating.

Methods

Participants

Participants were patients of Princess Margaret Hospital for Children (PMH) Eating Disorders Program (EDP). This is the only public specialist child and adolescent ED service in Western Australia (census population 2 331 500) [37]. The program offers outpatient and day-patient treatment, and inpatient treatment for medical stabilisation. The EDP accepts referrals of patients under age 16 and cares for patients up to gradual transition to adult services after age 18. At the study enrolment date, 14 April 2011, the EDP had 130 patients. At any given time, about eight EDP patients are in hospital for medical stabilisation and nutritional rehabilitation.

All 'active' patients of PMH EDP ($N = 115$), who met Diagnostic and Statistical Manual (DSM-IV) [38] criteria for an ED at initial assessment, were included. 'Active' refers to receiving treatment or follow-up of any kind at the study enrolment date. From the initial participant pool of 130, 7 patients were excluded who had not engaged following initial assessment and 8 patients were excluded as they did not meet criteria for an ED (generally had subthreshold eating problems).

Service model and provision

All patients are initially assessed through a comprehensive multidisciplinary process, including psychosocial diagnostic interview; paediatric medical and dietetic assessment; separate interviews of child and parents using child and parent informant versions of the Eating Disorder Examination (EDE) [39]; the Children's Depression Inventory (CDI) [40]; the Multidimensional Anxiety Scale for Children (MASC) [41]; and the Adolescent Dissociative Experiences Scale (A-DES) [42] self-report instruments. Information from the assessment is then reviewed in a multidisciplinary meeting, including the team psychiatrists, to determine a DSM-IV [38] ED diagnosis, any comorbid DSM-IV psychiatric diagnoses, and treatment plan. Further review by a team psychiatrist is readily available as needed, for example for diagnostic clarification, management planning, treatment of comorbid psychiatric disorders, and initiation and monitoring of psychotropic medication where necessary.

Patients are treated in a multidisciplinary team model, and each patient and family have a care coordinator. All patients are offered psychological therapy, including individual, group, and family therapy in various modalities. Weight restoration and physical monitoring are prioritised. Inpatient admissions for malnutrition are under the care of a paediatric gastroenterology team, with psychological medicine support, on a paediatric medicine ward, not a psychiatric ward. The goal of admission is to provide rapid, intensive nutritional rehabilitation to facilitate prompt return to family and community, often using nasogastric tube feeding. On occasion, provided that he or she is not at acute nutritional risk, a patient is admitted to a separate acute psychiatric ward for management of comorbid conditions and self-harm behaviours; close liaison is maintained with the ward clinical team regarding such patients.

The prescription of psychotropic medication usually follows psychiatric assessment by the EDP team consultant psychiatrist, psychiatry registrar or supervised medical officer. Occasionally, medications are initiated by paediatric staff. Some patients are referred already on medication prescribed by their general practitioner or psychiatrist. Within the EDP, all prescriptions are through a public hospital pharmacy at the same relatively low cost per medication per month, regardless of the medication or dosage, and further reduced for concession card holders. Cost to the patient is therefore not a major influence on prescribing practice.

Measures

Eating disorder examination

Child and parent informant versions of the clinician-administered structured EDE [39], widely considered the gold standard for assessing eating disorders, measured severity of eating disorder psychopathology based on the global score. Cronbach alpha reliability in the present study was 0.94.

Children's depression inventory

The 27-item CDI [40] is a well-established self-report measure of depressive symptoms with excellent reliability and construct validity, and has discriminant validity as demonstrated by evidence of its utility as a screening measure for depressive disorders [43]. Cronbach alpha reliability was 0.91.

Multidimensional anxiety scale for children

Anxiety symptoms were assessed with the self-report 39-item MASC, which has excellent psychometric properties [41]. Cronbach alpha reliability was 0.91.

Adolescent dissociative experiences scale

Dissociative symptoms were measured with the self-report 30-item A-DES, which has good reliability and validity, with increased scores corresponding to lifetime history of trauma [42]. Cronbach alpha reliability was 0.99.

Other sociodemographic and clinical features

These were extracted from psychological and medical records or an available clinical audit database. Children had been weighed wearing underwear and a hospital gown, using electronic scales accurate to 50 g. Height had been measured with the patient standing without shoes and socks, standing on a hard surface and using a Harpenden stadiometer, accurate to 1 mm. BMI z-scores had been calculated via Epi Info 7 [44] by entering the patient's age, height, and weight into the program. Z-scores were age- and sex-specific based on the Centers for Disease Control and Prevention [45,46] growth charts.

Procedure

The study received approval from the PMH Human Research Ethics Committee as a quality of care audit. A purpose designed paper form was used to collect information retrospectively from the medical file and psychiatric file of each patient, by reading through all case notes, correspondence, assessment materials, and medication charts. To test the clarity and ease of use of the form and to evaluate the inter-rater agreement for extracted data, JKM and EH both collected data from the same five randomly selected files; no discrepancies were found, yielding very high inter-rater reliability. Data collected included age, gender, date of assessment, duration of illness before referral, inpatient admissions, medical conditions, body mass index z score, history of self-harm or suicidal ideation or acts, binge eating history, EDE, CDI, MASC and A-DES scores; all of these are consistently and routinely recorded in a standardised assessment document for each new patient assessed by EDP. Further data collected included ECG, blood lipids, fasting blood glucose, and any extrapyramidal symptoms, hyponatraemia or QT_c prolongation; these were documented for some patients but not for others. Information collected about medication included prescriber, dose range, and total days of exposure, all of which were clearly documented for each patient; and indication, adverse effects, and reason for cessation, which were documented with a variable level of detail. Drug prescriptions by any prescriber within or external to the EDP were recorded, both prior to intake assessment at EDP, and subsequent to assessment, up until the date of the audit. PRN (pro re nata or "as required") medication for inpatients was not recorded. A hospital pharmacy database of all outpatient prescriptions was used to cross-check, but no missed medications were found.

Data were anonymised at collection with a study ID. The data collection team included a psychiatrist, advanced trainee in psychiatry, clinical psychologist, research psychologist, and mental health nurses, who all met to discuss standardisation of the data collection procedure. JKM (an advanced trainee in psychiatry) designed the coding procedure, performed all coding and entered all data into a spreadsheet. All data were re-checked against the original paper forms by JKM.

Statistical analysis

A series of analyses of variance (ANOVAs) for continuous outcomes and chi square tests of independence for categorical outcomes compared those prescribed (pre-referral and within EDP) versus not prescribed antidepressants, antipsychotics, and anxiolytics, respectively on a range of clinical characteristics across pre-referral, intake, and during service engagement. The 'other' psychotropic category was excluded from comparisons because of low frequency of use. The relationship between number of prescriptions and clinical characteristics was examined by way of ANOVAs and chi square testing. A logistic regression tested whether new binge onset (0 = no, 1 = yes) could be predicted from antipsychotic medication status (0 = no/prescribed antipsychotic after date of new binge onset, 1 = yes). All analyses were preliminary and exploratory, hence univariate analysis with no adjustment for multiple comparisons was used. Alpha was set at the conventional level of .05.

Results

Demographic characteristics

The sample included 115 patients, age 7 to 16 years, with 11 males and 104 females (90% female). The mean age at referral was 13 years (*SD* = 1.60). Average duration of engagement from referral up to the point of audit was 2 years (*SD* = 1.52 years; range = 25 days to 7 yrs 1 month).

Clinical characteristics

At intake, most met criteria for AN (*n* = 55, 48%; restricting subtype, *n* = 48, 42%; binge-purge subtype, *n* = 7, 6%) or EDNOS (*n* = 54, 47%), and a minority had BN (*n* = 6, 5%; purging subtype, *n* = 4, 3%; non-purging subtype, *n* = 2, 2%). The mean age of onset was 12 years (*SD* = 1.66) and the mean untreated duration of illness was 9 months (*SD* = 7.73). Forty-eight percent (*n* = 55) had a comorbid psychiatric diagnosis, most commonly an anxiety disorder (27%, *n* = 31) or major depressive episode (26%, *n* = 30). Two or more comorbid psychiatric diagnoses were present in 17% (*n* = 20). Twenty-seven percent (*n* = 31) had a comorbid medical diagnosis, the most frequent being asthma/atopic syndromes.

Psychometric assessments at intake showed above average depressive and anxiety symptoms, indicated by mean *t* scores of 56 (*SD* = 21.12, *n* = 109) on the CDI and 54 (*SD* = 13.22, *n* = 108) on the MASC. Using available data, the proportion with a *t* score ≥ 65 indicating clinically significant levels was 37% on the CDI and 24% on the MASC. Lifetime suicidal ideation was reported by 28% of cases (present, *n* = 32; absent, *n* = 74, 64%; unknown, *n* = 9, 8%). Lifetime deliberate self-harm was also common (present, *n* = 18, 16%; absent, *n* = 88, 77%; unknown, *n* = 9, 8%). Three cases reported a previous suicide attempt. During engagement with the ED service, a further 8% (*n* = 8) had new onset suicidal ideation or intent, 5% (*n* = 6) had new onset suicide attempts, and 16% (*n* = 19) had new onset deliberate self-harm. Sixty-five individuals (57%) had received inpatient treatment. The median number of admissions for the full sample of 115 patients was one (range 0 to 41) and median total bed days throughout service engagement was 15 (range 0 to 921).

Drug prescriptions

Psychotropic medication was prescribed to 52 of 115 patients (45%) pre-assessment or during engagement with PMH EDP. The youngest age at prescription was 10 years. Prescriptions were relatively infrequent for pre-adolescents compared to adolescents. The proportion of patients who were prescribed a psychotropic, by diagnosis, was 31/55 (56%) for AN, 4/6 (67%) for BN, and 17/54 (31%) for EDNOS.

Prescription frequencies prior to specialist service referral

Prior to referral, 9 cases (8%) were prescribed psychotropic medication. There were nine prescriptions, eight for antidepressants and one for lithium.

Prescription frequencies within the specialist eating disorder service

Forty-eight of the 115 patients (42%) were prescribed a new psychotropic medication during treatment within EDP. There were 138 prescriptions as some cases were prescribed multiple medications concurrently and/or sequentially. During engagement with EDP, 42 (37%) were prescribed antidepressants, 33 (29%) were prescribed anxiolytics or sedative/hypnotics, 25 (22%) were prescribed antipsychotics, and two (2%) were prescribed other psychotropic medications. Prescriptions were for 21 different psychotropics. The median time between assessment and prescription of psychotropic medication was 167 days (range 3 to 2012 days).

Medication classes

Antidepressants were the most common class prescribed either pre-referral or within the ED service. Overall (pre-referral and within EDP), antidepressants were prescribed in 47 of 115 patients (41%), followed by anxiolytics in 33 (29%), antipsychotics in 25 (22%), and other psychotropics in three (3%). The main indication for antidepressants was depression (Table 1).

Antidepressants

Fluoxetine was the most frequently prescribed antidepressant (see Table 1 for indication and dosage characteristics), comprising 39/60 (65%) of antidepressant prescriptions. Adverse effects were reported for 9/39 (23%) prescriptions. Although most were minor (sedation, dizziness, tremor), there was one case of new onset deliberate self-harm, two cases of small intentional overdose, and one case of large intentional overdose. (Here, and in all instances that follow, "small intentional overdose" is used when the admitting emergency department doctor described the overdose as "small" and no treatment or monitoring was required;

Table 1 Antidepressant prescriptions and indications in a specialist child and adolescent eating disorders program.

	Number of prescriptions		Indications											
Dosage/day (*M*, range)	**Pre-referral**	**During EDP**	**Depression mood**	**Depression & anxiety**	**Depression & OCD anxiety**	**OCD**	**Anxiety**	**Depression & OCD**	**OCD & anxiety**	**Depression & PTSD**	**Depression & insomnia**	**Anxiety & bulimic symptoms**	**Depression & bulimic symptoms**	**Unclear**
Amitriptyline (25 mg, NA)	-	1	-	-	-	-	-	-	-	-	1	-	-	-
Citalopram (32 mg, 20-60 mg)	-	6	3	2	-	-	-	1	-	-	-	-	-	-
Desvenlafaxine (83 mg, 50-100 mg)	-	3	3	-	-	-	-	-	-	-	-	-	-	-
Escitalopram (15 mg, 10-20 mg)	1	1	-	1	-	1	-	-	-	-	-	-	-	-
Fluoxetine (32 mg, 10-60 mg)	4	35	21	4	3	2	2	1	2	2	-	1	1	-
Fluvoxamine (150 mg, NA)	1	-	-	-	1	-	-	-	-	-	-	-	-	-
Mirtazapine (22 mg, 15-30 mg)	1	1	-	-	-	-	-	-	-	-	1	-	-	1
Moclobemide (150 mg, NA)	-	1	1	-	-	-	-	-	-	-	-	-	-	-
Sertraline (100 mg, NA)	1	-	1	-	-	-	-	-	-	-	-	-	-	-
Venlafaxine (168 mg, 150-225 mg)	-	4	2	1	1	-	-	-	-	-	-	-	-	-
Total	60		31 (52%)	8 (13%)	5 (8%)	3 (5%)	2 (3%)	2 (3%)	2 (3%)	2 (3%)	2 (3%)	1 (2%)	1 (2%)	1 (2%)

"large intentional overdose" is used when the admitting doctor described the overdose as "large" or inpatient medical treatment, cardiac or respiratory monitoring, pharmacological antidote, or intensive care was given). Fluoxetine was ceased in 15 instances, due primarily to either ineffectiveness or patient disengagement.

Twenty-one of 60 (35%) antidepressant prescriptions were for medications other than fluoxetine (see Table 1). Many prescriptions (38%, 8/21) occurred after a trial of fluoxetine. Five patients prescribed other antidepressant medications had adverse effects. A patient prescribed citalopram took a large overdose, while serotonin syndrome and new onset of suicidality and deliberate self-harm were noted in a patient prescribed moclobemide. One of the two patients prescribed mirtazapine developed new onset binge eating. Dizziness was reported with one patient prescribed sertraline. Medication was ceased in 8/21 instances (38%).

There was one case of hyponatraemia (plasma sodium 115 mmol/L) associated with fluoxetine treatment in an underweight 16 year-old male who had excessive water consumption; plasma sodium normalised with normalisation of water intake, while fluoxetine treatment continued.

Antipsychotics

The main indications for antipsychotic medications were agitation and anxiety (Table 2). All prescriptions were made during EDP treatment. There were 32 prescriptions for antipsychotics, 24/32 for quetiapine, 7/32 for olanzapine, and 1/32 for risperidone. Adverse events were reported in 41% (13/32) of prescription instances. Among these were nine cases prescribed quetiapine; one took a large overdose, there was clinical concern about precipitation or exacerbation of binge eating in two cases, one had extrapyramidal side effects while taking quetiapine 75 mg in combination with fluoxetine 20 mg and lorazepam 3 mg, one had QT_c prolongation, three reported somnolence, and one reported nightmares. In four cases there was clinical concern that olanzapine may have precipitated or exacerbated binge eating. Antipsychotic medication was ceased in 69% (22/32) of instances.

Anxiolytics and sedative-hypnotics

These were prescribed primarily for insomnia, anxiety, and agitation (Table 3). Lorazepam comprised more than half (28/46) of these prescriptions. Adverse effects were experienced by 13% (6/46) of those prescribed anxiolytics, all of whom were taking lorazepam. One adolescent took a small overdose, four reported somnolence, and one reported nausea. Medication was ceased in 83% of prescription instances (38/46).

Other medications

One patient was prescribed lithium pre-referral for a diagnosis of bipolar disorder. Lithium was ceased after EDP assessment with revision of the diagnosis. During EDP engagement, one patient was prescribed St John's wort by an external clinician for depression, and one was prescribed atomoxetine then dexamphetamine for attention deficit-hyperactivity disorder.

Pharmacotherapy vs. non-pharmacotherapy patient characteristics

Exploratory ANOVAs and chi square tests comparing those prescribed and not prescribed antidepressants on the clinical variables in Table 4 (results not presented), showed that the group prescribed antidepressant medication had significantly higher EDE, CDI, A-DES, Axis I comorbidity, binge eating presence, admissions, bed days, new onset deliberate self-harm and suicidality, and were less likely to have EDNOS (*ps* $< .05$). The group prescribed antipsychotic medication had significantly higher EDE, CDI, Axis I comorbidity, admissions, bed days, binge eating presence, and new onset deliberate self-harm and suicidality. Compared to those who did not receive anxiolytics, the group prescribed anxiolytics had higher EDE, CDI, Axis I comorbidity, admissions, bed days, binge eating presence, and new onset deliberate self-harm and suicidality, and were less likely to have EDNOS (*ps* $< .05$).

Number of prescriptions and polypharmacy

The total number of drugs prescribed per patient within PMH EDP ranged from 0 to 7. ANOVA and chi square analyses showed that of the clinical variables presented in Table 4, a higher number of prescriptions was associated with clinical severity (characterised by more severe eating and depressive symptomatology, Axis I comorbidity, onset of deliberate self-harm acts and suicidal ideation, presence of binge eating, and more admissions and bed days).

Concurrent prescriptions (i.e., having more than one prescription at a time) occurred during service engagement in 30% (34/115) of patients. The maximum number of concurrent prescriptions was four, with the following proportions: two drugs for 17% (19/115), three drugs for 10% (12/115), and four drugs for 3% (3/115). An antidepressant combined with an anxiolytic, an antipsychotic, or both, were the most common combinations.

Medication safety

Safety considerations studied included QT_c prolongation, ECG monitoring and metabolic monitoring for SGAs, deliberate overdose, and emergent suicidality with SSRIs. Another objective was to investigate the possibility of emergent binge eating with antipsychotics.

QT_c prolongation on ECG of clinical concern was recorded in two patients; both were nutritionally compromised, dehydrated female adolescent inpatients. The QT_c prolongation did not result in adverse clinical consequences. One patient was prescribed olanzapine,

Table 2 Antipsychotic prescriptions and indications in a specialist child and adolescent eating disorders program.

	Number of prescriptions		Indications											
Dosage/day (*M*, range)	**Pre-referral**	**During EDP**	**Anxiety**	**Agitation**	**Anxiety & agitation**	**Anxiety & insomnia**	**Depression & anxiety**	**Depression & PTSD**	**Depression & agitation**	**PTSD**	**Depression**	**Depression & insomnia**	**Depression & insomnia & affective dysregulation**	**OCD & anorexic ruminations**
Olanzapine (6.8 mg, 2.5-15 mg)	-	7	2	3	1	-	1	-	-	-	-	-	-	-
Quetiapine (56 mg, 12.5-200 mg)	-	24	7	4	3	2	1	1	1	1	1	1	1	1
Risperidone (1 mg, NA)	-	1	-	1	-	-	-	-	-	-	-	-	-	-
Total	32		9 (27%)	8 (24%)	4 (12%)	2 (6%)	2 (6%)	1 (3%)	1 (3%)	1 (3%)	1 (3%)	1 (3%)	1 (3%)	1 (3%)

Table 3 Anxiolytic prescriptions and indications in a specialist child and adolescent eating disorders program.

	Number of prescriptions		Indications							
Dosage/day (*M*, range)	**Pre-referral**	**During EDP**	**Insomnia**	**Anxiety**	**Anxiety & agitation**	**Agitation**	**Anxiety & insomnia**	**Depression & PTSD**	**PTSD**	**Unclear**
Clonazepam (2.3 mg, 1–4 mg)	-	4	-	-	2	1	1	-	-	-
Lorazepam (1.7 mg, 0.5-4 mg)	-	28	2	12	4	4	2	1	1	2
Melatonin (1.9 mg, 1.5-2 mg)	-	5	5	-	-	-	-	-	-	-
Nitrazepam (15 mg, 10–20 mg)	-	2	2	-	-	-	-	-	-	-
Temazepam (10 mg, 5–20 mg)	-	7	6	-	-	-	-	-	-	1
Total	46		15 (33%)	12 (26%)	6 (13%)	5 (11%)	3 (7%)	1 (2%)	1 (2%)	3 (7%)

clonazepam, nitrazepam and omeprazole, and had normal electrolytes. Medications were continued, and the mild QT_c prolongation of 469 ms resolved over three weeks as her nutritional state improved. The other was prescribed fluoxetine and recently commenced quetiapine, and had hypophosphataemia. Quetiapine was ceased, she was rehydrated and electrolytes were normalised, and the QTc prolongation of 500 ms resolved within 24 hours. Quetiapine was never reintroduced.

Only four of the 25 patients treated with a SGA had an ECG at baseline, and two had a repeat ECG within 2 weeks of initiation.

Table 4 Pre-referral, intake, and during service engagement characteristics of those prescribed none, one to two, or three or more psychotropic medications within a specialist child and adolescent eating disorders program.

		Number of prescriptions				
Time	**Characteristic**	**0 (*n* = 66)**	**1-2 (*n* = 27)**	**3+ (*n* = 22)**	***p***	**post hoc**
Pre-referral	Age at onset, yrs	12.79 (1.79)	12.81 (1.64)	12.95 (1.29)	ns	-
	Untreated duration of illness, mths	8.64 (7.61)	11.11 (7.98)	8.89 (7.76)	ns	-
	History of DSH/suicidal ideation	27% (16)	33% (8)	36% (8)	ns	-
	History of DSH acts	15% (9)	21% (5)	22% (4)	ns	-
	History of suicidal acts	3% (2)	0% (0)	5% (1)	ns	-
Intake	Age at referral, yrs	13.50 (1.76)	13.85 (1.49)	13.73 (1.60)	ns	-
	Primary diagnosis				ns	-
	AN	41% (27)	48% (13)	68% (15)	-	-
	non-AN	59% (39)	52% (14)	32% (7)	-	-
	(BN)	3% (2)	7% (2)	9% (2)	-	-
	(EDNOS)	56% (37)	44% (12)	23% (5)	-	-
	Axis I comorbidity	29% (19)	74% (20)	73% (16)	<.001	0 < exp; 1–2 > exp
	EDE	2.53 (1.57)	2.94 (1.59)	3.88 (1.58)	.003	1-2, 3+ > 0
	CDI *t* score	51.60 (21.87)	59.77 (17.80)	67.045 (18.33)	.008	3+ > 0
	MASC *t* score	52.94 (13.47)	53.24 (11.66)	59.10 (13.22)	ns	-
	ADES	1.95 (1.71)	2.16 (1.80)	2.57 (2.17)	ns	-
	BMI *z* score	−1.50 (1.38)	−1.60 (1.20)	−1.76 (.96)	ns	-
EDP	Inpatient admissions	0.48 (.71)	2.04 (2.28)	6.82 (8.82)	<.001	3+ > 0, 1-2
	Inpatient bed days	11.67 (18.59)	59.96 (82.69)	166.05 (218.58)	<.001	3+ > 0, 1-2
	DSH new onset	2% (1)	20% (5)	59% (13)	<.001	0 < exp; 3+ > exp
	Suicidality new onset	3% (2)	15% (4)	36% (8)	<.001	0 < exp; 3+ > exp
	Presence of objective binge episodes	24% (16)	38% (10)	68% (15)	.001	3+ > exp

Data are presented as means (standard deviations) or percentages (number) and are based on available data only (i.e., missing or unknown data excluded). Chi square post hoc analyses indicate whether cell counts are lower or higher than would be expected based on equivalent count distributions. ADES = Adolescent Dissociative Experiences Scale; AN = anorexia nervosa; BN = bulimia nervosa; BMI = body mass index; CDI = Children's Depression Inventory; DOI = duration of illness; DSH = deliberate self-harm; EDE = Eating Disorder Examination; EDNOS = eating disorders not otherwise specified; EDP = eating disorders program; exp = expected cell count; MASC = Multidimensional Anxiety Scale for Children. Missing data for some individuals; available data: EDE $n = 111$, CDI $n = 109$, MASC $n = 108$, ADES $n = 91$, DSH new onset, $n = 110$.

Self-harm by overdose was observed in 11% (6/52) of patients prescribed a psychotropic drug, with one taking an overdose on two separate occasions. Although there were no permanent sequelae, three instances involved large, potentially dangerous dosages.

In patients prescribed SGAs, none had monitoring of blood glucose or lipids at any time.

There were no completed suicides in the cohort (or in previous active cases since program inception). Of 106 evaluable patients, 3/42 (7%) prescribed antidepressants with an FDA black box warning label of suicidal risk (fluoxetine, sertraline, paroxetine, citalopram, escitalopram, fluvoxamine) experienced suicidality onset within 3 months of initiation, and overall 14/106 (13%) had suicidality onset at some time.

Eighty-three percent (96/115) of patients were binge abstinent at intake, and 19% (22/115) of the entire sample developed new binge eating during treatment in the EDP. An exploratory logistic regression showed that medication status reliably distinguished between those with and without new binge onset, $\chi^2(1) = 3.93$, $p = .047$. The odds ratio of new binge onset was 3.5 times as large for a patient prescribed antipsychotic medication than the odds for a patient not prescribed antipsychotic medication. Of the six patients with new binge onset after SGA initiation, three were prescribed olanzapine and three quetiapine. The exposure time before recorded binge onset ranged from 7 to 667 days ($M = 260$ days exposure, $SD = 235$ days).

Discussion

To the best of our knowledge, this is the first retrospective case note study of psychotropic drug prescribing in an Australian specialist child and adolescent ED program. Forty-five percent of patients were prescribed psychotropic medication. In our sample, 48% had one or more comorbid Axis I psychiatric diagnoses, consistent with reported high comorbidity [47,48]. Those with psychiatric comorbidity were significantly more likely to be prescribed medication. There was a significant relationship between prescribing (including number of prescriptions) and disease severity and number and total length of hospital admissions. Adverse effects of medication were commonly recorded and somewhat higher for antipsychotic medications (39%) than antidepressants (23%). Most of these adverse effects were minor, although there were a number of instances of non-fatal self-harm by overdose of medication. Deliberate overdose of prescribed medication was relatively frequent. The study showed a very preliminary association between emergent binge eating and antipsychotic use in this population, which may be explained by mechanisms linking SGAs and appetite dysregulation [49]. Before being accepted, this finding needs replication to establish that it is not reflective of sampling variability or a Type I error.

The prevalence of psychotropic prescription in this study was higher than reported by Gowers et al. [36] or Rossi et al. [35]. It is difficult to compare services operating in different countries, which probably have different patient populations, service resources, and care philosophies. In our sample 57% received inpatient treatment at some time compared with 41% in Gowers et al. [36]. These figures are not directly comparable, as different services have different criteria for admission, but may suggest a more severely unwell population in our study. Gowers et al. also reported a prevalence of 23% for comorbid psychiatric disorders, less than half the prevalence for our sample. The study designs differed, for example, Gowers et al. reported on prescribing during a 12-month period for all subjects, whereas we reported prescribing during the full period of engagement with the EDP, which averaged 24 months.

The medication dosages used were low to medium for antipsychotics. For antidepressants, most dosages were low to medium, but a few patients were on higher doses of selective serotonin uptake inhibitors, in line with usual clinical practice for adults with bulimia nervosa. No conclusions can be drawn about effectiveness or safety of dosages from the data.

Patients within our service were prescribed more benzodiazepines, such as lorazepam, than reported by Gowers et al. [36]: 29% of total prescriptions were for benzodiazepines, often for a short period. There were no cases of benzodiazepine abuse or other serious adverse effects. Severe and persistent insomnia was a common, distressing symptom in our patient population. Insomnia was noted as a consequence of malnutrition in a classic starvation experiment [50], though clinical literature on insomnia in EDs is lacking. We speculate that the rate of benzodiazepine prescription may reflect the clinical difficulties of managing acute re-feeding on a busy general paediatric ward without specialist mental health nursing and with limited resources to provide structured support for EDP patients: anxiety, agitation, and insomnia are common complaints in this setting.

Patients with EDs constitute a highly distressed, high-risk population, with prevalent suicidal attempts and ideation and deliberate self-harm. Among adults, 3% to 20% with AN and 25% to 35% with BN report a history of attempted suicide; completed suicide is more common in AN than BN [15,16]. Exact rates among children and adolescents are unknown. In our study, 11% of patients prescribed medication (6/52 patients) self-harmed by overdose on their prescribed psychotropic medication. Attention to prescribing medications of lower risk in overdose, limiting amount dispensed, observing medication being swallowed to reduce potential for hoarding, and engaging patients and families in maintaining safe medication storage are commonsense measures.

There are no data to indicate whether suicidality risk increases with SSRIs in a paediatric ED population; however, given there is a heightened risk in youth with anxiety and depressive problems to age 25 years, and that anxiety and depressive comorbidity is common in ED populations, this is an important safety concern. Of 20 patients who developed suicidality during service engagement, three of the 18 evaluable who had onset date recorded were within three months of SSRI initiation. Routine clinical monitoring for suicidality in ED populations is imperative, and future investigation of suicidality risk with SSRIs in paediatric ED patients is warranted.

Routine monitoring of metabolic parameters in patients prescribed antipsychotic medications is recommended by Australian guidelines [51]. Hyperlipidaemia is a common complication of antipsychotic therapy even in underweight young patients with EDs [19]. The PMH protocol for SGAs specifies regular monitoring of metabolic parameters; monitoring of weight and blood pressure is universal due to the close medical monitoring of EDP patients, but clinician compliance with monitoring of blood lipids and glucose was lacking. Compliance with ECG monitoring for QT_c prolongation in patients prescribed SGAs was low. This problem of translating evidence-based guidelines into routine clinical care is not unique to our service; low compliance with metabolic monitoring has been reported internationally [52]. An Australian specialist youth service has recently reported on barriers and enabling factors for metabolic monitoring within a first episode psychosis clinic [52] and showed substantial improvement in screening and monitoring after a package of interventions [53].

Limitations of this study include a retrospective audit design; adverse effects of medication may be under-recorded when pharmacovigilance occurs via spontaneous reporting [54]. This is likely to be particularly true for binge eating, which tends to be concealed. The retrospective design led to limitations due to variability in documentation; for example, if a prescriber documented "anxiety"

Table 5 Proposal for prescribing psychotropic medication for children and adolescents with eating disorders.

Principle	Key elements
1. Adjunctive treatment in selected patients	a. In context of comprehensive medical and psychological assessment and treatment, including weight restoration
	b. For relief of persistent distressing symptoms
	c. For treatment of comorbid psychiatric disorders
2. Informed consent	a. Patient and family/carers
	b. Discuss rationale, potential benefits, potential risks, alternative treatment options, data available
	c. Choice of medication informed by individual characteristics
	d. Documentation
3. Record baseline information	a. Identify target symptoms
	b. Document level of baseline symptoms and social/occupational function
	c. Use appropriate pre and post rating scales
	d. Screen for suicidality and binge eating
	e. Baseline investigations e.g. electrolytes, ECG, fasting lipids and fasting blood sugar prior to prescribing SGAs
4. Treat	a. Start at low doses, increase cautiously
	b. Safe prescription and storage to reduce harm from intentional overdose
	c. Enlist patient and family in adherence and monitoring
5. Monitor	a. Monitor treatment response clinically and using appropriate rating scales
	b. Monitor for adverse effects
	1. Screen for binge eating and suicidality
	2. Examination for extrapyramidal adverse effects of SGAs
	3. Monitor for SGAs with ECG, serum lipids, fasting blood sugar, weight, any other measures specific to the drug
6. Review	a. Regular review of balance of benefit and risk
	b. Continue if effective and tolerated, cease if ineffective or poorly tolerated
	c. Minimise polypharmacy
	d. Maintain emphasis on non-pharmacological treatments
	e. Review appropriateness as patient's nutritional state changes
7. Audit	a. Collect and share data on prescription, effectiveness and adverse effects
	b. Implement service-wide procedures that facilitate good prescribing and monitoring practices and allow data collection

as an indication for medication, it was not always clear whether the patient met criteria for a particular DSM-IV anxiety disorder at that time. Comorbid Axis I diagnoses were assigned clinically without the administration of gold standard structured interviews, which reduces reliability. We classified deliberate overdose of prescription medication as an adverse effect related to that medication; this methodology may differ from that used by other authors. No conclusions can be drawn about efficacy of psychotropic medications in managing EDs. Our results may differ from the prescription of medication in other ED treatment settings. In particular, because all medications were supplied at standard PBS charges, these findings may not generalise to other settings in which high cost to the patient may limit off-label use of antipsychotic medications. Analyses are preliminary and exploratory, with many variables, and occurred in the context of an observational design with a sample size pre-determined by the "active" caseload; in future replications due attention will need to be given to statistical power and controlling the Type 1 error rate. Chi-square analyses must be interpreted tentatively as sometimes data were unevenly distributed across cells, leading to violations in expected cell counts. Nonetheless, the presented results correlating prescribing practices to severity and complexity of presentation have clinical validity. Adherence to prescribed medication could not be formally evaluated due to the retrospective audit design; therefore, safety and risk data may underestimate actual risk. We enrolled only patients who were "active", that is, receiving some form of treatment or follow up at the study commencement date. To maximise current clinical relevance, we chose to study only the current group, as prescribing practices and medications available have changed over the 10 years since the EDP's inception; however, this led to a potential source of bias by excluding patients who had dropped out of treatment, who may have different characteristics.

Conclusions

Our hope is that this study will provide a template for future studies, which may include the follow up of this cohort, as well as multicentre collaboration examining the efficacy and utility of psychotropic medication in managing paediatric EDs, with larger samples and a prospective design. Given the difficulty of conducting large randomised controlled trials of medication in this patient population [55], reports of actual prescribing practices, medication safety, and treatment outcomes in a naturalistic setting are of value. Understanding the prevalence and indications of psychotropic use is essential to considering their place in clinical practice and implications for service provision, including treatment and safety monitoring. We propose some principles to guide prescription of psychotropics for children and adolescents with eating disorders (Table 5).

Abbreviations

A-DES: Adolescent dissociative experiences scale; AN: Anorexia nervosa; ANOVAs: Analyses of variance; BN: Bulimia nervosa; CDI: Children's depression inventory; DSM-IV: Diagnostic and statistical manual; ECG: Electrocardiogram; EDE: Eating disorder examination; EDs: Eating disorders; EDNOS: EDs not otherwise specified; EDP: Eating disorders program; MASC: Multidimensional anxiety scale for children; OCD: Obsessive-compulsive disorder; PMH: Princess margaret hospital for children; PRN: Pro re nata or "as required"; SGAs: Second generation antipsychotics; SSRIs: Selective serotonin reuptake inhibitors..

Competing interests

The authors report no conflicts of interest. The authors alone are responsible for the content and writing of the paper.

Authors' contributions

All authors contributed to the design and implementation of the study, reviewed and edited drafts of the manuscript, and read and approved the final draft. JKM undertook the literature review, conducted a proportion of the medical record reviews, coded and entered the data, contributed to the quality control and data interpretation, contributed to the initial draft, and edited the final draft. HJW conducted a proportion of the medical record reviews, conducted the quality control, data analysis and interpretation, and contributed to the initial draft. EH conducted the major proportion of medical record reviews and contributed to the initial draft. JM had a significant role in study design and data interpretation, and was involved in revising the manuscript critically. TN conducted a proportion of the medical record reviews and made particular contributions to data interpretation. All authors read and approved the final manuscript.

Acknowledgements

We would like to thank the clinicians of the PMH EDP who assisted with the project, especially Charmaine Ainsworth, Dawn Hopkins, and Annabel Izumi; and Sarah D'Andrea for the initial draft of the audit form. We are grateful to Professor David Forbes for his comments on the manuscript. Thanks to Mr David Moore for invaluable technical support. We express our gratitude to the National Eating Disorders Collaboration for its sponsorship of the entire publication fee.

Author details

[1]Princess Margaret Hospital for Children, Perth, Australia. [2]Centre for Clinical Interventions, Perth, Australia. [3]The School of Paediatrics and Child Health, University of Western Australia, Perth, Australia. [4]The School of Psychology and Speech Pathology, Curtin University, Perth, Australia. [5]The School of Psychiatry and Clinical Neurosciences, University of Western Australia, Perth, Australia.

References

1. Wade T, Bergin J, Tiggemann M, Bulik C, Fairburn CG: **Prevalence and long-term course of eating disorders in an adult Australian cohort.** *Aust N Z J Psychiatry* 2006, **40**:121–128.
2. Treasure J, Claudino AM, Zucker N: **Eating disorders.** *Lancet* 2010, **375**:583–593.
3. Van den Eynde F, Treasure J: **Neuroimaging in eating disorders and obesity: implications for research.** *Child Adolesc Psychiatr Clin N Am* 2009, **18**:95–115.
4. Chui HT, Christensen BK, Zipursky RB, Richards BA, Hanratty MK, Kabani NJ, Mikulis DJ, Katzman DK: **Cognitive function and brain structure in females with a history of adolescent-onset anorexia nervosa.** *Pediatrics* 2008, **122**:e426–e437.
5. Steinhausen H-C: **Outcome of eating disorders.** *Child Adolesc Psychiatr Clin N Am* 2009, **18**:225–242.
6. American Psychiatric Association: *Practice guideline for the treatment of patients with eating disorders. 3rd edn.* Washington: American Psychiatric Association; 2006.
7. Beumont P, Hay P, Beumont D, Birmingham L, Derham H, Jordan A, Kohn M, McDermott B, Marks P, Mitchell J, *et al:* **Australian and New Zealand clinical practice guidelines for the treatment of anorexia nervosa.** *Aust N Z J Psychiatry* 2004, **38**:659–670 [Erratum appears in Aust N Z J Psychiatry. 2004 Nov-Dec;38(11-12):987].

8. National Institute for Clinical Excellence: ***Eating Disorders.*** NICE clinical guideline: Core Interventions in the Treatment and Management of Anorexia Nervosa, Bulimia Nervosa and Related Eating Disorders; 2004. Available at www.nice.org.uk/CG9.
9. Aigner M, Treasure J, Kaye W, Kasper S: **Disorders WTFoE: World Federation of Societies for Biological Psychiatry (WFSBP) Guidelines for the Pharmacological Treatment of Eating Disorders.** *World J Biol Psychiatry* 2011, **12:**400–443.
10. Powers PS, Bruty H: **Pharmacotherapy for eating disorders and obesity.** *Child Adolesc Psychiatr Clin N Am* 2009, **18:**175–187.
11. Correll CU, Kratochvil CJ, March JS: **Developments in pediatric psychopharmacology: focus on stimulants, antidepressants, and antipsychotics.** *J Clin Psychiatry* 2011, **72:**655–670.
12. Holtkamp K, Konrad K, Kaiser N, Ploenes Y, Heussen N, Grzella I, Herpertz-Dahlmann B: **A retrospective study of SSRI treatment in adolescent anorexia nervosa: insufficient evidence for efficacy.** *J Psychiatr Res* 2005, **39:**303–310.
13. Walsh BT, Kaplan AS, Attia E, Olmsted MP, Parides M, Carter JC, Pike KM, Devlin MJ, Woodside B, Roberto CA, Rockert W: **Fluoxetine after weight restoration in anorexia nervosa: A randomized controlled trial.** *JAMA* 2006, **295:**2605–2612.
14. Hammad TA, Laughren T, Racoosin J: **Suicidality in pediatric patients treated with antidepressant drugs.** *Arch Gen Psychiatry* 2006, **63:**332–339.
15. Franko DL, Keel PK: **Suicidality in eating disorders: occurrence, correlates, and clinical implications.** *Clin Psychol Rev* 2006, **26:**769–782.
16. Bulik CM, Thornton L, Pinheiro AP, Plotnicov K, Klump KL, Brandt H, Crawford S, Fichter MM, Halmi KA, Johnson C, *et al:* **Suicide attempts in anorexia nervosa.** *Psychosom Med* 2008, **70:**378–383.
17. Cantor C, Neulinger K: **The epidemiology of suicide and attempted suicide among young Australians.** *Aust N Z J Psychiatry* 2000, **34:**370–387.
18. Hay PJ, Claudino AM: **Clinical psychopharmacology of eating disorders: a research update.** *Int J Neuropsychopharmacol* 2012, **15:**209–222.
19. Norris ML, Spettigue W, Buchholz A, Henderson KA, Gomez R, Maras D, Gaboury I, Ni A: **Olanzapine use for the adjunctive treatment of adolescents with anorexia nervosa.** *J Child Adolesc Psychopharmacol* 2011, **21:**213–220.
20. Correll CU, Manu P, Olshanskiy V, Napolitano B, Kane JM, Malhotra AK: **Cardiometabolic risk of second-generation antipsychotic medications during first-time use in children and adolescents.** *JAMA* 2009, **302:**1765–1773 [Erratum appears in JAMA. 2009 Dec 2;302(21):2322].
21. Fazeli PK, Calder GL, Miller KK, Misra M, Lawson E, Meenaghan E, Lee H, Herzog D, Klibanski A: **Psychotropic medication use in anorexia nervosa between 1997 and 2009.** *Int J Eat Disord* 2012, **45**(8):6–970.
22. Cooke RA, Chambers JB, Singh R, Todd GJ, Smeeton NC, Treasure J, Treasure T: **QT interval in anorexia nervosa.** *Br Heart J* 1994, **72:**69–73.
23. Ritchie B, Norris ML: **QTc prolongation associated with atypical antipsychotic use in the treatment of adolescent-onset anorexia nervosa.** *Journal of the Canadian Academy of Child and Adolescent Psychiatry* 2009, **18:**60–63.
24. Nielsen J, Graff C, Kanters JK, Toft E, Taylor D, Meyer JM: **Assessing QT interval prolongation and its associated risks with antipsychotics.** *CNS Drugs* 2011, **25:**473–490.
25. Brewerton TD, Shannon M: **Possible clozapine exacerbation of bulimia nervosa.** *Am J Psychiatry* 1992, **149:**1408–1409.
26. Bromel T, Blum WF, Ziegler A, Schulz E, Bender M, Fleischhaker C, Remschmidt H, Krieg JC, Hebebrand J: **Serum leptin levels increase rapidly after initiation of clozapine therapy.** *Mol Psychiatry* 1998, **3:**76–80.
27. Crockford DN, Fisher G, Barker P: **Risperidone, weight gain, and bulimia nervosa.** *Canadian Journal of Psychiatry - Revue Canadienne de Psychiatrie* 1997, **42:**326–327.
28. Mehler C, Wewetzer C, Schulze U, Warnke A, Theisen F, Dittmann RW: **Olanzapine in children and adolescents with chronic anorexia nervosa. A study of five cases.** *Eur Child Adolesc Psychiatry* 2001, **10:**151–157.
29. Theisen FM, Linden A, Konig IR, Martin M, Remschmidt H, Hebebrand J: **Spectrum of binge eating symptomatology in patients treated with clozapine and olanzapine.** *J Neural Transm* 2003, **110:**111–121.
30. Theisen FM, Cichon S, Linden A, Martin M, Remschmidt H, Hebebrand J: **Clozapine and weight gain.** *Am J Psychiatry* 2001, **158:**816.
31. McKnight RF, Park RJ: **Atypical antipsychotics and anorexia nervosa: a review.** *Eur Eat Disord Rev* 2010, **18:**10–21.
32. Eddy KT, Dorer DJ, Franko DL, Tahilani K, Thompson-Brenner H, Herzog DB: **Diagnostic crossover in anorexia nervosa and bulimia nervosa: implications for DSM-V.** *Am J Psychiatry* 2008, **165:**245–250.
33. Graae F, Milner J, Rizzotto L, Klein RG: **Clonazepam in childhood anxiety disorders.** *J Am Acad Child Adolesc Psychiatry* 1994, **33:**372–376.
34. Watson HJ: **Combined psychological and pharmacological treatment of pediatric anxiety disorders.** In *Handbook of child and adolescent anxiety disorders.* Edited by McKay D, Storch EA. New York: Springer Publishing; 2011:379–402.
35. Rossi G, Balottin U, Rossi M, Chiappedi M, Fazzi E, Lanzi G: **Pharmacological treatment of anorexia nervosa: a retrospective study in preadolescents and adolescents.** *Clin Pediatr (Phila)* 2007, **46:**806–811.
36. Gowers S, Claxton M, Rowlands L, Inbasagaran A, Wood D, Yi I, Hugo P, Clark-Stone S, Bryant-Waugh R, Nicholls D, Ayton A: **Drug prescribing in child and adolescent eating disorder services.** *Child and Adolescent Mental Health* 2010, **15:**18–22.
37. Australian Bureau of Statistics: ***Australian demographic statistics, March 2011.*** ABS, Canberra: cat. no. 3101.0; 2011. www.abs.gov.au.
38. American Psychiatric Association: *Diagnostic and statistical manual of mental disorders, 4th edition, text revised. 4th edn.* Washington, DC: American Psychiatric Association; 2000.
39. Fairburn CG, Cooper Z: **The Eating Disorder Examination.** In *Binge eating: nature, assessment and treatment.* 12th edition. Edited by Fairburn CG, Wilson GT. New York: Guilford Press; 1993:317–360.
40. Kovacs M: *Manual of the Children's Depression Inventory.* New York: Multi-Health Systems; 1992.
41. March JS, Parker JD, Sullivan K, Stallings P, Conners CK: **The Multidimensional Anxiety Scale for Children (MASC): factor structure, reliability, and validity.** *J Am Acad Child Adolesc Psychiatry* 1997, **36:**554–565.
42. Armstrong JG, Putnam FW, Carlson EB, Libero DZ, Smith SR: **Development and validation of a measure of adolescent dissociation: The Adolescent Dissociative Experiences Scale.** *J Nerv Ment Dis* 1997, **185:**491–497.
43. Timbremont B, Braet C, Dreessen L: **Assessing depression in youth: Relation between the Children's Depression Inventory and a structured interview.** *J Clin Child Adolesc Psychol* 2004, **33:**149–157.
44. *Centers for Disease Control and Prevention:* ***Epi Info 7 (Version 7.1.0.6) [Computer Program].*** ; 2012. http://wwwn.cdc.gov/epiinfo/html/downloads.htm.
45. *Clinical growth charts.* http://www.cdc.gov/growthcharts/clinical_charts.htm.
46. *Centers for Disease Control and Prevention:* ***Clinical growth charts. Retrieved August 15, 2012.*** ; 2010. http://www.cdc.gov/growthcharts/clinical_charts.htm.
47. Hudson JI, Hiripi E, Pope HG Jr, Kessler RC: **The prevalence and correlates of eating disorders in the National Comorbidity Survey Replication.** *Biol Psychiatry* 2007, **61:**348–358.
48. Swanson SA, Crow SJ, Le Grange D, Swendsen J, Merikangas KR: **Prevalence and correlates of eating disorders in adolescents. Results from the national comorbidity survey replication adolescent supplement.** *Arch Gen Psychiatry* 2011, **68:**714–723.
49. Gebhardt S, Haberhausen M, Krieg J-C, Remschmidt H, Heinzel-Gutenbrunner M, Hebebrand J, Thiesen FM: **Clozapine/olanzapine-induced recurrence or deterioration of binge eating-related eating disorders.** *J Neural Transm* 2007, **114:**1091–1095.
50. Keys A, Brozek J, Henschel A, Mickelson O, Taylor HL: *The biology of human starvation (2 vols).* Minneapolis, Minnesota: University of Minnesota Press; 1950.
51. Lambert TJR, Chapman LH: **Consensus Working Group: Diabetes, psychotic disorders and antipsychotic therapy: a consensus statement.** *Med J Aust* 2004, **181:**544–548.
52. Hetrick S, Alvarez-Jimenez M, Parker A, Hughes F, Willet M, Morley K, Fraser R, McGorry PD, Thompson A: **Promoting physical health in youth mental health services: ensuring routine monitoring of weight and metabolic indices in a first episode psychosis clinic.** *Australas* 2010, **18:**451–455.
53. Thompson A, Hetrick SE, Alvarez-Jiménez M, Parker AG, Willet M, Hughes F, Gariup M, Gomez DL, McGorry PD: **Targeted intervention to improve monitoring of antipsychotic-induced weight gain and metabolic disturbance in first episode psychosis.** *Aust N Z J Psychiatry* 2011, **45:**740–748.
54. Hazell L, Shakir SAW: **Under-reporting of adverse drug reactions : a systematic review.** *Drug Saf* 2006, **29:**385–396.
55. Norris ML, Spettigue W, Buchholz A, Henderson KA, Obeid N: **Factors influencing research drug trials in adolescents with anorexia nervosa.** *Eat Disord* 2010, **18:**210–217.

4

The ethics of neuromodulation for anorexia nervosa: a focus on rTMS

Alina Coman[1,2*], Finn Skårderud[1,3], Deborah L Reas[1] and Bjørn M Hofmann[2]

Abstract

Objective: Recently there has been emerging clinical and research interest in the application of deep brain stimulation (DBS) and repetitive transcranial magnetic stimulation (rTMS) to the treatment of anorexia nervosa (AN). To our knowledge, few studies have discussed ethical aspects associated with the increased use of neuromodulation in AN, some of which are quite specific to AN, despite the rapid development and dissemination of these new technologies.

Method: We provide a brief overview of three published rTMS studies for AN and discuss ethical issues involved in the use of neuromodulation for AN.

Results: In contrast to neurosurgery or DBS, rTMS is a less invasive technique, with less associated risk, and thus has greater potential to become a more widespread augmentation or add-on therapy for AN. New therapeutic procedures are promising, yet they raise ethical questions regarding informed consent and patient selection. Illness-specific issues surrounding authenticity and autonomy are important to consider, ensuring an ethical approach to treatment for patients with AN.

Discussion: We argue that ethical investigations for neuromodulation techniques are timely and important, and discussions should go beyond the immediate goals of patient safety, consent, and risk and benefit, to consider broader ethical concepts such as authenticity and autonomy.

Review

Recently, the US National Institute of Mental Health (NIMH) has moved towards a conceptualization of AN as a disorder of neurocircuitry which can be elucidated with modern tools and technological advances, especially genomics and neuroimaging [1]. At present, the aetiology and pathophysiology of AN are not completely known, yet genetic and neuroimaging studies are revealing greater insight into the underlying neural correlates which might be involved in the aetiology of AN. To date, neuroimaging, especially fMRI studies, suggest alterations in the dorsolateral prefrontal cortex area (DLPFC), insular, parietal and anterior cingulated cortex, all of which are areas involved in emotional processing, processing of reward, and body perception [2,3]. Traditionally, study paradigms used in neuroimaging have focused on investigating response to food and body stimuli, and illness-specific brain activity patterns related to symptoms. As has been acknowledged, underweight status is an ever-present confounder in investigations of AN, and while some studies indicate the presence of pre-existing traits [4] other studies indicate the existence of a scar effect due to underweight status or malnutrition [5]. At present, knowledge about the relationship between brain activity and illness, as informed by neuroimaging technologies, is correlational, yet findings are typically used as a rationale for the application of neuromodulation techniques to the treatment of AN. Neuromodulation techniques include invasive methods such as neurosurgery or deep brain stimulation (DBS), or non-invasive brain stimulation (NIBS), including repetitive transcranial stimulation (rTMS). Neuroimaging is seen as a promising tool to improve the efficacy of these techniques, especially rTMS by helping identify an appropriate stimulation target, which is considered to be a current main limitation [6].

* Correspondence: alina.coman@medisin.uio.no
[1]Regional Eating Disorders Service (RASP), Division of Mental Health and Addiction, Oslo University Hospital-Ullevål, P.O. Box 4956 Nydalen, Oslo N-0424, Norway
[2]Centre for Medical Ethics, University of Oslo, P.O. Box 1130, Blindern, Oslo N-0318, Norway
Full list of author information is available at the end of the article

Data demonstrating efficacy of neuromodulation methods for treating psychiatric disorders in general is accumulating, with a growing consensus towards the application of neuromodulation such as rTMS in treating depression, for example [7]. The invasive nature of these interventions, especially neurosurgery and DBS, and the inherent ethical considerations render these forms of treatment a last-resort for a subgroup of treatment-resistant patients. Anorexia nervosa is associated with high mortality rates [8] and a subgroup of patients experiences a chronic outcome [9]. As such, neuromodulation techniques have been increasingly proposed for the treatment of severe and long-standing AN proven refractory to standard treatment [10]. Such neuromodulation techniques are often not stand-alone treatment but they are used as additional or augmentation treatment in combination with behavioural training or other forms of therapy [11].

Some studies have shown positive results and provide proof-of-concept for AN as a disorder of brain circuitry, yet the mechanisms underlying neuromodulation techniques are not completely known. For AN, the evidence base for rTMS and DBS remains limited. Lipsman et al. [12] offer a thorough historical overview of the literature on the frequency and effects of neurosurgery. The lack of understanding neurocircuitry and the lack of specificity in targets of stimulation has made some critics advocate for 'neuromodesty' [13] and emphasize the necessity to investigate ethical aspects associated with neuromodulation. History has shown that it is important to stay vigilant and prevent misuse of these techniques in order to avoid negative experiences and attitudes that could deprive patients of therapeutic help [6].

We feel that rapid advances and new research priorities have arguably introduced a paradigm shift in defining and treating AN, making a renewed discussion of associated ethical concerns timely and important [11,12,14]. Some have argued that elucidating important ethical concerns is vital, especially since new technologies are often approved and implemented without critical appraisal [15] and the promise of neuroscience might, for some, have a "seductive" allure [16]. This appears to be also the case for psychotropic medication that is still recommended to a group of patients with AN despite known adverse effects and lack of data supporting their efficacy [17].

Brain-based interventions, even neurosurgery for AN, are not new [18]. Some have argued that although techniques such as DBS or rTMS represent recent therapeutic advances, the relevant ethical challenges they pose have been previously addressed in the bioethical literature for other medical or psychological treatments [13]. However, whereas specific ethical issues related to DBS have been discussed more broadly for other psychiatric disorders [19-21], and recently for AN [22], few debates have focused on rTMS. Further, existing ethical evaluations of rTMS for other psychiatric disorders have focused predominantly on safety issues alone [6].

This article can be seen as a first step in the endeavor to shed light on specific ethical issues that the use of neuromodulation techniques pose for patients suffering from AN. Although some issues pertain to neuromodulation techniques at-large, we focus mainly on rTMS. Clinically speaking, we feel a focus on rTMS is timely and important, as this procedure is less invasive and might be applied less severe patients, thereby not constituting a 'last-resort' treatment, but possibly functioning as an additional or augmentation treatment which is more widely accessible to treatment providers. In contrast, DBS is a more invasive treatment with greater challenges to issues of safety, long-term effects and informed consent, and its use will most probably be guided by restrictive regulations.

Neuromodulation techniques for AN: rTMS studies

Repetitive transcranial magnetic stimulation induces repetitive stimulation to cortical tissue with the help of magnetic field pulses from a magnetic coil placed outside the head. It either suppresses (at low frequency, 1 Hz) or excites (at higher frequency, 20 Hz) cortical activity, and its effect can propagate beyond the site of stimulation to a network of brain regions. The only Food and Drug Administration (FDA) approved therapeutic use of TMS is for stimulating the dorsolateral prefrontal cortex (DLPFC) for medication-resistant depression. However, the therapeutic efficacy data for depression is limited, partly because stimulation of DLPFC is based on a vague understanding of which specific mechanisms are stimulated, considering that DLPFC is connected with many other brain areas [23].

There are six studies that explore the effects of rTMS on bulimic disorders and findings are inconsistent, with some studies showing placebo effects while other reporting significant changes [10]. Three studies, of which one is a single case study, explore effects of rTMS for symptoms of AN. Table 1 provides a brief overview of clinical details and outcome for the three studies for AN. Initial findings are promising, yet mixed [24-26]. No studies have yet assessed the duration of improvement in symptoms beyond one month, or the longer-term and secondary effects of these interventions, and future studies will need to establish for which patients these interventions work best. Randomized controlled studies, which are underway in several countries including the UK and France, are necessary to delineate specific effects of rTMS and confirm the proof-of-concept for rTMS as a method which affects disturbed neural circuitry for reward and self-regulation [25]. Thus far, however, the use of these methods is exploratory and mostly confined to research settings and has not been routinely implemented as a therapeutic technique in the clinics.

Table 1 rTMS studies in anorexia nervosa

Authors (year)	N	Patient characteristics	Treatment	Primary outcome
Kamolz et al. (2008) [24]	1	Gender: female Age: 24 yrs. BMI: 12.4 DOI: app. 4 yrs.	Treatment of comorbid depression in a female patient with AN. 1st cycle included 10 sessions within 16 days of high frequency rTMS to the left dorsolateral prefrontal cortex. 2nd cycle included 6 sessions. 3rd cycle included 10 sessions. Continuation therapy included twice weekly rTMS sessions for 8 weeks.	Improvement in depression was observed, as well as weight gain and fewer ED symptoms. After 1st cycle, HAM-D scores decreased from 28 to 14. After 2nd cycle, HAM-D scores decreased from 18 to 10. After 3rd cycle, HAM-D scores decreased 18 to 11. During continuation therapy, HAM-D scores remained between 8 and 10. BMI increased to approximately 16 kg/m^2 after 12 weeks of rTMS.
Van den Eynde et al. (2013) [25]	10	Gender: female Mean age: 25 yrs. (18-44) Mean BMI: 15.7 (13.8-17.8) DOI: 10 yrs (3–30)	Delivered 1 session of high frequency rTMS to the left dorsolateral prefrontal cortex. ED-related experiences were measured pre-post following exposure to visual and food stimuli	1 patient dropped out prematurely due to discomfort. On the visual analogue scale, significant reductions in feeling fat, feeling full, and anxiety, with a non-significant trend for decreased urge to exercise. No significant changes in mood, tension, hunger, "urge to eat" or "urge to restrict". No reduction in cortisol levels, but found to be cardiac safe, as measured by blood pressure and heart rate.
McClelland et al. (2013) [26]	2	Patient A Gender: female Age: 23 yrs. BMI: 15.7 DOI: 12 yrs. Patient B Gender: female Age: 52 BMI: 16.4 DOI: 35 yrs.	Delivered 19–20 sessions of high frequency rTMS, applied to the left dorsolateral prefrontal cortex. Within-session changes in ED-related experiences were measured. BMI, ED symptoms, and depression measured at pre-treatment, post-treatment, and 1-month follow-up.	Patient A No change in weight at post-treatment or at 1-month follow-up. EDE-Q scores (except Eating Concern) were significantly lower at post-treatment and improvements were maintained at FUP. Some improvement in depression was observed. Patient B No change in weight at post-treatment or 1-month follow-up. Improvements in EDE-Q scores and depression were observed.

Note: rTMS = repetitive transcranial magnetic stimulation; BMI = body mass index (kg/m^2); DOI = duration of illness; HAM-D = Hamilton Depression Scale; EDE-Q = Eating Disorder Examination-Questionnaire, FUP = follow-up period.

Ethical issues in neuromodulation for AN

In the treatment of AN, ethical discussions have mostly focused on clinical issues related to underweight, malnutrition, and the capacity to refuse treatment. However, with the increased use of brain interventions for treating AN, other ethical concerns specific to the application of (mechanical) brain interventions need elaboration.

Ethical assessment of the use of neuromodulation is often based on four principles: respect for autonomy, beneficence, non-maleficence, and justice. Table 2 provides an overview of the application of these ethical principles to the case of rTMS in AN. The following section summarizes and relates these aspects to principalism, as this is the most influential approach in bioethics.

Balancing non-maleficence and beneficence

So far, the risks associated with participating in rTMS are low; however, since there is no evidence for the long-term effects and efficacy of rTMS, the risk-benefit ratio is difficult to assess [21]. Hence, utilitarian analysis fails to provide clear guidance in decision-making, and the beneficence is unclear. A pilot study for rTMS showed reductions in feeling of fatness and fullness, and anxiety, but fewer changes in mood, tension or urge to exercise [25]. In the future, it will also be relevant to establish criteria for evaluating effectiveness. If rTMS is proven effective and alleviates symptoms, it is relevant to establish the criteria for patient inclusion that should be adopted before neuromodulation is recommended, and establish the patient group for whom rTMS is relevant. In Van den Eynde's study [25], the group of participants investigated was heterogeneous, and included individuals with different duration of disorders, which make it hard to know whether neuromodulatory interventions are more effective for less severe patients or chronic patients. Difficulties and disagreement over the definition of severity, e.g., in terms of BMI-alone, level of impairment, or other eating-related or general psychopathology, has thus far rendered the assessment of beneficence complicated.

Table 2 rTMS in AN and relevant ethical considerations

Ethical principle	Threats pertinent for rTMS in AN
Non-maleficence (do no harm)	Risks
	Side-effects and long-term effects
Beneficence (do well)	Effectiveness
	Patient selection
Respect for autonomy	Informed consent
	(Emotional and cognitive) capacity issue due to underweight
	Comorbidity, mortality, resistance to treatment
Justice	Patient selection, Resource allocation, Research deprivation

Related to this argument, illness duration and refractoriness to treatment is often invoked as a rationale for neuromodulation [12]. Some have argued that moderate or a less severe illness might in fact be more responsive to brain interventions [27]. In AN, chronicity is typically seen after a period of 10 years [28]. Treating only patients with a long duration of illness may do injustice to individuals with a shorter duration of illness [27]. Thus ensuring a favorable risk-benefit ratio has also a moral aspect where issues of safety have to be balanced with the desire to help a group of patients who are not helped by other methods. This poses problems for autonomy and informed consent.

Respect for autonomy

Respect for autonomy is usually ensured by proper informed consent. At present, rTMS (and DBS) interventions for AN are often a last–resort treatment for patients who do not respond to other treatments. It has often been underlined in the ethics literature that patients participating in such last-resort exploratory research or treatment trials are "desperate" for a solution. As such, this subgroup of treatment refractory patients may be "overly motivated' to participate in exploratory research and to expose themselves to risks [13]. This poses challenges to the capacity of these patients to fully understand the nature of intervention and implications of participation. Depression can affect perception of risks associated with participating in research [19], although some argue that depression in itself is not enough to compromise judgment [29]. For AN, the condition of severe underweight poses some additional ethical considerations of competency and non-maleficence. Severe underweight can lead to involuntary hospitalization and forced feeding based on the assumption that individuals lack cognitive or emotional capacity to make decisions [30]. Offering neuromodulation treatment to patients who are emaciated or malnourished poses inherent ethical dilemmas given the potential incapacity associated with underweight status.

While some rTMS studies conducted so far have excluded severely underweight patients, protecting them from harm, other studies have included patients with a BMI from 12.3.

Chronicity of illness, underweight and willingness to participate in last resort interventions, be it proven or experimental, can raise questions about the validity of informed consent. The validity of a consent coming from a person that is severely underweight, refractory to treatment, yet willing to undergo brain interventions, can be questioned. Assessing the validity of such consent will be dependent on objective and established criteria for competence. However, it is also dependant on the kind of policy adopted, either a restrictive, paternalistic attitude or a permissive one "permitting people to make unencumbered decision about how to govern their own lives", and on how low the competence bar is set [13]. In cases where the competence bar is set low, it is essential to disclose to the participant all known and unknown information about the intervention in order to ensure informed consent.

The "overtly motivated," possibly depressed patient is a general ethical concern. However, in AN, a lack of motivation and reluctance to engage in treatment has more often been the case. Especially pharmacological treatment, for example, antipsychotic medication such as olanzapine, is associated with higher drop-out than cognitive [31] and cognitive-behavioural treatment [32]. Further, the drop-out rate for adults with AN is higher (40%) than for adolescents in family therapy, in which the drop-out rates fall around 10-20% [32]. However, reluctance to medication might be explained by fears of weight gain, which can be a secondary effect of olanzapine [33]. Although it remains yet unknown how patients view neuromodulatory treatments, rTMS has been shown to reduce feelings of fullness or fatness, and to lessen anxiety, which may have greater appeal. In this case, the concern is rather, when the patient is motivated, how to proceed ethically. Given the current limited status of knowledge of neurocorrelates for AN, of the efficacy of mechanisms for brain stimulation and long-term effects, critics have drawn attention to the fact that neuromodulation means little. To proceed ethically would mean an invitation to "hyper disclosure" [13].

Another threat to autonomous participation in neuromodulatory interventions is the risk for *therapeutic misconception*, adopting the belief that participating in research will alleviate suffering. Informed consent should therefore aim to avoid misunderstanding, and facilitate autonomy, by making explicit the current experimental nature of the research, and ensure that the patient is explicitly informed about what rTMS can offer and not offer.

It is also possible that investigator bias, or simply the desire to understand the relation between the brain and illness, or to alleviate intense suffering, leads to overstatements of the current state of knowledge and this can impede cautious proceeding [13]. Especially in light of the high mortality and morbidity rate, AN may challenge the therapists' clinical judgment and bias them to recommend the available new treatments, despite an evidence base which is still evolving. On the other hand, any negative attitudes or bias against brain interventions may encourage therapists to withhold treatment from patients [6].

Justice

Critics have drawn attention to the need to balance ethical concerns and (over) protection of rights that has sometimes led to "research deprivation" [34]. This is perhaps especially applicable to children and adolescents with AN, with a consideration of young individuals' agency [35] and the need to proceed cautiously.

Researchers have already pointed to the perplexities of providing sound scientific evidence for medicated treatment and how consideration for safety by including the adult population entails high drop-out and biases samples [32]. This has made researchers inclined to advocate intensification of interventions at early stages of the disorder instead of conducting more randomized studies [32]. Others have warranted a more detailed and critical re-evaluation of the meaning and criteria for resistance to treatment [36], as it is an often-invoked argument for use of neuromodulation techniques but little described in the studies [12].

Autonomy and beyond: authenticity

Whether such interventions are proven effective in the future and the medical risks low, it will still be necessary to provide adequate care and attention to the individual and also longer-term follow-up. Resistance to standard treatment is often invoked by patients on the grounds of threats to authenticity, where aspects of AN are seen as integrative of the self and therefore the patient is less willing to change [37]. All treatments, medical or psychological, can be said to change aspects of the self, and to either threaten or contribute to the development of what is conceived as "authentic", although this concept is contested [38]. Although the understanding of authenticity and the role of this concept in treatment is still poorly understood, studies show that threats to authenticity are experienced by patients although mostly in the beginning of the treatment as grounds to refuse treatment [37]. Although concerns for authenticity appear to be amenable to change over time, and should not just be taken at face-value as a valid reason to respect patients' refusal of treatment, an ethical approach to treatment requires nevertheless a consideration of patients' concerns with authenticity.

Technological assisted treatment, as with rTMS, touches on broader debates about the nature and meaning of symptoms and neuromodulatory techniques. As mentioned earlier, the results from early trials of rTMS seem to show reductions in feelings of fullness and fatness. Yet patients may be reluctant to address ideas regarding overconcern of shape and weight, which may be intertwined with the subjective meaning of the illness ascribed by the patient [39]. For example, feelings of fatness have been shown to be related to expressing emotions of sadness or disgust that are displaced on the body, and depend on context [40]. Preoccupation with the body, restriction, purging can be seen as concrete representation of psychological states, a tendency some have termed 'psychological equivalence' [41].

Importantly, differentiating between the meaning of symptoms according to the patient and the aetiology of symptoms demands clinical skills from the therapists. It is feasible that recommending a neuromodulation technique might alienate the patient by rendering important and ego-syntonic symptoms reducible to defect neuronetworks. Earlier studies show that although biological framing of the disorder can reduce self-blame, it can also disturb self-understanding and the perception of volition seen as significant for recovery [42,43]. Therefore the therapist is in a position to address participants concerns about authenticity and agency when they jointly determine treatment goals [37].

A complementary criterion: individual experience, cultural and social aspects.

The risk-benefit calculations must be based on assessing effectiveness both at the group level but also at the individual level [44]. At present, it remains uncertain how patients might experience these technologies and whether they present threats to authenticity. We argue that this should be done not only based on quantitative measures of benefit, but should be complemented by a first-person account of the role such technologies play in the life of the sufferer. For example, such first-person accounts have been shown to be a contribution to the debate about medication of children with ADHD [38]. The answers to these questions could ensure a complete ethical evaluation and ethical approach to the use of neurotechnologies, and prevent "clinical push" and technological enthusiasm which may create stigma that would deprive sufferers of therapeutic benefit [6].

Lastly, ethical perspectives may be influenced by cultural and societal values. While the media is increasingly presenting the brain as a "capital that should be optimized" [45], and the brain becomes an integrated, although not dominant part of our self-understanding [43,46], the public may become more cautious about brain interventions as neuromodulation techniques have a controversial history [6]. Such social and cultural values might also be impacted by the specific features of the disorder, and attention to context is warranted [13]. Limited knowledge exists regarding factors, which might impede or encourage acceptability of neuromodulation interventions for both sufferers, health professionals and the general public [14].

Conclusions

This article can be seen as a first step in the attempt to shed light on specific ethical issues that the use of neuromodulation techniques pose for patients with AN. Although promising, findings are mixed and future studies are warranted to demonstrate their efficacy. The risks for rTMS are currently low and thus further experimental trials can proceed and ensure consistent evidence for the efficacy of the neuromodulation techniques. However, considering the current limited knowledge, careful attention to context and practice should follow. Ethical issues such as careful informed consent and clinical sensitivity have to be taken into account when gaining this knowledge and applying these techniques. Further, if these methods prove effective, it is nevertheless relevant that patients, families, caregivers, treatment providers, and the public-at-large are involved in discussions regarding potential ethical dilemmas.

In this article, we have applied a principle-based approach as described by Beauchamp and Childress [47]. Other perspectives exist and could have been followed; for example, a deontological approach would have highlighted human worth and dignity. However, our approach addressed concerns for authenticity and meaning without reference to intention-based ethical theories. The utilitarian perspective has been covered by the principle of beneficence. Various types of utilitarianism exist, but they are all faced with challenges when the knowledge on risks and benefits is vague, uncertain, or absent. Correspondingly, procedural approaches, such as discourse ethics [48] and "accountability for reasonableness" [49,50] are relevant, especially when assessing health care interventions under uncertainty. However, they may face challenges in AN as the persons themselves may refuse to be participants in the discourse and deliberation.

In conclusion, we argue that investigations of neurostimulation techniques such as rTMS in AN go beyond establishing efficacy to a broader phenomenological, first-person understanding of how technologies affect users' lives. As such, future studies and ethical debates about the efficacy and acceptability of these methods should therefore investigate attitudes both among health providers and patients. Finally, considering that research on neurobiology of AN will most likely continue to rapidly develop in concert with NIMH research priorities, concomitant ethical debates should follow in parallel with such developments.

Competing interests

The authors declare that they have no competing interests.

Authors' contributions

AC drafted the manuscript, completed the literature search and analysis of the material. DR contributed to developing the manuscript, presentation of review material, as well as revising for intellectual content and language editing. FS and BH contributed to validation and developing of ideas, and were involved in approval of final draft of the paper. All authors read and approved the final manuscript.

Acknowledgements

The work on this paper has been supported by internal funds from the Regional Eating Disorder Unit, Department of Mental Health and Addiction, Oslo University Hospital, Ullevål. We also want to thank the peer-reviewers for valuable comments.

Author details

[1]Regional Eating Disorders Service (RASP), Division of Mental Health and Addiction, Oslo University Hospital-Ullevål, P.O. Box 4956 Nydalen, Oslo N-0424, Norway. [2]Centre for Medical Ethics, University of Oslo, P.O. Box 1130, Blindern, Oslo N-0318, Norway. [3]Institute of Special Needs Education, University of Oslo, Sognsveien 250, Oslo N-0863, Norway.

References

1. Insel T: *Mental illness Defined as Disruption in Neural Circuits*; 2011. [updated 2011National Institute of Mental Health]; Available from: http://www.nimh.nih.gov/about/director/2011/mental-illness-defined-as-disruption-in-neural-circuits.shtml.
2. Pietrini F, Castellini G, Ricca V, Polito C, Pupi A, Faravelli C: **Functional neuroimaging in anorexia nervosa: a clinical approach.** *Eur Psychiatry* 2011, **26**(3):176–182.
3. Uher R, Brammer MJ, Murphy T, Campbell IC, Ng VW, Williams SCR, Treasure J: **Recovery and chronicity in anorexia nervosa: brain activity associated with differential outcomes.** *Biol Psychiatry* 2003, **54**(9):934–942.
4. Kaye WH, Wagner A, Fudge JL, Paulus M: **Neurocircuity of eating disorders.** In *Behavioral Neurobiology of Eating Disorders.* 6th edition. Edited by Adan RAH, Kaye WH. Heidelberg: Springer Berlin; 2011:37–57.
5. Pruis TA, Keel PK, Janowsky JS: **Recovery from anorexia nervosa includes neural compensation for negative body image.** *Int J Eat Dis* 2012, **45**(8):919–931.
6. Horvath JC, Perez JM, Forrow L, Fregni F, Pascual-Leone A: **Transcranial magnetic stimulation: a historical evaluation and future prognosis of therapeutically relevant ethical concerns.** *J Med Ethics* 2011, **37**(3):137–143.
7. Slotema CW, Dirk Blom J, Hoek HW, Sommer IEC: **Should we expand the toolbox of psychiatric treatment methods to include repetitive transcranial magnetic stimulation (rTMS)? a meta-analysis of the efficacy of rTMS in psychiatric disorders.** *J Clin Psychiatry* 2010, **71**(7):873.
8. Arcelus J, Mitchell AJ, Wales J, Nielsen S: **Mortality rates in patients with anorexia nervosa and other eating disorders: a meta-analysis of 36 studies.** *Arch Gen Psychiatry* 2011, **68**(7):724.
9. Steinhausen HC: **The outcome of anorexia nervosa in the 20th century.** *Am J Psychiatry* 2002, **159**(8):1284–1293.
10. McClelland J, Bozhilova N, Campbell I, Schmidt U: **A systematic review of the effects of neuromodulation on eating and body weight: evidence from human and animal studies.** *Eur Eat Disord Rev* 2013, **21**(6):436–455.
11. Kadosh RC, Levy N, O'Shea J, Shea N, Savulescu J: **The neuroethics of non-invasive brain stimulation.** *Curr Biol* 2012, **22**(4):R108–R111.
12. Lipsman N, Woodside DB, Giacobbe P, Lozano AM: **Neurosurgical treatment of anorexia nervosa: review of the literature from leucotomy to deep brain stimulation.** *Eur Eat Disord Rev* 2013, **21**(6):428–435.
13. Morse SJ: **New therapies, old problems, or a plea for neuromodesty.** *AJOB Neuroscience* 2012, **3**(1):60–64.
14. Mendelsohn D, Lipsman N, Bernstein M: **Neurosurgeons' perspectives on psychosurgery and neuroenhancement: a qualitative study at one center.** *J Neurosurg* 2010, **113**(6):1212–1218.
15. Jeanne L, Shannon B: **Why the FDA can't protect the public.** *BMJ* 2010, **341**(7780):966–968.
16. Weisberg DS, Keil FC, Goodstein J, Rawson E, Gray JR: **The seductive allure of neuroscience explanations.** *J Cogn Neurosci* 2007, **20**(3):470–477.
17. Fazeli PK, Calder GL, Miller KK, Misra M, Lawson EA, Meenaghan E, Lee H, Herzog D, Klibanski A: **Psychotropic medication use in anorexia nervosa between 1997 and 2009.** *Int J Eat Disord* 2012, **45**(8):970–976.
18. Sifneos PE: **A case of anorexia nervosa treated succesfully by leucotomy.** *Am J Psychiatry* 1952, **109**(5):356–360.
19. Fisher CE, Dunn LB, Christopher PP, Holtzheimer PE, Leykin Y, Mayberg HS, Lisanby SH, Appelbaum PS: **The ethics of research on deep brain stimulation for depression: decisional capacity and therapeutic misconception.** *Ann NY Acad Sci* 2012, **1265**(1):69–79.
20. Glannon W: **Stimulating brains, altering minds.** *J Med Ethics* 2009, **35**(5):289–292.
21. Pisapia JM, Halpern CH, Muller UJ, Vinai P, Wolf JA, Whiting DM, Wadden TA, Baltuch GH, Caplan AL: **Ethical considerations in deep brain stimulation for the treatment of addiction and overeating associated with obesity.** *AJOB Neuroscience* 2013, **4**(2):35–46.
22. Wu H, Van Dyck-Lippens PJ, Santegoeds R, van Kuyck K, Gabriels L, Lin G: **Deep-brain stimulation for anorexia nervosa.** *World Neurosurg* 2013, **80**(3):S29–S.
23. Fox MD, Buckner RL, White MP, Greicius MD, Pascual-Leone A: **Efficacy of transcranial magnetic stimulation targets for depression is related to intrinsic functional connectivity with the subgenual cingulate.** *Biol Psychiatry* 2012, **72**(7):595–603.
24. Kamolz S, Richter D-PMM, Schmidtke A, Fallgatter AJ: **Transkranielle magnetstimulation gegen komorbide depression bei anorexie.** *Nervenarzt* 2008, **79**(9):1071–1073.
25. Van den Eynde F, Guillaume S, Broadbent H, Campbell IC, Schmidt U: **Repetitive transcranial magnetic stimulation in anorexia nervosa: a pilot study.** *Eur Psychiatry* 2013, **28**(2):98–101.
26. McClelland J, Bozhilova N, Nestler S, Campbell IC, Jacob S, Johnson-Sabine E, Schmidt U: **Improvements in symptoms following neuronavigated repetitive transcranial magnetic stimulation (rTMS) in severe and enduring anorexia nervosa: findings from two case studies.** *Eur Eat Disord Rev* 2013, **21**(6):500–506.
27. Kuhn J, Gaebel W, Klosterkoetter J, Woopen C: **Deep brain stimulation as a new therapeutic approach in therapy-resistant mental disorders: ethical aspects of investigational treatment.** *Eur Arch Psychiatr Clin Neurosci* 2009, **259**(2):135–141.
28. Strober M, Freeman R, Morrell W: **The long-term course of severe anorexia nervosa in adolescents: survival analysis of recovery, relapse, and outcome predictors over 10ΓÇô15 years in a prospective study.** *Int J Eat Dis* 1997, **22**(4):339–360.
29. Appelbaum PS: **Assessment of patients' competence to consent to treatment.** *N Engl J Med* 2007, **357**(18):1834–1840.
30. Tan J, Hope T: **Treatment refusal in anorexia nervosa: a challenge to current concepts of capacity.** In *Empirical Ethics in Psychiatry.* Edited by Widdershoven G, McMillan J, Hope T, Scheer LS. Oxford: Oxford University Press; 2008:187–210.
31. Dahlgren CL, Lask B, Landrø N-I, Rø O: **Developing and evaluating cognitive remediation therapy (CRT) for adolescents with anorexia nervosa: a feasibility study.** *Clin Child Psychol Psychiatry* 2013. 1359104513489980.
32. Halmi K: **The perplexities of conducting randomized, double-blind, placebo-controlled treatment trials in anorexia nervosa patients.** *Am J Psychiatr* 2008, **165**(10):1227–1228.
33. Bissada H, Tasca G, Barber AM, Bradwejn J: **Olanzapine in the treatment of low body weight and obsessive thinking in women with anorexia nervosa: a randomized, double-blind, placebo-controlled trial.** *Am J Psychiatr* 2008, **165**(10):1281–1288.
34. Arnold LE, Stoff DM, Cook E Jr, Cohen DJ, Kruesi M, Wright C, Hattab J, Graham P, Zametkin A, Castellanos FX, *et al*: **Ethical issues in biological psychiatric research with children and adolescents.** *J Am Acad Child Adolesc Psychiatry* 1995, **34**(7):929–939.
35. Singh I: **Victimology versus character: new perspectives on the use of stimulant drugs in children.** *J Med Ethics* 2013, **39**(6):372–373.
36. Abbate-Daga G, Amianto F, Delsedime N, De-Bacco C, Fassino S: **Resistance to treatment and change in anorexia nervosa: a clinical overview.** *BMC psychiatry* 2013, **13**(1):294.
37. Hope T, Tan J, Stewart A, Fitzpatrick R: **Anorexia nervosa and the language of authenticity.** *Hastings Cent Rep* 2011, **41**(6):19–29.
38. Singh I: **Not robots: children's perspectives on authenticity, moral agency and stimulant drug treatments.** *J Med Ethics* 2013, **39**(6):359–366.
39. Habermas T: **On the uses of history in psychiatry: diagnostic implications for anorexia nervosa.** *Int J Eat Dis* 2005, **38**(2):167–182.
40. Espeset EMS, Nordbø RHS, Gulliksen KS, Skarderud F, Geller J, Holte A: **The concept of body image disturbance in anorexia nervosa: an empirical inquiry utilizing patients' subjective experiences.** *Eat Disord* 2011, **19**(2):175–193.
41. Skårderud F, Sommerfeldt B, Fonagy P: **Den reflekterende kroppen. Mentalisering og spiseforstyrrelser.** *Nord J of Child Adol Psychother* 2012, **2**:6–21.
42. Easter MM: **Not all my fault: genetics, stigma, and personal responsibility for women with eating disorders.** *Social Sci Med* 2012, **75**(8):1408–1416.
43. Coman A, Skårderud F, Hofmann BM: **A disorder of a vulnerable self: anorexia nervosa patients' understanding of disorder and self in the context of fMRI brain scanning.** *EHPP* 2013, **15**(2):120–134.
44. Schermer M: **Ethical issues in deep brain stimulation.** *Frontiers in Integrative Neuroscience* 2011, **5**(17).
45. O'Connor C, Rees G, Joffe H: **Neuroscience in the public sphere.** *Neuron* 2012, **74**(2):220–226.
46. Pickersgill M, Cunningham-burley S, Martin P: **Constituting neurologic subjects: neuroscience, subjectivity and the mundane significance of the brain.** *Subjectivity* 2011, **4**:346–365.
47. Beauchamp TL, Childress JF: *Principles of bioethical ethics.* New York: Oxford University Press; 2013.
48. Habermas J: *Moral Consciousness and Communicative Ethics Cambridge.* Cambridge: MIT Press; 1990.
49. Daniels N: **Accountability for reasonable limits to care.** In *Policy Challenges in Modern Health Care.* Edited by Mechanic D, Rogut L, Colby D, Knickman J. New Brunswick: NJ: Rutgers University Press; 2005:228–248.
50. Daniels N, Sabin JE: **Accountability for reasonableness: an update.** *BMJ* 2008, **337**:228–248.

The current status of suicide and self-injury in eating disorders: a narrative review

Katrina Kostro[1*], Jessica B Lerman[2] and Evelyn Attia[1,2]

Abstract

The aim of this paper is to review recent literature on suicide and self-injury in eating disorders (ED) including anorexia nervosa (AN), bulimia nervosa (BN), and binge eating disorder (BED). Among psychiatric diagnoses, EDs are associated with increased mortality rates, even when specialized treatment is available. Of the mortalities that are reported in individuals with EDs, suicide is among the most commonly reported causes of death. Additionally, suicidal and non-suicidal self-injurious behaviors occur frequently in this clinical population. A literature search was undertaken using the databases of Medline/PubMed and PsycInfo to identify papers describing suicidality in individuals with ED diagnoses. The authors identified studies and review articles published between 2005-2013 (inclusive) that describe the relationship between EDs and suicide, and associated behaviors including self-injurious behaviors, or non-suicidal self-injury (NSSI). The initial search resulted in 1095 papers that met the *a priori* search criteria. After careful review, 66 papers were included. The majority of papers described clinical cohorts that were studied longitudinally. The diagnosis described most frequently in selected studies was AN. There are limited current data about the prevalence of suicide and NSSI among individuals with EDs. Among the published studies that focus specifically on the relationship between EDs and suicidality, most describe AN in more detail than other EDs. Nonetheless, rates of mortality, and specifically rates of suicide, are undeniably high in ED populations, as are the rates of self-harm. Therefore, it is critical for clinicians and caretakers to carefully evaluate these patients for suicide risk and to refer promptly for appropriate treatment.

Keywords: Anorexia nervosa, Bulimia nervosa, Binge eating disorder, Eating disorders, Suicidality, Suicide, Mortality, Self-injury, Non-suicidal self-injury, Review

Background

Eating disorders (ED), including anorexia nervosa (AN) and bulimia nervosa (BN), are serious psychiatric illnesses with high rates of morbidity and mortality. Studies of clinical samples, mostly from specialized programs in Europe and North America, have described high rates of suicidal behaviors and completed suicides associated with EDs, and have helped increase clinical awareness about the seriousness of these psychiatric disorders [1-6]. A comprehensive review published in 2006 by Franko and Keel describes findings from 1985-2004 [7]. This review highlighted findings of high suicide rates among individuals with AN, and contrasted these with individuals with BN, whose rates of suicide did not appear to be elevated. Conversely, the review reported that non-lethal suicide attempts occurred in 25-35% of BN patients, compared with a rate of 3-20% of AN patients [7]. The review also described common clinical correlates of suicidality in EDs, including comorbid diagnoses such as depression, self-injurious behaviors such as bingeing and purging, a history of substance abuse, and a history of childhood abuse.

Considering the consistent finding of high risk of suicidality in this population, it is important for researchers and clinicians to continue to examine the risk factors and associations with the prevalence of suicidality in individuals with EDs. This narrative review aims to update the previous review by Franko and Keel [7], and to extend the scope to include non-suicidal self-injury (NSSI). The authors included NSSI in this review as these behaviors are commonly reported in EDs and were not included in many earlier reports of suicidality in this clinical population. The authors aimed to include publications that described all ED diagnosis groups, including binge eating disorder (BED) and eating disorder not otherwise specified (EDNOS), as many earlier reviews focused primarily on AN and BN. The

* Correspondence: katrinakostro@gmail.com
[1]Columbia University Medical Center, New York, NY, USA
Full list of author information is available at the end of the article

authors aimed to describe the available data, including their quality and scope and to identify areas in need of additional study.

Review

Methods

The authors performed a literature search between July and December 2013, using the databases of Medline/PubMed and PsycInfo, to review papers published between January 1, 2005 and December 31, 2013, describing suicidality and self-injury in individuals with ED diagnoses. The start date for the search interval was selected because the most recently published comprehensive review on similar subject matter described studies published between 1985-2004. Twenty advanced searches were undertaken, combining ED key words with suicidality key words. The first and second key words of each search were required to appear in the article title or abstract. The ED key words used were: "eating disorders"; "anorexia nervosa"; "bulimia nervosa"; "binge eating disorder"; or "eating disorder not otherwise specified". Each of the five ED terms was paired with a second key word of the following key words: "suicide"; "mortality"; "self-injurious behavior"; or "non-suicidal self-injury". Additionally, the authors conducted four searches, combining the ED key words "avoidant/restrictive food intake disorder" and "ARFID" with each of the four selected second key words to identify any recent literature that may have been published in anticipation or soon following the release of DSM-5 in May 2013.

Articles were included in this review if studies included information about the relationship between suicidality or self-injury and individuals with ED diagnoses including AN, BN, BED, EDNOS and ARFID. Articles were excluded if they did not present data about suicidality or self-injury in EDs, or if they did not identify and discuss a specific relationship between EDs and suicidality or self-injury. Only articles in English were reviewed. The articles were reviewed by all authors of this paper.

Results

Quality appraisal of included papers

The literature search of suicidality and EDs produced overlapping lists of published studies and review articles. The initial search resulted in 1095 papers that met the *a priori* search criteria (Figure 1). Seventy-four duplicate articles were removed, as were 69 articles written in languages other than English, and 886 papers were excluded due to failure to include data regarding suicidality in EDs. The authors ultimately identified 66 papers that met the inclusion criteria and present them in Table 1 including information about study type, sample size, age group and gender. The literature search results are highlighted in narrative text organized by ED diagnosis and then by general features relevant to risk of suicidality and EDs.

The literature included variation regarding methodology, sample size, length of follow-up, and diagnostic criteria that may account for the variability among studies. Overall, the authors found that data on the prevalence of suicidality in EDs have focused mainly on AN. Interpretation of the more limited data about BN is difficult because information regarding initial ED diagnosis is rarely available and diagnostic cross-over from AN to BN is high, with estimated cross-over rates ranging from 20-50% [10]. Additionally, many studies examined predictors of poor outcome in EDs but did not specify predictors of mortality. Furthermore, the cause of patient deaths, including death by suicide, was not always readily available, and thus limited the ability to interpret study findings. Also, there were few studies assessing the cause of mortality in patients with BN, BED, and other EDs not otherwise specified.

Anorexia nervosa

Until recently, the majority of research regarding increased mortality risk conferred by EDs, including risk of suicidality, has focused on AN. Across ED diagnoses, recent studies examining the characteristics of suicide attempts among individuals with AN, BN, and individuals without EDs, found higher Standardized Mortality Ratios (SMR) in AN than in BN, ranging from 6.2 to 10.6 [34,39,52]. SMR represents the observed number of deaths divided by the expected number of deaths in a certain group, and thus represents the estimated risk of death in a group compared to individuals from the general population, matched by age and gender. A clinical cohort study published by Bulik et al. in 2008 reported suicide attempts approaching approximately 17% in the AN population [14]. According to Guillaume et al., the odds ratio (OR) for suicide attempts in AN compared to other ED diagnoses showed that AN patients were more likely to have made a serious attempt (OR 3.4, 95% CI 1.4-7.9) [34]. The results also showed that the AN group with suicide attempts had a higher expectation of dying (OR 3.7, 95% CI 1.1-13.5) based on scores from The Suicidal Intent Scale, a 15-item scale that assesses the severity of suicidal intention associated with suicide attempts [34]. Huas et al. concluded that in AN patients with a lifetime history of suicide attempt, risk of death was multiplied by 2.6 [38].

Reported rates of suicide attempts in AN are high, and there are also data confirming completed suicides in individuals with AN. Huas et al. reported that suicide was the second highest cause of death (17%, n = 7) in a clinical cohort with AN, 28.4% of which had committed at least one suicide attempt [38]. Papadopoulos et al. found that the SMR of observed deaths caused by suicide in a study population defined by having been admitted at least once for treatment of AN, compared to expected

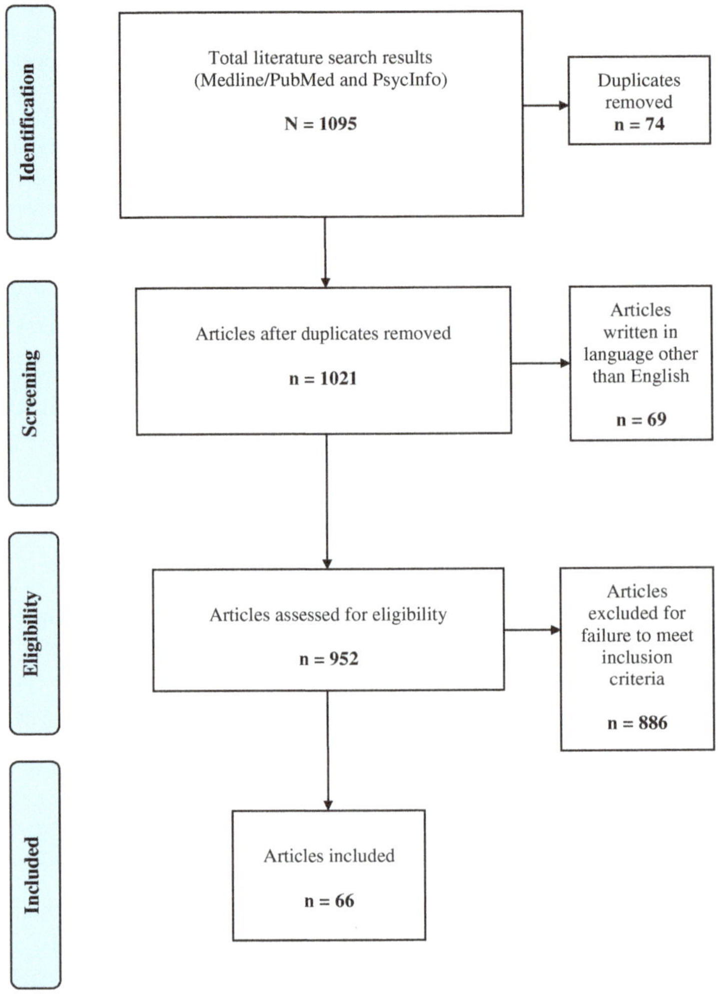

Figure 1 Flow chart of included studies.

suicide deaths in the general population, was 13.6 (95% CI 10.9-16.8) [45]. The SMR was only exceeded in this sample by deaths due to psychoactive substance use (SMR 18.9, 95% CI 10.0-32.3) and those caused primarily by AN (SMR 650.0, 95% CI 462.2-888.6) [45]. In a study that analyzed eight years of follow-up data from 147 outpatients with AN, and combined these data with those from 10 additional studies that included follow-up data from other samples, Signorini et al. reported 5.3% overall mortality rate, including 1.2% death due to suicide [56]. In a meta-analysis of 36 studies published between 1966-2010 that included mortality rates in individuals with EDs, Arcelus et al. found a SMR of 5.9 for the AN sample, in which one in five individuals who died had committed suicide [10].

While overall mortality risk, including risk of death by suicide, appears to be significantly higher in AN, compared to risk in individuals with BN and BED [11], there are significant differences in rates of suicidality between AN subtypes: 7.4% of AN-restricting subjects reported at least one suicide attempt, whereas approximate rates are between 20 and 30% for other AN subtypes [36]. Selby et al. conducted a two-part cohort study investigating suicidality and associated "provocative behaviors" among AN subtypes including: restricting, purging, binge-purging, and history of BN [55]. The study found in both cohorts (n = 787 and replicated n = 249) that suicidal behavior in AN may be the result of these associated behaviors defined by the AN subtypes. Repetitive experience with behaviors such as binge eating and self-induced vomiting may be a route to suicidal behavior in bingeing and/or purging subtypes, while the exposure to pain through starvation

Table 1 Papers describing suicide and/or self-injury associated with eating disorders

Author *N = 66*	Study design *n = 70*	Sample size *n = 54*	ED diagnoses *n = 67*	Age group *n = 55*	Gender *n = 52*
Ahrén-Moonga, [8]	Clinical cohort with controls	105*	AN, BN	Adults	Females
Ajetunmobi, [1]	Community cohort	111504*	ED	Adults	Mixed
Anestis, [9]	Clinical cohort	127	BN	Adults	Females
Arcelus, [10]	Review/meta-analysis	-	AN, BN, EDNOS	-	-
Berkman, [11]	Review/meta-analysis	-	AN, BN, BED	-	-
Birmingham, [12]	Clinical cohort	954	AN, BN, EDNOS	Adults	Females
Bodell, [13]	Community cohort	364	AN, BN, EDNOS	Adults	Females
Bulik, [14]	Clinical cohort	432	AN, BN	Adolescents and adults	Mixed
Button [15]	Clinical cohort	1892	AN, BN, EDNOS	Adults	Females
Carano, [16]	Clinical cohort	80	BED	Adults	Mixed
Chen, [17]	Clinical cohort	135	AN, BN, BED	Adults	Females
Claes, [18]	Clinical cohort	70*	AN, BN	Adults	Females
Claes, [19]	Clinical cohort	130	AN, BN, EDNOS	Adults	Males
Crow, [20]	Clinical cohort	1885	AN, BN, EDNOS	Adults	-
Dancyger, [21]	Review/meta-analysis	-	AN, BN, EDNOS	Adolescents	-
Erdur, [22]	Clinical cohort	169*	AN	Adolescents and adults	Females
Favaro, [23]	Clinical cohort	934	AN, BN, ED	Adults	Females
Favaro, [24]	Clinical cohort	95	BN	Adults	-
Fedorowicz, [25]	Clinical cohort	968*	AN, BN, EDNOS	Adolescents and adults	Females
Fennig, [26]	Clinical cohort	46	AN, BN	Adolescents	Females
Fichter, [27]	Clinical cohort	103	AN	Adolescents and adults	Females
Fischer, [28]	Clinical cohort	80	BN	Adolescents	Mixed
Forcano, [29]	Clinical cohort with controls	172	AN	Adults	Females
Forcano, [30]	Clinical cohort	566	BN, EDNOS	Adults	Females
Foulon, [2]	Clinical cohort	304	AN	Adolescents and adults	Mixed
Franko, [5]	Clinical cohort	246	AN, BN	Adolescents and adults	Females
Franko, [7]	Review/meta-analysis	-	AN, BN	-	-
Fujimori, [31]	Clinical cohort with controls	200	ED	Adults	Females
Grucza, [32]	Community cohort	910	BED	Adults	Mixed
Gueguen, [33]	Clinical cohort	1009*	AN	Adults	Mixed
Guillaume, [34]	Clinical cohort with controls	1563*	AN, BN	Adults	Mixed
Harris, [35]	Review/meta-analysis	-	AN, BN, BED, EDNOS	-	-
Herpertz-Dahlmann, [36]	Review/meta-analysis	-	AN, BN, BED, EDNOS	-	-
Hoek, [37]	Review/meta-analysis	-	AN, BN	-	-
Huas, [38]	Clinical cohort	601*	AN	Adults	Females
Huas, [39]	Clinical cohort with controls	258*	BN	Adolescents and adults	Females
Latzer, [40]	Review/meta-analysis	-	AN	-	-
Liang, [41]	Clinical cohort with controls	316	AN, BN, EDNOS	Adolescents and adults	Females
Millar, [42]	Clinical cohort	524	AN	Adolescents and adults	Females
Muehlenkamp, [43]	Clinical cohort	422*	AN, BN, BED, EDNOS	Adults	Females
Muehlenkamp, [44]	Clinical cohort	131	BN	Adults	Females
Nickel, [3]	Community cohort	813	BN	Adolescents and adults	Females
Papadopoulos, [45]	Clinical cohort	6009*	AN	Adolescents and adults	Females

Table 1 Papers describing suicide and/or self-injury associated with eating disorders *(Continued)*

Papadopoulos, [46]	Clinical cohort	5251	AN	Adolescents and adults	Females
Peebles, [47]	Clinical cohort	1432	ED	Adolescents and adults	Mixed
Peterson, [48]	Clinical cohort	489	BN	Adolescents and adults	Females
Pisetsky, [4]	Clinical cohort	13035	AN, BN, BED	Adults	Females
Pompili, [49]	Review/meta-analysis	-	AN, BN	-	-
Preti, [50]	Review/meta-analysis	-	AN, BN, BED	-	-
Rigaud, [51]	Clinical cohort	484*	AN	Adolescents and adults	Mixed
Rosling, [52]	Clinical cohort	201*	AN, BN	Adolescents and adults	Mixed
Ross, [6]	Community cohort with controls	440	ED	Adolescents	Mixed
Ruuska, [53]	Clinical cohort	57	AN, BN	Adolescents	Females
Schroeder, [54]	Clinical cohort with controls	69	AN, BN	Adults	Females
Selby, [55]	Clinical cohort	787	AN	Adolescents and adults	Mixed
	Clinical cohort	249	AN	Adolescents and adults	Mixed
Signorini, [56]	Clinical cohort	2240	AN	Adults	Females
Silber, [57]	Review/meta-analysis	-	AN, BN	-	-
Smink, [58]	Review/meta-analysis	-	AN, BN, BED, EDNOS	-	-
Smink, [59]	Review/meta-analysis	-	AN, BN, BED, EDNOS	-	-
Smith, [60]	Clinical cohort	204	BN	Adolescents and adults	Females
	Community cohort	171	-	Adolescents and adults	Mixed
	Community cohort	467	-	Adolescents and adults	Mixed
	Community cohort	512	-	Adolescents and adults	Mixed
Steinhausen, [61]	Review/meta-analysis	-	AN, BN	-	-
Steinhausen, [62]	Review/meta-analysis	-	BN	-	-
Suokas, [63]	Clinical cohort with controls	2450	AN, BN, BED	adults	Mixed
Svirko, [64]	Review/meta-analysis	-	AN, BN, EDNOS	-	-
Tozzi, [65]	Clinical cohort	1021	AN, BN, EDNOS	Adolescents and adults	Mixed
Vansteelandt, [66]	Clinical cohort	59	AN, BN	Adults	Females

Note. All ED diagnoses are based on DSM-IV. The following abbreviations are used: AN = anorexia nervosa; BN = bulimia nervosa; BED = binge eating disorder; ED = eating disorders, general; EDNOS = eating disorder not otherwise specified.
*inpatient.

from restriction may lead to suicidal behavior in restricting subtypes [29,51,55].

Other factors that have been specifically examined in relation to suicidality in populations with AN include patients' age at assessment, pregnancy and gender. Arcelus et al. found that the age of the patient at the time of ED assessment is a significant predictor of mortality, including death by suicide [10]. Pregnancy has also been examined in relation to suicidality and AN. In a population-based analysis, 5251 females with AN were evaluated, comparing suicide rates between a parous and a nulliparous group [46]. Suicide was the most common cause of death in both groups. The SMR for suicide in the parous group was 6.3 (95% CI 2.7-12.3) compared to 16.1 in the nulliparous group (95% CI 1.8-21.4), and in fact, childbearing was associated with 65% lower general mortality in AN [46]. While few studies evaluate AN in the male population due to the small sample sizes, Gueguen et al. conducted a longitudinal cohort study comparing 23 men with AN to 601 women with AN and found that men with AN were less likely to have a history of a suicide attempts compared to women with AN (4% vs. 29%; $p = 0.01$) [33].

Bulimia nervosa

Previously, data have shown that mortality rates in general are lower in populations with a diagnosis of BN than in populations with a diagnosis of AN, but few data have specified rates of suicidality in BN. For example, the meta-analysis from Arcelus et al. and a longitudinal study from Franko et al. both examined the mortality rates for BN: Arcelus et al. found a weighted mortality rate of 1.7 (95% CI 1.09-2.44) per 1000 person-years, compared to a weighted mortality rate of 5.1 for AN [10], and Franko's findings were similar [5], but neither of these reports mentioned suicide as a cause of death in the BN population. One study that did look at suicide in BN found that characteristics of suicide attempts did not significantly differ between BN and controls with no ED diagnosis [34].

With regard to completed suicides in BN, findings are mixed. Rates of suicide in both the BN and control samples from Guillaume et al. were altogether lower than in patients with AN [34]. A meta-analysis by Preti et al. reported that in BN, suicide as the cause of death was present in roughly the same proportion as that seen in AN [50]. Crow and colleagues reported a larger percentage of death due to suicide in a BN sample (0.9%) versus an AN sample (0.6%) [20]. Overall, however, the literature indicates that the number of completed suicides among BN appears to be low in comparison to AN.

Some studies have focused on suicidal ideation and suicide attempts, as opposed to completed suicides, and have found that, consistent with the earlier findings of Franko and Keel, suicide attempts are more prevalent in BN populations than in AN populations [7]. Investigating the risk for suicidality between patients with AN, BN and EDNOS, Bodell and colleagues found that BN was significantly associated with suicidality independent of risk predicted by comorbid disorders, while neither AN nor EDNOS were found to be uniquely associated with suicidality [13]. In a meta-analysis by Fedorowicz and colleagues, BN was most strongly associated with suicide attempts or suicidal ideation, followed by AN-binge/purge subtype [25]. Ahrén-Moonga and colleagues investigated the prevalence of suicide plans and/or thoughts, as well as history of suicide attempts in inpatients with EDs, and found a higher prevalence of suicide attempts associated with BN compared with AN ($p < 0.02$) [8]. Forcano et al. found a lifetime prevalence of suicide attempts to be 26.9% ($n = 152$, 95% CI 23.2-30.5) in a sample of 566 BN outpatients [30]. More recently published data from Smith et al. found that approximately one-third of women with a diagnosis of BN have had at least one suicide attempt [60]. There are fewer published data on adolescents with BN than on adults, but a diagnosis of BN in adolescents does appear to raise the risk of increased suicidality and self-harm. For example, in a study that looked at 80 adolescents with BN, 25% reported having attempted suicide or engaging in self-injurious behavior [28]. A study comparing adolescents with AN to adolescents with BN found that the BN group had significantly more suicidal ideation than the AN group [53].

Binge eating disorder and other categories of eating disorders

Less is known about the prevalence of suicidality in populations with a specific diagnosis of BED, or in individuals previously diagnosed with EDNOS according to DSM-IV, or other categories of illness described in the DSM-5 such as ARFID. BED was described in DSM-IV but identified as a formal diagnostic category only recently with the publication of DSM-5. The authors identified few studies that specifically examine suicide associated with BED. Among collected data from community samples, subjects with BED have shown elevated odds for suicide attempts [4,32]. In a thorough examination of all deaths reported among a clinical cohort of 2450 individuals with EDs and a control population, followed for up to 15 years (average length of follow-up was 8.7 years), Suokas et al. identified that four deaths occurred among the 171 individuals with broadly defined BED, one of which was due to suicide [63]. Pisetsky et al. reported that 19% of a sample that met criteria for a narrow diagnosis of BED, and 59% of a sample that met for a broad diagnosis of BED, had a lifetime prevalence of at least one suicide attempt [4]. No results were produced from literature searches using ED key words "avoidant/restrictive food intake disorder" or the acronym "ARFID".

Other risk factors of suicidality in eating disorders

The literature described by Franko and Keel in their 2006 review as well as more recent publications identified in this review consistently emphasize the clinical importance of identifiable risk factors associated with suicidality in EDs. Individual studies have identified a range of factors that may be associated with increased risk of suicidality and/or associated behaviors among individuals with EDs. Illness severity [26], co-occurring psychiatric illnesses including borderline personality disorder [17] and substance abuse [25], excessive exercise [60], and alexithymia [16] have been mentioned as possible risk factors. With regard to age groups, Dancyger and Fomari found that across ED diagnoses, adolescents demonstrate a strong relationship between suicidal behavior and completed suicides [21]. Dancyger and Fomari's review concluded with an emphasis on the importance of clinical awareness to the heightened risk of suicide in the adolescent ED population, the treatment for which may present to be challenging as it requires careful coordination between clinicians, parents, and the young adult patients themselves.

Self-injurious behaviors

In addition, data from reviews, clinical longitudinal investigations, and community cohort studies, show significant associations between EDs and self-injurious behaviors [18,23,60,64,65]. Self-injurious behaviors, which may include compulsive behaviors (e.g., hair pulling, nail biting, skin picking, self-biting) and impulsive self-injurious behaviors (e.g., cutting, burning, self-hitting, banging, scratching), are sometimes referred to as NSSI because the individuals engaging in the behaviors are doing so with the intention of physical self-harm, but without suicidal intent [23]. However, these behaviors, considered on a spectrum of self-destructive behaviors, may be associated with risk of suicidality [23,65].

Data on the relationship between self-injury and EDs indicate that self-injury has a higher prevalence in ED patients with a history of BN, binge eating, or purging behaviors. Tozzi et al. focused specifically on laxative abuse and found in samples of AN and BN that the function of laxative abuse included both a method of purging as well as a form of self-harm [65]. In a case study of 70 female inpatients with EDs, Claes et al. found that 38.6% engaged in NSSI [18]. Of the NSSI and ED group, a significantly higher portion of individuals with BN engaged in NSSI than did individuals with AN ($p < 0.05$) [18]. Ahrén-Moonga and colleagues found that 36.8% of a group of 38 ED patients engaged in self-injury [8]. Fourteen of the patients also reported suicidal ideation or plans, and 10 patients had a history of suicide attempts. Consistent with other studies [18,23,60,64,65], these data show a higher prevalence of self-injury—as well as suicide attempts—in BN compared with AN ($p < 0.05$ and 0.02, respectively) [8].

Other factors that appear to positively influence the relationship between EDs and self-injury include depression, impulsivity, obsessive-compulsiveness, affect dysregulation, dissociation, self-criticizing cognitive style, and need for control, as well as affective lability and previous suicidal behavior or attempts [9,53,64]. Consistent with previous reports, the current review found support for a strong association between EDs and self-injury among individuals with EDs who report a history of trauma and abuse, including verbal, emotional, neglectful, physical, sexual, and/or substance abuse [8,18,24,43,47]. Furthermore, one study that looked specifically at the relationship between pregnancy and self-injury in an ED sample found that, while the majority of women with EDs experience improved ED symptoms during pregnancy, some women in this sample, particularly those diagnosed with binge eating pathology or subclinical ED diagnoses, had a risk of experiencing escalated pathological behaviors during pregnancy [35].

These additional risk factors that may co-occur with or even result in self-injury seem to correlate with more severe ED pathology among ED individuals. In a longitudinal follow-up study, Peterson et al. found that young-adult BN patients who engaged in NSSI at baseline showed an association with increased purging at follow-up eight months after initial presentation [48]. The results also showed that negative urgency at baseline was a significant predictor of NSSI and BN symptoms at follow-up. Fujimori and colleagues found that among individuals with EDs, those who reported self-injury had higher Eating Disorder Inventory scores, signifying greater severity of ED symptoms, than those without self-injury ($p < 0.001$) [31]. In Muehlenkamp and colleagues' study of 422 inpatient ED females, 34.6% of participants engaged in NSSI [43]. This investigation revealed that no specific ED diagnosis was associated with self-injury more commonly than another, but the ED types that specifically include binge or purge behaviors (e.g. AN-BP and BN) were associated with a significantly higher number of types of NSSI including cutting, scratching, bruising, and burning, compared to individuals with other ED types (X^2 (16) = 32.94, $P < 0.01$) [43]. In an all-male ED sample ($N = 130$), Claes and colleagues found that 20.8% reported engaging in NSSI [19]. The NSSI group showed significantly more ED symptoms and had an overall more severe presentation than the non-self-injurious ED males. While there was no significant difference in the rate of NSSI occurring among the three ED diagnostic groups in the sample (AN, BN, and EDNOS), there was a tendency for a higher rate of NSSI among the BN group [19].

Self-injurious behaviors are especially common among adolescents with ED symptoms. Even among adolescents without specific ED diagnoses, results indicate that students who engage in NSSI display significantly more eating pathology, including increased body dissatisfaction and bulimic tendencies (especially binge eating), than their non-NSSI peers [6]. Peebles et al. conducted a chart review of 1432 adolescent ED patients over a nine-year period and found that 40.8% of the sample reported engaging in self-injury [47]. Of those ED adolescents reporting self-injury, females were more likely than males to engage in self-harm behaviors, the most common of which was cutting (85.2%). In this sample, there was also a strong association between self-injury and history of abuse ($p < 0.05$) [47].

Conclusion

As a group, despite the variation in the content of the existing literature, the 66 publications described in this narrative review support the finding of a consistently high prevalence of suicidality associated with EDs. Specifically, AN is consistently associated with high rates of suicide, especially in the context of significantly elevated SMRs for adolescents and young adults. Contrary to previous findings, some recent studies have found that suicide risk appears elevated in BN as well, although there is more variability in the literature on BN study findings; this may be due to sample differences across studies, including the possibility that some individuals with BN may have a history of AN. Self-injurious behaviors are frequent in EDs, with higher rates among EDs that include binge and purge behaviors. Self-injurious behaviors, which may or may not include suicidal intent, are especially high among adolescents with EDs. Furthermore, recent investigations on individuals who engage in rigorous physical exercise are important because they suggest that over-exercise – often considered a self-injurious behavior among ED individuals – may pose additional risk beyond the physical consequence of the activity itself. Over-exercise may change pain sensation and in turn affect individuals' acquired capability for suicide. Based on these findings, individuals with EDs, including those with BN symptoms, who engage in over-exercise, may be at higher risk for suicide. These data underscore the importance of assessing for suicide risk not just in individuals with AN, where suicide rates have long been recognized as elevated, but also in individuals presenting with BN and other ED symptoms. Ultimately, there are a number of risk factors associated with suicidality, which may occur across ED diagnoses. Clinicians must pay close attention to these factors, including chronicity of illness, comorbid diagnoses, history of abuse, and self-injurious behaviors, as occurrence of these factors may increase the potential risk of suicidality.

Limitations

There are several limitations with regard to this review's assessment of the prevalence of suicidality and self-injury in EDs. Methodologically, the review is narrative without a quantitative aggregation of data. While all authors read the reviews that resulted in the literature search, the reviewing of only papers in English limited the quantity of literature search results reviewed. Additionally, the authors' search for the DSM-5's newly described diagnosis ARFID produced no results. Perhaps future published data will include the prevalence of suicidality in EDs, including ARFID, corresponding to newly described criteria in the DSM-5. Ultimately, while more standardized investigation is necessary, multiple studies have clearly found a high risk of mortality, including risk of suicide and self-injurious behaviors, among patients with EDs.

Abbreviations

AN: Anorexia nervosa; ARFID: Avoidant/restrictive food intake disorder; BED: Binge eating disorder; BN: Bulimia nervosa; CI: Confidence interval; ED: Eating disorder; EDNOS: Eating disorder not otherwise specified; NSSI: Non-suicidal self-injury; OR: Odds ratio; SMR: Standardized mortality ratio.

Competing interests

The authors declare that they have no competing interests. Dr. Attia receives research support from Eli Lilly and Co. Publication of this manuscript was supported by *Beyondblue*.

Authors' contributions

All authors carried out the literature search, contributed to the development of this review, and drafted the manuscript. All authors read and approved the final manuscript.

Author details

[1]Columbia University Medical Center, New York, NY, USA. [2]Weill Cornell Medical College, New York, NY, USA.

References

1. Ajetunmobi O, Taylor M, Stockton D, Wood R: **Early death in those previously hospitalised for mental healthcare in Scotland: a nationwide cohort study, 1986-2010.** *BMJ Open* 2013, **3**(7):1–9.
2. Foulon C, Guelfi JD, Kipman A, Adès J, Romo L, Houdeyer K, Marquez S, Mouren MC, Rouillon F, Gorwood P: **Switching to the bingeing/purging subtype of anorexia nervosa is frequently associated with suicidal attempts.** *Eur Psychiatry* 2007, **8:**513–519.
3. Nickel MK, Simek M, Lojewski N, Muehlbacher M, Fartacek R, Kettler C, Bachler E, Egger C, Rother N, Buschmann W, Pedrosa Gil F, Kaplan P, Mitterlehner FO, Anvar J, Rother WK, Loew TH, Nickel C: **Familial and sociopsychopathological risk factors for suicide attempt in bulimic and in depressed women: prospective study.** *Int J Eat Disord* 2006, **39**(5):410–417.
4. Pisetsky EM, Thornton LM, Lichtenstein P, Pedersen NL, Bulik CM: **Suicide attempts in women with eating disorders.** *J Abnorm Psychol* 2013, **122**(4):1042–1056.
5. Franko DL, Keshaviah A, Eddy KT, Krishna M, Davis MC, Keel PK, Herzog DB: **A longitudinal investigation of mortality in anorexia nervosa and bulimia nervosa.** *Am J Psychiatry* 2013, **170**(8):917–925.
6. Ross S, Heath NL, Toste JR: **Non-suicidal self-injury and eating pathology in high school students.** *Am J Orthopsychiatry* 2009, **79**(1):83–92.
7. Franko DL, Keel PK: **Suicidality in eating disorders: occurrence, correlates, and clinical implications.** *Clin Psychol Rev* 2006, **26**(6):769–782.
8. Ahrén-Moonga J, Holmgren S, von Knorring L, Af Klinteberg B: **Personality traits and self-injurious behaviour in patients with eating disorders.** *Eur Eat Disord Rev* 2008, **16**(4):268–275.
9. Anestis MD, Silva C, Lavender JM, Crosby RD, Wonderlich SA, Engel SG, Joiner TE: **Predicting nonsuicidal self-injury episodes over a discrete period of time in a sample of women diagnosed with bulimia nervosa: an analysis of self-reported trait and ecological momentary assessment based affective lability and previous suicide attempts.** *Int J Eat Disord* 2012, **45**(6):808–811.
10. Arcelus J, Mitchell AJ, Wales J, Nielsen S: **Mortality rates in patients with anorexia nervosa and other eating disorders: a meta-analysis of 36 studies.** *Arch Gen Psychiatry* 2011, **68**(7):724–731.
11. Berkman ND, Lohr KN, Bulik CM: **Outcomes of eating disorders: a systematic review of the literature.** *Int J Eat Disord* 2007, **40**(4):293–309.
12. Birmingham CL, Su J, Hlynsky JA, Goldner EM, Gao M: **The mortality rate from anorexia nervosa.** *Int J Eat Disord* 2005, **38**(2):143–146.
13. Bodell LP, Joiner TE, Keel PK: **Comorbidity-independent risk for suicidality increases with bulimia nervosa but not with anorexia nervosa.** *J Psychiatr Res* 2013, **47**(5):617–621.
14. Bulik CM, Thornton L, Pinheiro AP, Plotnicov K, Klump KL, Brandt H, Crawford S, Fichter MM, Halmi KA, Johnson C, Kaplan AS, Mitchell J, Nutzinger D, Strober M, Treasure J, Woodside DB, Berrettini WH, Kaye WH: **Suicide attempts in anorexia nervosa.** *Psychosom Med* 2008, **70**(3):378–383.
15. Button EJ, Chadalavada B, Palmer RL: **Mortality and predictors of death in a cohort of patients presenting to an eating disorders service.** *Int J Eat Disord* 2010, **43**(5):387–392.
16. Carano A, De Berardis D, Campanella D, Serroni N, Ferri F, Di Iorio G, Acciavatti T, Mancini L, Mariani G, Martinotti G, Moschetta FS, Di Giannantonio M: **Alexithymia and suicide ideation in a sample of patients with binge eating disorder.** *J Psychiatr Pract* 2012, **18**(1):5–11.
17. Chen EY, Brown MZ, Harned MS, Linehan MM: **A comparison of borderline personality disorder with and without eating disorders.** *Psychiatry Res* 2009, **170**(1):86–90.
18. Claes L, Vandereycken W: **Is there a link between traumatic expriences and self-injurious behaviors in eating-disordered patients?** *Eat Disord* 2007, **15**(4):305–315.
19. Claes L, Jimenez-Murcia S, Aguera Z, Castro R, Sanchez I, Manuel Menchon J, Fernandez-Aranda F: **Male eating disorder patients with and without non-suicidal self-injury: A comparison of psychopathological and personality features.** *Eur Eat Disord Rev* 2012, **20**(4):335–338.
20. Crow SJ, Peterson CB, Swanson SA, Raymond NC, Specker S, Eckert ED, Mitchell JE: **Increased mortality in bulimia nervosa and other eating disorders.** *Am J Psychiatry* 2009, **166**(12):1342–1346.
21. Dancyger IF, Fornari VM: **A review of eating disorders and suicide risk in adolescence.** *ScientificWorldJournal* 2005, **5:**803–811.
22. Erdur L, Kallenbach-Dermutz B, Lehmann V, Zimmermann-Viehoff F, Köpp W, Weber C, Deter HC: **Somatic comorbidity in anorexia nervosa: First results of a 21-year follow-up study on female inpatients.** *Biopsychosoc Med* 2012, **6**(1):4.
23. Favaro A, Ferrara S, Santonastaso P: **Self-injurious behavior in a community sample of young women: relationship with childhood abuse and other types of self-damaging behaviors.** *J Clin Psychiatry* 2007, **68**(1):122–131.

24. Favaro A, Santonastaso P, Monteleone P, Bellodi L, Mauri M, Rotondo A, Erzegovesi S, Maj M: **Self-injurious behavior and attempted suicide in purging bulimia nervosa: associations with psychiatric comorbidity.** *J Affect Disord* 2008, **105**(1-3):285–289.
25. Fedorowicz VJ, Falissard B, Foulon C, Dardennes R, Divac SM, Guelfi JD, Rouillon F: **Factors associated with suicidal behaviors in a large French sample of inpatients with eating disorders.** *Int J Eat Disord* 2007, **40**(7):589–595.
26. Fennig S, Hadas A: **Suicidal behavior and depression in adolescents with eating disorders.** *Nord J Psychiatry* 2010, **64**(1):32–39.
27. Fichter MM, Quadflieg N, Hedlund S: **Twelve-year course and outcome predictors of anorexia nervosa.** *Int J Eat Disord* 2006, **39**(2):87–100.
28. Fischer S, le Grange D: **Comorbidity and high-risk behaviors in treatment-seeking adolescents with bulimia nervosa.** *Int J Eat Disord* 2007, **40**(8):751–753.
29. Forcano L, Alvarez E, Santamaría JJ, Jimenez-Murcia S, Granero R, Penelo E, Alonso P, Sánchez I, Menchón JM, Ulman F, Bulik CM, Fernández-Aranda F: **Suicide attempts in anorexia nervosa subtypes.** *Compr Psychiatry* 2011, **52**(4):352–358.
30. Forcano L, Fernández-Aranda F, Alvarez-Moya E, Bulik C, Granero R, Gratacòs M, Jiménez-Murcia S, Krug I, Mercader JM, Riesco N, Saus E, Santamaría JJ, Estivill X: **Suicide attempts in bulimia nervosa: personality and psycho-pathological correlates.** *Eur Psychiatry* 2009, **24**(2):91–97.
31. Fujimori A, Wada Y, Yamashita T, Choi H, Nishizawa S, Yamamoto H, Fukui K: **Parental bonding in patients with eating disorders and self-injurious behavior.** *Psychiatry Clin Neurosci* 2011, **65**(3):272–279.
32. Grucza RA, Przybeck TR, Cloninger CR: **Prevalence and correlates of binge eating disorder in a community sample.** *Compr Psychiatry* 2007, **48**(2):124–131.
33. Gueguen J, Godart N, Chambry J, Brun-Eberentz A, Foulon C, Divac Phd SM, Guelfi JD, Rouillon F, Falissard B, Huas C: **Severe anorexia nervosa in men: comparison with severe AN in women and analysis of mortality.** *Int J Eat Disord* 2012, **45**(4):537–545.
34. Guillaume S, Jaussent I, Olié E, Genty C, Bringer J, Courtet P, Schmidt U: **Characteristics of suicide attempts in anorexia and bulimia nervosa: a case-control study.** *PLoS One* 2011, **6**(8):e23578.
35. Harris AA: **Practical advice for caring for women with eating disorders during the perinatal period.** *J Midwifery Womens Health* 2010, **55**(6):579–586.
36. Herpertz-Dahlmann B: **Adolescent eating disorders: definitions, symptomatology, epidemiology and comorbidity.** *Child Adolesc Psychiatr Clin N Am* 2009, **18**(1):31–47.
37. Hoek HW: **Incidence, prevalence and mortality of anorexia nervosa and other eating disorders.** *Curr Opin Psychiatry* 2006, **19**(4):389–394.
38. Huas C, Caille A, Godart N, Foulon C, Pham-Scottez A, Divac S, Dechartres A, Lavoisy G, Guelfi JD, Rouillon F, Falissard B: **Factors predictive of ten-year mortality in severe anorexia nervosa patients.** *Acta Psychiatr Scand* 2011, **123**(1):62–70.
39. Huas C, Godart N, Caille A, Pham-Scottez A, Foulon C, Divac SM, Lavoisy G, Guelfi JD, Falissard B, Rouillon F: **Mortality and its predictors in severe bulimia nervosa patients.** *Eur Eat Disord Rev* 2013, **21**(1):15–19.
40. Latzer Y, Hochdorf Z: **Dying to be thin: attachment to death in anorexia nervosa.** *ScientificWorldJournal* 2005, **5**:820–827.
41. Liang KY, Meg Tseng MC: **Impulsive behaviors in female patients with eating disorders in a university hospital in northern Taiwan.** *J Formos Med Assoc* 2011, **110**(9):607–610.
42. Millar HR, Wardell F, Vyvyan JP, Naji SA, Prescott GJ, Eagles JM: **Anorexia nervosa mortality in Northeast Scotland, 1965-1999.** *Am J Psychiatry* 2005, **162**(4):753–757.
43. Muehlenkamp JJ, Claes L, Smits D, Peat CM, Vandereycken W: **Non-suicidal self-injury in eating disordered patients: a test of a conceptual model.** *Psychiatry Res* 2011, **188**(1):102–108.
44. Muehlenkamp JJ, Engel SG, Wadeson A, Crosby RD, Wonderlich SA, Simonich H, Mitchell JE: **Emotional states preceding and following acts of non-suicidal self-injury in bulimia nervosa patients.** *Behav Res Ther* 2008, **47**(1):83–87.
45. Papadopoulos FC, Ekbom A, Brandt L, Ekselius L: **Excess mortality, causes of death and prognostic factors in anorexia nervosa.** *Br J Psychiatry* 2009, **194**(1):10–17.
46. Papadopoulos FC, Karamanis G, Brandt L, Ekbom A, Ekselius L: **Childbearing and mortality among women with anorexia nervosa.** *Int J Eat Disord* 2013, **46**(2):164–170.
47. Peebles R, Wilson JL, Lock JD: **Self-injury in adolescents with eating disorders: correlates and provider bias.** *J Adolesc Health* 2011, **48**(3):310–313.
48. Peterson CM, Fischer S: **A prospective study of the influence of the UPPS model of impulsivity on the co-occurrence of bulimic symptoms and non-suicidal self-injury.** *Eat Behav* 2012, **13**(4):335–341.
49. Pompili M, Girardi P, Tatarelli G, Ruberto A, Tatarelli R: **Suicide and attempted suicide in eating disorders, obesity and weight-image concern.** *Eat Behav* 2006, **7**(4):384–394.
50. Preti A, Rocchi MB, Sisti D, Camboni MV, Miotto P: **A comprehensive meta-analysis of the risk of suicide in eating disorders.** *Acta Psychiatr Scand* 2011, **124**(1):6–17.
51. Rigaud D, Tallonneau I, Brindisi MC, Vergès B: **Prognosis in 41 severely malnourished anorexia nervosa patients.** *Clin Nutr* 2012, **31**(5):693–698.
52. Rosling AM, Sparén P, Norring C, von Knorring AL: **Mortality of eating disorders: a follow-up study of treatment in a specialist unit 1974-2000.** *Int J Eat Disord* 2011, **44**(4):304–310.
53. Ruuska J, Kaltiala-Heino R, Rantanen P, Koivisto AM: **Psychopathological distress predicts suicidal ideation and self-harm in adolescent eating disorder outpatients.** *Eur Child Adolesc Psychiatry* 2005, **14**(5):276–281.
54. Schroeder M, Eberlein C, de Zwaan M, Kornhuber J, Bleich S, Frieling H: **Lower levels of cannabinoid 1 receptor mRNA in female eating disorder patients: association with wrist cutting as impulsive self-injurious behavior.** *Psychoneuroendocrinology* 2012, **37**(12):2032–2036.
55. Selby EA, Smith AR, Bulik CM, Olmsted MP, Thornton L, McFarlane TL, Berrettini WH, Brandt HA, Crawford S, Fichter MM, Halmi KA, Jacoby GE, Johnson CL, Jones I, Kaplan AS, Mitchell JE, Nutzinger DO, Strober M, Treasure J, Woodside DB, Kaye WH, Joiner TE Jr: **Habitual starvation and provocative behaviors: two potential routes to extreme suicidal behavior in anorexia nervosa.** *Behav Res Ther* 2010, **48**(7):634–645.
56. Signorini A, De Filippo E, Panico S, De Caprio C, Pasanisi F, Contaldo F: **Long-term mortality in anorexia nervosa: a report after an 8-year follow-up and a review of the most recent literature.** *Eur J Clin Nutr* 2007, **61**(1):119–222.
57. Silber TJ: **Ipecac syrup abuse, morbidity, and mortality: isn't it time to repeal its over-the counter status?** *J Adolesc Health* 2005, **37**(3):256–260.
58. Smink FR, van Hoeken D, Hoek HW: **Epidemiology, course, and outcome of eating disorders.** *Curr Opin Psychiatry* 2013, **26**(6):543–548.
59. Smink FR, van Hoeken D, Hoek HW: **Epidemiology of eating disorders: incidence, prevalence and mortality rates.** *Curr Psychiatry Rep* 2012, **14**(4):406–414.
60. Smith AR, Fink EL, Anestis MD, Ribeiro JD, Gordon KH, Davis H, Keel PK, Bardone-Cone AM, Peterson CB, Klein MH, Crow S, Mitchell JE, Crosby RD, Wonderlich SA, le Grange D, Joiner TE Jr: **Exercise caution: over-exercise is associated with suicidality among individuals with disordered eating.** *Psychiatry Res* 2013, **206**(2–3):246–255.
61. Steinhausen HC: **Outcome of eating disorders.** *Child Adolesc Psychiatr Clin N Am* 2009, **18**(1):225–242.
62. Steinhausen HC, Weber S: **The outcome of bulimia nervosa: findings from one-quarter century of research.** *Am J Psychiatry* 2009, **166**(12):1331–1341.
63. Suokas JT, Suvisaari JM, Gissler M, Löfman R, Linna MS, Raevuori A, Haukka J: **Mortality in eating disorders: A follow-up study of adult eating disorder patients treated in tertiary care, 1995-2010.** *Psychiatry Res* 2013, **210**(3):1101–1106.
64. Svirko E, Hawton K: **Self-injurious behavior and eating disorders: the extent and nature of the association.** *Suicide Life Threat Behav* 2007, **37**(4):409–421.
65. Tozzi F, Thornton LM, Mitchell J, Fichter MM, Klump KL, Lilenfeld LR, Reba L, Strober M, Kaye WH, Bulik CM, Price Foundation Collaborative Group: **Features associated with laxative abuse in individuals with eating disorders.** *Psychosom Med* 2006, **68**(3):470–477.
66. Vansteelandt K, Claes L, Muehlenkamp J, De Cuyper K, Lemmens J, Probst M, Vanderlinden J, Pieters G: **Variability in affective activation predicts non-suicidal self-injury in eating disorders.** *Eur Eat Disord Rev* 2013, **21**(2):143–147.

6

The cognitive-interpersonal maintenance model of anorexia nervosa revisited: a summary of the evidence for cognitive, socio-emotional and interpersonal predisposing and perpetuating factors

Janet Treasure* and Ulrike Schmidt

Abstract

Aim: To describe the evidence base relating to the Cognitive-Interpersonal Maintenance Model for anorexia nervosa (AN).

Background: A Cognitive-Interpersonal Maintenance Model maintenance model for anorexia nervosa was described in 2006. This model proposed that cognitive, socio-emotional and interpersonal elements acted together to both cause and maintain eating disorders.

Method: A review of the empirical literature relating to the key constructs of the model (cognitive, socio-emotional, interpersonal) risk and maintaining factors for anorexia nervosa was conducted.

Results: Set shifting and weak central coherence (associated with obsessive compulsive traits) have been widely studied. There is some evidence to suggest that a strong eye for detail and weak set shifting are inherited vulnerabilities to AN. Set shifting and global integration are impaired in the ill state and contribute to weak central coherence. In addition, there are wide-ranging impairments in socio-emotional processing including: an automatic bias in attention towards critical and domineering faces and away from compassionate faces; impaired signalling of, interpretation and regulation of emotions. Difficulties in social cognition may in part be a consequence of starvation but inherited vulnerabilities may also contribute to these traits. The shared familial traits may accentuate family members' tendency to react to the frustrating and frightening symptoms of AN with high expressed emotion (criticism, hostility, overprotection), and inadvertently perpetuate the problem.

Conclusion: The cognitive interpersonal model is supported by accumulating evidence. The model is complex in that cognitive and socio-emotional factors both predispose to the illness and are exaggerated in the ill state. Furthermore, some of the traits are inherited vulnerabilities and are present in family members. The clinical formulations from the model are described as are new possibilities for targeted treatment.

Keywords: Anorexia nervosa, Model, Complex intervention, Eating disorder

* Correspondence: janet.treasure@kcl.ac.uk
Department of Psychological Medicine, King's College London, Institute of Psychiatry, The Basement, P059, 103 Denmark Hill, London SE5 8AF, UK

Background

Treatment for anorexia nervosa (AN) has focused on remediating the eating and weight symptoms. Historically, inpatient care was used but the NICE guidelines recommended outpatient care in the first instance. In the early phase of adolescent AN, mobilising the parents to restore a normal eating pattern is effective [1-3]. Nevertheless a sizeable proportion of patients (30-60%) fail to change their behaviour. In adult patients, particularly if the duration of illness has lasted over 3 years, change is more difficult [4].

Premorbid vulnerabilities contribute to a poor response to treatment. Cognitive rigidity and obsessive compulsive traits [5] and social communication difficulties are associated with a poorer outcome from AN [6]. Furthermore, secondary consequences of malnutrition that accumulate over time contribute to treatment resistance. A starved brain, for instance, is less plastic and hence responds less well to talking treatments which require changes to be made in reflective cognitive functions.

Features such as these led us to develop a cognitive-interpersonal maintenance model for AN. The essential features of this model were that there were predisposing factors such as obsessive compulsive features and anxious avoidance (particularly of close relationships) increased the vulnerability to AN and that these contributed also to the maintenance of the disorder because they fostered pro anorexia nervosa beliefs and behaviours. These traits cause problems relating to others and, in addition, the highly visible eating disorders (ED) symptoms and behaviors have a profound effect on other people and lead them to react in ways which in turn serve to maintain the disorder. Thus, interpersonal relationships become entangled with the disorder in a complex manner.

The predictions from this model were that obsessive compulsive and anxious avoidant traits would be intermediate phenotypes increasing the risk of the disorder developing and that social processing and interpersonal interactions might be problematic. It follows that treatment for AN would therefore need to be a complex form of intervention with multiple interacting components. The Medical Research Council (MRC) has developed guidelines on the development of complex interventions as it is acknowledged that they entail unique challenges [7]. A key step is to develop a strong theoretical understanding in order to target the processes and outcomes that are integral to recovery. Developing the theoretical framework is an ongoing process and the model may need to be adjusted as new evidence emerges.

The aim of this paper is to examine the evidence relating to the cognitive interpersonal model. First, we scrutinise and synthesise the literature on genes, molecules, cells, circuits, physiology, behavior and self report measures relating to the cognitive phenotype (OCPD traits) and the anxious, avoidant, social emotional phenotype. We then summarise the evidence relating interpersonal aspects of the illness. Lastly, we describe how clinical formulations and treatments follow from the model.

Premorbid traits

In the original model, obsessive compulsive traits (OCP) traits were considered to be a key vulnerability factor [8] [9] contributing to maintenance through pro anorexia nervosa beliefs and behaviours. Cognitive processing styles such as set shifting and central coherence [10-12] underpin these traits and have been the subject of highly active examination.

Set shifting

Behavioural studies

People with EDs (AN and BN) have moderate to large sized problems with set shifting in a range of tasks (as summarised in a systematic review see [13]). After recovery, these inefficiencies remain in an attenuated form [14,15]. Adolescents with anorexia nervosa are also less impaired [16-19]. This suggests that set shifting may be accentuated as a consequence of the illness. The alternative explanation is that individuals with less pronounced problems in this area are more likely to recover and that these serve as moderating factors. First degree relatives (sisters, twins, parents) of people with eating disorders also perform poorly on some tasks (WCST) [15,20].

Furthermore, in a study by Kothari et al., (2012), children (aged 8) of women with EDs perform poorly on a set shifting task [21]. In summary reduced set shifting is a feature of AN in the acute state. Furthermore, this trait is also present in first degree relatives which suggests that it might be an inherited vulnerability for AN. It is less pronounced after recovery (see Figure 1) suggesting that it is accentuated by starvation.

What do we know about the underpinning biology of set shifting?

Set shifting tasks involve increased frontal and parietal and decreased striatal activation in AN [22] and BN [23]. One interpretation is that these tasks may involve more cognitive effort in people with EDs.

Set shifting difficulties are a generic risk factor for other forms of psychopathology. It appears to result from a biological vulnerability in corticostriatal circuits. Set shifting in rodents [24] and in primates is associated with frontal lobe function [25]. An inbred mouse model (BTBR) has problems in set shifting [26,27], Thus, set shifting inefficiencies seen in EDs may be linked to genetic factors that control brain development.

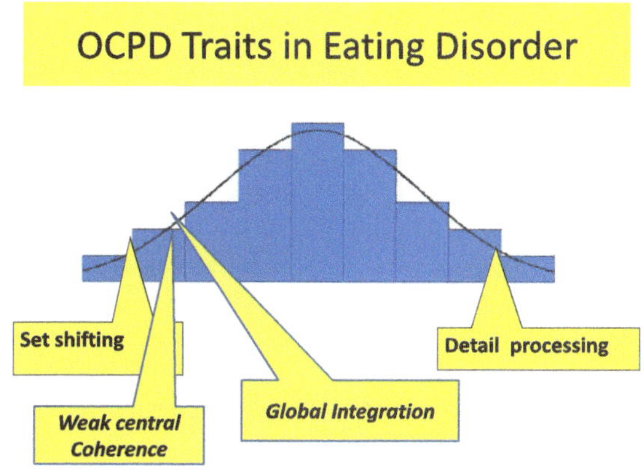

Figure 1 Obsessive compulsive personality traits. Legend A diagrammatic representation of traits related to obsessive compulsive personality disorder (OCPD) in eating disorders . Those that are mainly present in the acute, starved state are shown in italics.

Central coherence

Weak central coherence (an inability to see the forest for the trees) is thought to arise from an imbalance between global and detail processing and is common in people with EDs. People with EDs have a moderate to large superiority in detail processing tasks in the acute state [15,28] and after recovery [11,15,29,30]. Superior detail processing is also found to a degree in first degree relatives (sisters) [11,15,31]. This suggests that a strong focus on detail might be an inherited vulnerability of AN.

Global integration is poor in acute AN, and it may be a consequence of low weight [29]. Therefore, with starvation the balance between global and detail processing which contributes to central coherence is reduced (Figure 1). Moreover, the accentuated set shifting problems in the acute state reduce the flexible switching between the global/detail processing. Thus, weak central coherence may be a secondary consequence of the illness contributing to the maintenance of the illness by impeding adaptation to environmental demands.

Clinical formulation relating to obsessive compulsive traits

A causal and maintenance model derived from the evidence described above is shown in Figure 2. Although people with EDs, in general, have good cognitive abilities with superior attention to detail they show problems in set shifting. Both of these appear to be an inherited traits. These traits in the child make them more susceptible to societal rules and their eye for detail makes aspects of appearance more salient. The traits mean that once dieting behaviour is started (triggered by stress for example), it is undertaken meticulously and the rules and rituals become embedded as rigid habits. Attention

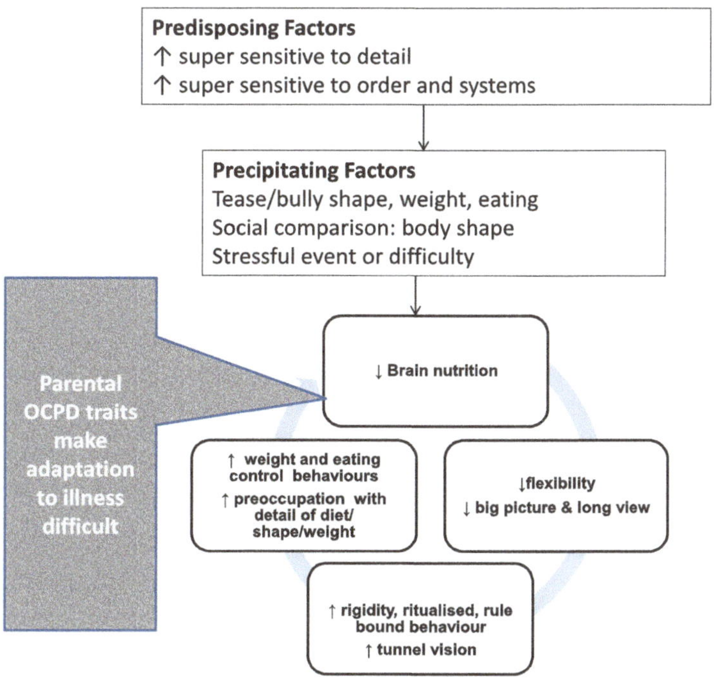

Figure 2 A diagrammatic formulation of obsessive compulsive personality disorder (OCPD) traits. Legend. A diagrammatic formulation of obsessive compulsive personality disorder (OCPD) traits showing how they predispose to, and increase, the vulnerability to precipitating factors and also perpetuate the disorder. The grey box indicates how shared familial traits may contribute to the perpetuation of the problem.

to the detail of weight control rules and inflexibility leads to success in the goal of weight loss. This, because of starvation, in turn, impacts on brain function reducing global integration and central coherence and so the focus is further narrowed to the dieting behaviour which become even more habitual. A vicious circle which maintains the disorder develops.

Parents and other family members may share some of these obsessive compulsive traits. These may lead to over controlling parenting (Corfield et al. submitted) which can increase risk particularly in those with the ss form of the serotonin transporter gene [32,33]. Also these traits in parents and other family members may make the process of adjustment and management of the ED behaviours more difficult. A battle for control can ensue as both sides defend their rules, often losing sight of the bigger picture and the longer view of life. This unhelpful reaction inhibits flexible adjustment and serves to maintain ED behaviours.

Anxiety, avoidance (social and emotional) behaviours

Anxious avoidance of emotions, in particular those aroused by social encounters, insecure attachments, was the second feature within the model considered to be present before the illness. Social avoidance can be a core feature of people with EDs. For example, a personal account of the illness by a medical practitioner described the illness in one word: "isolation" [34]. Difficulties relating to others predate the onset of the illness, can be accentuated by the illness and sometimes persist despite recovery.

People with AN are more likely than controls to report an impoverished social network before the onset of the illness (e.g. having no close friends in childhood; [33,35] fewer social activities [36] and less social support [37]). In part, this relates to temperamental characteristics, as people with EDs are inhibited and shy with internalising problems [38]. Loneliness, feelings of inferiority and high levels of social anxiety [39] are also reported.

In cases ascertained in adolescence, social problems predated the illness in 20% of cases and informed the prognosis, such that cases with social deficits prior to onset at age 15, were found to be impaired 18 years later at follow-up [6,40]. Experiences of teasing, bullying and criticism, often pertaining to weight/shape and eating, are found before the illness [41]. During the illness social networks are often reduced [42,43]. In addition, a sense of inferiority in relationship to others can persist post recovery [44]. Thus, a wide variety of behavioural features support the model, in that an avoidant social phenotype is of relevance to the onset and prognosis. In the next section we examine the form of this social phenotype in more detail. A variety of experimental paradigms have been used to examine factors that may underpin social avoidance in people with EDs, [45] including attention, emotional expression and interpretation and theory of mind.

Attentional mechanisms

People with AN differ from healthy controls in that they have an attentional bias towards negative facial expressions such as anger [46-48] criticism [49] and dominance (Cardi et al. submitted) but not towards positive facial expressions such as happiness [46] and compassion [49]. Also, people with AN have been found to direct their gaze less at the face and eyes [50]. These traits remain present, albeit in an attenuated form, in the recovered state and in first degree relatives (twins, parents) (Kanakam et al. submitted Goddard et al. submitted). These findings suggest that there is increased attention to social threat and a decreased attention to social reward and that this may be an inherited vulnerability.

Interpretation of social signals

Accurate reading of the intentions and emotions of others is necessary for effective social communication. People with AN have impairments in this domain. A systematic review and meta analysis concluded that people with AN have impairments in recognizing facial emotions, [51]. In contrast, people with BN have little or no impairment in facial emotion recognition [52], and may be better than healthy controls at recognizing negative emotions [53]. In AN, interpreting emotional meaning from the voice [54,55], body movement [56] and from films [54] is also impaired. For the most part, these impairments are less marked after recovery, suggesting that they may be starvation, state effects. There is little evidence that these traits are part of an inherited vulnerability as they are not present in first degree relatives (twins, parents) (Kanakam et al. submitted Goddard et al. submitted).

Signaling emotions

The ability to signal one's own intentions and emotions to others is an important component of effective social communication and people with AN also have impairments in this domain. In a study that examined emotional expression and experience of people with AN, it was found that when watching sad or funny films, people with AN expressed little facial emotional expression and were also less attentive, e.g. turning away more, when watching sad films. This lack of reciprocity and attention contrasts with their self reported emotional reactions which were intense [57]. Also, when people with AN were engaged in a therapeutic emotional skills training video game, they had minimal facial displays of anger and yet on self report measures they had high levels of anger [58]. This suggests that there is inhibited emotional expression and reduced mirroring of emotion.

This has not been examined after recovery and in family members.

Understanding the mind of another

The most sophisticated aspect of social communication is the ability to understand the mental processes of other people, so called 'theory of mind'. A proportion of people with AN have problems with theory of mind tasks such as cartoons, which require understanding of implicit thoughts rather than explicit words spoken [59,60]. This has not been examined after recovery and in family members.

A related concept is that of social perception, which denotes "a person's ability to ascertain social cues from behaviour provided in a social context", which includes, but is not limited to, emotion cues. Social perception abilities are preserved in ED patients, but those with restricting AN have difficulty in identifying degree of intimacy in social relationships (Renwick et al., submitted).

Understanding the self

Finally the perception and understanding of self is an additional component of the social cognition domain that has found to be disturbed in anorexia nervosa. The most widely studied concept in this domain is alexithymia. Sisters of people with anorexia nervosa also have problems in this area which suggests that it might be an additional endophenotype [61]. Abnormalities in other paradigms which measure aspects of interoception such as the rubber hand illusion have also been found [62].

The traits relating to social processing are displayed in Figure 3.

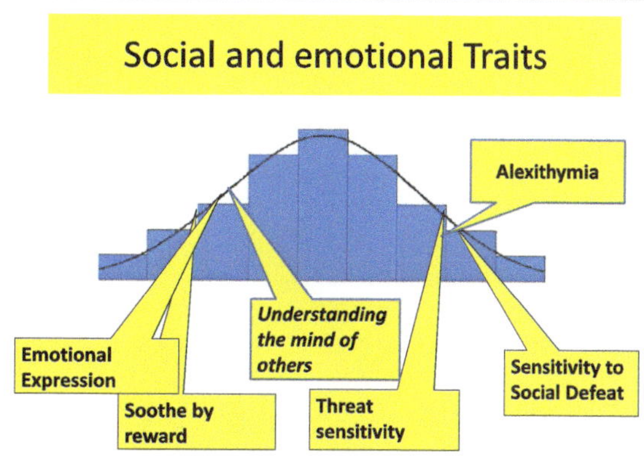

Figure 3 Social processing traits. Legend. A diagrammatic representation of social processing traits in eating disorders. Those that are mainly present in the acute starved state are shown in italics.

What do we know about the underpinning biology of social processes

Brain activation during social processing in AN differs from that seen in the comparison population. The evoked potential to faces (implicitly and explicitly presented) was reduced both in the acute state and after weight restoration [63]. Two groups have used a task in which moving shapes representing social or non-social/mechanical interactions are shown. Adults (partially recovered) [64] and adolescents (in both the acute phase of AN and after weight restoration (> 100 days treatment)) did not show the expected increase in activation in social processing circuits. On the other hand there was normal activation to emotional faces after recovery AN [65]. Thus, it is possible that some of the anomalies in the brain response to social processing tasks in AN, result from the illness state and are resolved with full recovery but this needs further study.

It is not surprising that social cognition is impaired in the acute state, as this form of cognition requires higher levels of processing. An illustration of this is the social brain hypothesis of Dunbar and colleagues. This theory is based on the observations that throughout the animal and bird kingdoms, social complexity is related to brain size [66,67]. The shrunken, starved brain of AN may not have the functional capacity to optimally participate in the sophisticated communication developed in humans [68]. Moreover, oxytocin functioning, a hormone which is central to aspects of social communication, appears to be disturbed in AN. In the acute state, oxytocin is reduced both peripherally [69] and in the brain [70]. Even after recovery, however, oxytocin released after a test meal is reduced [71].

Clinical formulation

The balance of evidence is that there are both predisposing inefficiencies in this system and secondary problems acquired as a consequence of the illness. A causal and maintenance model derived from the evidence described above is shown in Figure 4.

Negative self evaluation, internalising strategies and reduced social processing skills predispose to the development of the illness. This is perhaps due to an increased sensitivity to social hierarchies and to negative judgments from others (particularly teasing and criticism about shape, weight or eating) or by the desire to belong and be accepted by attaining social norms (internalisation of thinness). By starving the brain and reducing high level brain function, the symptoms themselves decrease social processing abilities which leads to further withdrawal from social pursuits and poor confidence in situations that require social problem solving abilities [72]. This allows the ED thoughts and behaviours, used to control the biological homeostatic forces, to dominate brain function. The ED becomes the only friend and a vicious circle develops.

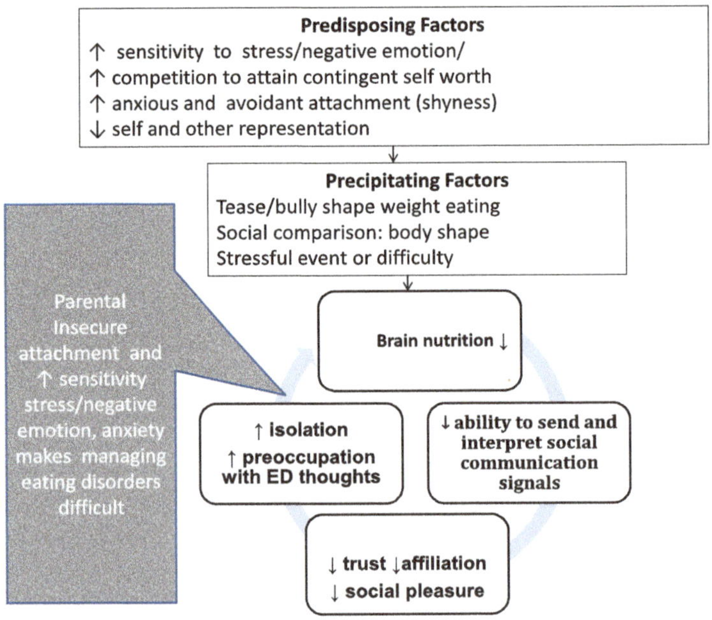

Figure 4 A diagrammatic formulation of social processing traits. Legend. A diagrammatic formulation of social processing traits showing how they predispose to and increase the vulnerability to precipitating factors and also perpetuate the disorder. The grey box indicates how shared familial traits may contribute to the perpetuation of the problem.

There is a small amount of evidence suggesting that some of these traits run in families. This may make social communication in the family more difficult and allow the isolation of AN to take a greater hold.

Interpersonal relationships

In the initial prototype of the model, the key interpersonal maintaining factors were thought to be high expressed emotion, criticism, hostility and over protection. Systematic reviews of this concept suggest that these behaviours are present and impact on the response to treatment and outcome [73] (Duclos in press). Accommodating and enabling behaviours [74-78] have been added as behavioural reactions that maintain the illness, another vicious circle.

A formulation for carers showing the interface with eating disorder symptoms is shown in Figure 5. There may be shared OCPD and anxiety traits which become pronounced in the face of the symptoms of anorexia nervosa. This may lead to high expressed emotion (criticism, over protection) and accommodating behaviour which fuels further symptoms.

Adaptations to the model on the basis of new evidence

The new clinical and behavioural evidence has clarified the model. Although the original key concepts remain, the model has become somewhat more complex as some of the risk factors (strong detail, set shifting and social communication difficulties) appear to be familial vulnerability traits and so have a wider effect by causing a maladaptive response by family members. Also social communication deficits develop or are accentuated as a result of starvation which means that interpersonal relationships become more difficult. Thus, three interlocking formulations relating to cognitive, emotional and interpersonal style may be needed to encapsulate the illness and plan treatment.

Translational treatment implications

Psycho education

This model is a useful heuristic to help patients and their families understand the illness, the role that they can play in causing the illness to persist and how treatment can be managed and directed. Firstly, patients and their families can be helped to understand the many factors that contribute to the illness and which become entwined in a complex manner when the symptoms themselves either alter brain function and so make the individual less capable of change or cause others to react in ways that maybe unhelpful.

Patients and family members may find it helpful to know that the strength in detail, can become problematic when combined with weakened set shifting in the ill state. Also, when patients and families understand how their automatic attention and interpretation mode is biased towards the negative, they can appreciate that

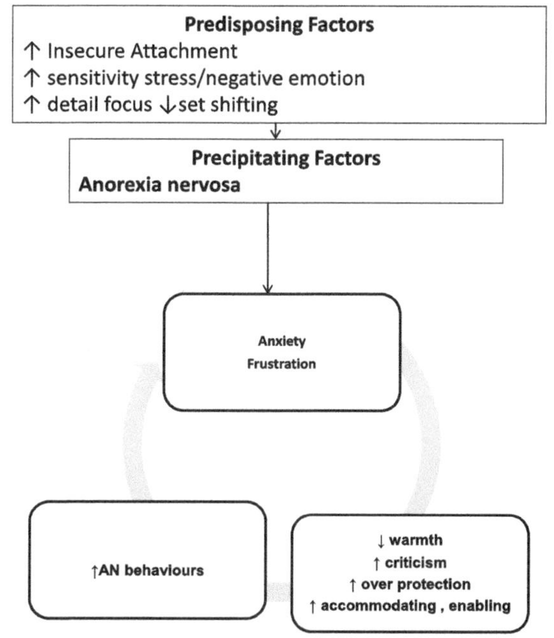

Figure 5 A diagrammatic formulation of carers involvement within the maintenance of an eating disorder. Legend. A diagrammatic formulation of how carers own vulnerabilities, insecure attachment, anxiety and OCPD traits predispose to more difficulties coping with the eating disorder leading to anxiety and distress which in turn are associated with high expressed emotion, or accommodation to eating disorder symptoms which act to maintain the disorder.

their judgments about themselves and the world may be skewed. Furthermore, painful miscommunication can occur because social communication is attenuated by starvation induced, inefficient brain function. Thus their ability to have a balanced appraisal of the emotional state and intentions of themselves and others is weakened.

Therapeutic relationship

A common ingredient of many forms of psychotherapy used to treat people with EDs, is the development of a good working alliance and reflective listening to help the individual obtain a more realistic and holistic view of the world and themselves. However, one or three hours a week of therapy is a minimal input compared to the 20 hours a week or more of contact time that most parents/carers have with their offspring [79]. Thus, if families can be helped to develop more effective forms of social communication, this may help them facilitate a restoration of nutritional balance.

In our experience families and therapists find that this conceptualization and explanation of the brain based factors underpinning ED behaviours with an emphasis on the cognitive and social facets of the illness, rather than food alone, can build a more collaborative, inclusive approach. This serves as the rationale to explain why it is helpful to reduce the critical and dominating communication style, which is an understandable reaction to the frustrations of the illness, and instead use a style which elicits a positive self concept by increasing warmth and listening and selectively attending to healthy behaviours rather than anorexia talk. Teaching parents the basic skills of motivational interviewing (MI), such as reflective listening with affirmations and differential attention to "change talk" fosters this communication style. The complex reflections, which are a key part of MI, are a form of theory of mind intervention, in that they seek to encapsulate the gist of the other person's beliefs motivations and drives. Carers (professional and family members) can model high quality listening and communication. Affirmations serve to allow the individual with an ED to have a positive self image in mind. Improving communication within the family can be generalised to a wider social network. We have found that it is possible for carers to develop high levels of these skills.

Specific interventions

We have developed a talking therapy (Maudsley Model of Anorexia Nervosa, MANTRA) based on the cognitive-interpersonal model of AN. This manual-based treatment has been pilot-tested in a case series [80] and a small randomized controlled trial [81]. However, like all forms of talking treatments MANTRA targets complex aspects of brain function which are impaired with a severe and /or chronic form of illness. To improve outcomes further, adjunctive strategies may be needed which use interventions that target some of these brain mechanisms more directly. Examples of these include attention training protocols that have been used to modify threat-related attentional biases in anxiety disorders [82,83] (Renwick et al., in press). The use of pharmacological approaches to supplement psychological interventions for EDs may be of value. For example, oxytocin may enhance the effectiveness of social interventions [84] and promote affiliation and the formation of positive bonding. Finally, neuromodulatory treatments which improve focal brain activation may also have potential [85].

Conclusion

We have summarised and evaluated the new evidence relating to the cognitive interpersonal model of AN. The key concepts of the model have been clarified and the constructs relating to cognitive, socio-emotional and interpersonal relationships have been more clearly defined, including aspects that pertain to all ED and those that are specific to AN. Primary strengths in detail and vulnerabilities in social and emotional processing may increase the potency of social pressures during adolescence a critical stages of development. These in combination with reduced set shifting allow the illness to take a hold. The secondary consequences of the illness (intra and interpersonal) accentuate these difficulties and cause the illness to persist. There are three sub formulations within the model which can be used to guide treatment. Involving close others, irrespective of individual's age, is helpful as social and interpersonal reactions are central to the model. New treatments specifically targeted to aspects of the model may improve outcomes.

Competing interests
The authors declare that they have no competing interests.

Authors' contribution
Both authors have contributed to the manuscript and have read and approved the final draft.

References

1. Fisher CA, Hetrick SE, Rushford N: **Family therapy for anorexia nervosa.** *Cochrane Database Syst Rev* 2010(4):CD004780. Epub 2010/04/16.
2. Lock J, Le Grange D, Agras WS, Moye A, Bryson SW, Jo B: **Randomized clinical trial comparing family-based treatment with adolescent-focused individual therapy for adolescents with anorexia nervosa.** *Arch Gen Psychiatry* 2010, **67**(10):1025–1032. Epub 2010/10/06.
3. Stiles-Shields C, Hoste RR, Doyle PM, Le Grange D: **A review of family-based treatment for adolescents with eating disorders.** *RRCT* 2012, **7**(2):133–140. Epub 2012/02/23.
4. Treasure J, Russell G: **The case for early intervention in anorexia nervosa: theoretical exploration of maintaining factors.** *Br. J. Psychiatry: J Ment Sci.* 2011, **199**(1):5–7. Epub 2011/07/02.
5. Crane AM, Roberts ME, Treasure J: **Are obsessive-compulsive personality traits associated with a poor outcome in anorexia nervosa? A systematic review of randomized controlled trials and naturalistic outcome studies.** *Int J Eat Disorder* 2007, **40**(7):581–588. Epub 2007/07/04.
6. Anckarsater H, Hofvander B, Billstedt E, Gillberg IC, Gillberg C, Wentz E, *et al*: **The sociocommunicative deficit subgroup in anorexia nervosa: autism spectrum disorders and neurocognition in a community-based, longitudinal study.** *Psychol Med* 2012, **42**(9):1957–1967. Epub 2011/12/22.
7. Craig P, Dieppe P, Macintyre S, Michie S, Nazareth I, Petticrew M: **Developing and evaluating complex interventions: the new Medical Research Council guidance.** *BMJ* 2008, **337**:a1655. Epub 2008/10/01.
8. Anderluh MB, Tchanturia K, Rabe-Hesketh S, Treasure J: **Childhood obsessive-compulsive personality traits in adult women with eating disorders: defining a broader eating disorder phenotype.** *Am. J. Psych* 2003, **160**(2):242–247. Epub 2003/02/04.
9. Jacobi C, Hayward C, De Zwaan M, Kraemer HC, Agras W: **Coming to Terms With Risk Factors for Eating Disorders: Application of Risk Terminology and Suggestions for a General Taxonomy.** *Psychol Bull* 2004, **130**(1):19–65.
10. Roberts ME, Tchanturia K, Treasure JL: **Exploring the neurocognitive signature of poor set-shifting in anorexia and bulimia nervosa.** *J Psychiatr Res* 2010, **44**(14):964–970.
11. Roberts ME, Tchanturia K, Treasure JL: **Is attention to detail a similarly strong candidate endophenotype for anorexia nervosa and bulimia nervosa?** *World J Biol Psychiat: J World Federation Soc Bio Psyc* 2012. Epub 2012/01/24.
12. Kanakam N, Treasure J: **A review of cognitive neuropsychiatry in the taxonomy of eating disorders: State, trait, or genetic?** *Cogn Neuropsychiatry* 2012. Epub 2012/09/22.
13. Alexander-Bloch A, Lambiotte R, Roberts B, Giedd J, Gogtay N, Bullmore E: **The discovery of population differences in network community structure: new methods and applications to brain functional networks in schizophrenia.** *Neuroimage* 2012, **59**(4):3889–900. Epub 2011/11/29.
14. Tchanturia K, Davies H, Roberts M, Harrison A, Nakazato M, Schmidt U, *et al*: **Poor cognitive flexibility in eating disorders: examining the evidence using the Wisconsin Card Sorting Task.** *PLoS One* 2012, **7**(1):e28331. Epub 2012/01/19.
15. Tenconi E, Santonastaso P, Degortes D, Bosello R, Titton F, Mapelli D, *et al*: **Set-shifting abilities, central coherence, and handedness in anorexia nervosa patients, their unaffected siblings and healthy controls: exploring putative endophenotypes.** *J World Federation Soc Bio Psyc* 2010, **11**(6):813–23. Epub 2010/05/22.
16. McAnarney ER, Zarcone J, Singh P, Michels J, Welsh S, Litteer T, *et al*: **Restrictive anorexia nervosa and set-shifting in adolescents: a biobehavioral interface.** *J Adolescent Health: Pub Soc Adolescent Med* 2011, **49**(1). Epub 2011/06/28.
17. Buhren K, Mainz V, Herpertz-Dahlmann B, Schafer K, Kahraman-Lanzerath B, Lente C, *et al*: **Cognitive flexibility in juvenile anorexia nervosa patients before and after weight recovery.** *J Neural Transm* 2012. Epub 2012/05/31.
18. Stedal K, Rose M, Frampton I, Landro NI, Lask B: **The neuropsychological profile of children, adolescents, and young adults with anorexia nervosa.** *Arch Clin Neuropsych: J Nat Acad Neuropsych* 2012, **27**(3):329–37. Epub 2012/03/15.
19. Shott ME, Filoteo JV, Bhatnagar KA, Peak NJ, Hagman JO, Rockwell R, *et al*: **Cognitive Set-Shifting in Anorexia Nervosa.** *Eur Eat Disord Rev: J Eating Disorders Assoc* 2012. Epub 2012/04/12.
20. Holliday J, Tchanturia K, Landau S, Collier D, Treasure J: **Is impaired set-shifting an endophenotype of anorexia nervosa?** *Am J Psychiatry* 2005, **162**:2269–2275.
21. Kothari R, Solmi F, Treasure J, Micali N: **The neuropsychological profile of children at high risk of developing an eating disorder.** *Psychol Med* 2012:1–12. Epub 2012/10/02.
22. Zastrow A, Kaiser S, Stippich C, Walther S, Herzog W, Tchanturia K, *et al*: **Neural correlates of impaired cognitive-behavioral flexibility in anorexia nervosa.** *Am. J. Psych* 2009, **166**(5):608–16. Epub 2009/02/19.
23. Marsh R, Steinglass JE, Gerber AJ, Graziano O'Leary K, Wang Z, Murphy D, *et al*: **Deficient activity in the neural systems that mediate self-regulatory control in bulimia nervosa.** *Arch Gen Psychiatr* 2009, **66**(1):51–63. Epub 2009/01/07.
24. Chase EA, Tait DS, Brown VJ: **Lesions of the orbital prefrontal cortex impair the formation of attentional set in rats.** *Eur J Neurosci* 2012, **36**(3):2368–75. Epub 2012/06/08.
25. Stoet G, Snyder LH: **Neural correlates of executive control functions in the monkey.** *Trends Cogn Sci* 2009, **13**(5):228–34. Epub 2009/04/14.
26. Meyza KZ, Defensor EB, Jensen AL, Corley MJ, Pearson BL, Pobbe RL, *et al*: **The BTBR T(+)tf/J mouse model for autism spectrum disorders-in search of biomarkers.** *Behav Brain Res* 2012. Epub 2012/09/11.
27. Amodeo DA, Jones JH, Sweeney JA, Ragozzino ME: **Differences in BTBR T + tf/J and C57BL/6J mice on probabilistic reversal learning and stereotyped behaviors.** *Behav Brain Res* 2012, **227**(1):64–72. Epub 2011/11/08.
28. Lopez C, Tchanturia K, Stahl D, Booth R, Holliday J, Treasure J: **An examination of the concept of central coherence in women with anorexia nervosa.** *Int J Eating Disorders* 2008, **41**(2):143–52. Epub 2007/10/17.
29. Harrison A, Tchanturia K, Naumann U, Treasure J: **Social emotional functioning and cognitive styles in eating disorders.** *Br J Clin Psychol* 2012, **51**(3):261–79. Epub 2012/07/19.
30. Lopez C, Tchanturia K, Stahl D, Treasure J: **Weak central coherence in eating disorders: a step towards looking for an endophenotype of eating disorders.** *J Clin Exp Neuropsyc* 2009, **31**(1):117–25. Epub 2008/07/09.
31. Kanakam N, Raoult C, Collier D, Treasure J: **Set shifting and central coherence as neurocognitive endophenotypes in eating disorders: A preliminary investigation in twins.** *World J Biol Psychia: J World Federation Soc Bio Psych* 2012. Epub 2012/05/29.
32. Karwautz A, Wagner G, Waldherr K, Nader I, Fernandez-Aranda F, Estivill X, *et al*: **Gene-environment interaction in anorexia nervosa: Relevance of non-shared environment and the serotonin transporter gene.** *Mol Psych* 2011, **16**(6):590–2.
33. Fairburn CG, Cooper Z, Doll HA, Welch SL: **Risk factors for anorexia nervosa: three integrated case-control comparisons.** *Arc Gen Psych* 1999, **56**(5):468–76. Epub 1999/05/08.
34. McKnight R, Boughton N: **A patient's journey. Anorexia nervosa.** *BMJ* 2009, **339**:b3800. Epub 2009/09/26.
35. Karwautz A, Rabe-Hesketh S, Hu X, Zhao J, Sham P, Collier DA, *et al*: **Individual-specific risk factors for anorexia nervosa: a pilot study using a discordant sister-pair design.** *Psych Med* 2001, **31**(2):317–29. Epub 2001/03/10.

36. Krug I, Penelo E, Fernandez-Aranda F, Anderluh M, Bellodi L, Cellini E, *et al*: **Low social interactions in eating disorder patients in childhood and adulthood: A multi-centre European case control study.** *J Health Psych* 2012, **2012**:2012. Epub 2012/04/12.
37. Kim Y-R, Heo SY, Kang H: **Song Kj, Treasure J. Childhood risk factors in Korean women with anorexia nervosa: Two sets of case–control studies with retrospective comparisons.** *Int J Eating Disorders.* 2010, **43**(7):589–95.
38. Adambegan M, Wagner G, Nader IW, Fernandez-Aranda F, Treasure J, Karwautz A: **Internalizing and externalizing behaviour problems in childhood contribute to the development of anorexia and bulimia nervosa-a study comparing sister pairs.** *Eu Eating Disorders Rev: J Eating Disorders Assoc* 2012, **20**(2):116–20. Epub 2011/08/10.
39. Swinbourne J, Hunt C, Abbott M, Russell J, St Clare T, Touyz S: **The comorbidity between eating disorders and anxiety disorders: prevalence in an eating disorder sample and anxiety disorder sample.** *Aust Nz J Psychia* 2012, **46**(2):118–31. Epub 2012/02/09.
40. Wentz E, Gillberg IC, Anckarsater H, Gillberg C, Rastam M: **Adolescent-onset anorexia nervosa: 18-year outcome.** *Br. J. Psychiatry: J Men Sci* 2009, **194**(2):168–74. Epub 2009/02/03.
41. Menzel JE, Schaefer LM, Burke NL, Mayhew LL, Brannick MT, Thompson JK: **Appearance-related teasing, body dissatisfaction, and disordered eating: A meta-analysis.** *Body Image* 2010, **7**(4):261–70. Epub 2010/07/27.
42. Adenzato M, Todisco P, Ardito RB: **Social cognition in anorexia nervosa: evidence of preserved theory of mind and impaired emotional functioning.** *PLoS One* 2012, **7**(8):e44414. Epub 2012/09/07.
43. Tiller JM, Sloane G, Schmidt U, Troop N, Power M, Treasure JL: **Social support in patients with anorexia nervosa and bulimia nervosa.** *Int J Eating disorders* 1997, **21**(1):31–8. Epub 1997/01/01.
44. Oldershaw A, Dejong H, Hambrook D, Broadbent H, Tchanturia K, Treasure J, *et al*: **Emotional Processing Following Recovery from Anorexia Nervosa.** *Eu Eating Disorders Rev: J Eating Disorders Assoc* 2012. Epub 2012/01/14.
45. Zucker NL, Losh M, Bulik CM, LaBar KS, Piven J, Pelphrey KA: **Anorexia nervosa and autism spectrum disorders: guided investigation of social cognitive endophenotypes.** *Psychol Bull* 2007, **133**(6):976–1006. Epub 2007/10/31.
46. Cserjesi R, Vermeulen N, Lenard L, Luminet O: **Reduced capacity in automatic processing of facial expression in restrictive anorexia nervosa and obesity.** *Psychia Res* 2011, **188**(2):253–7. Epub 2011/01/07.
47. Harrison A, Sullivan S, Tchanturia K, Treasure J: **Attentional bias, emotion recognition and emotion regulation in anorexia: state or trait?** *Bio Psychia* 2010, **68**(8):755–61.
48. Harrison A, Sullivan S, Tchanturia K, Treasure J: **Emotional functioning in eating disorders: attentional bias, emotion recognition and emotion regulation.** *Psychol Med* 2010, **40**(11):1887–97. Epub 2010/01/28.
49. Cardi V, Matteo RD, Corfield F, Treasure J: **Social reward and rejection sensitivity in eating disorders: An investigation of attentional bias and early experiences.** *World J Biol Psychia: J World Federation Soc Bio Psychia* 2012. Epub 2012/03/20.
50. Watson KK, Werling DM, Zucker NL, Platt ML: **Altered social reward and attention in anorexia nervosa.** *Front Psychol* 2010, **1**:36. Epub 2010/01/01.
51. Oldershaw A, Hambrook D, Stahl D, Tchanturia K, Treasure J, Schmidt U: **The socio-emotional processing stream in Anorexia Nervosa.** *Neurosci Biobehav Rev* 2011, **35**(3):970–88. Epub 2010/11/13.
52. Dejong H, Van den Eynde F, Broadbent H, Kenyon MD, Lavender A, Startup H, *et al*: **Social cognition in bulimia nervosa: A systematic review.** *Eu Psychia: J Assoc Eu Psychia* 2011. Epub 2011/09/17.
53. Kenyon M, Samarawickrema N, Dejong H, Van den Eynde F, Startup H, Lavender A, *et al*: **Theory of mind in bulimia nervosa.** *Int J Eating Disorders.* 2012, **45**(3):377–84. Epub 2012/01/04.
54. Oldershaw A, Hambrook D, Tchanturia K, Treasure J, Schmidt U: **Emotional theory of mind and emotional awareness in recovered anorexia nervosa patients.** *Psychosom Med* 2010, **72**(1):73–9. Epub 2009/12/10.
55. Kucharska-Pietura K, Nikolaou V, Masiak M, Treasure J: **The recognition of emotion in the faces and voice of anorexia nervosa.** *Int J Eating Disorders.* 2004, **35**(1):42–7. Epub 2004/01/06.
56. Zucker N, Moskovich A, Bulik CM, Merwin R, Gaddis K, Losh M, *et al*: **Perception of affect in biological motion cues in anorexia nervosa.** *Int J Eating Disorders.* 2012. Epub 2012/10/31.
57. Davies H, Schmidt U, Stahl D, Tchanturia K: **Evoked facial emotional expression and emotional experience in people with anorexia nervosa.** *Int J Eating Disorders.* 2011, **44**(6):531–9. Epub 2010/10/20.
58. Claes L, Jimenez-Murcia S, Santamaria JJ, Moussa MB, Sanchez I, Forcano L, *et al*: **The facial and subjective emotional reaction in response to a video game designed to train emotional regulation (playmancer).** *Eu Eating Disorders Rev: J Eating Disorders Assoc* 2012, **20**(6):484–9. Epub 2012/10/26.
59. Russell TA, Schmidt U, Doherty L, Young V, Tchanturia K: **Aspects of social cognition in anorexia nervosa: affective and cognitive theory of mind.** *Psychiatry Res* 2009, **168**(3):181–5. Epub 2009/05/27.
60. Gillberg IC, Billstedt E, Wentz E, Anckarsater H, Rastam M, Gillberg C: **Attention, executive functions, and mentalizing in anorexia nervosa eighteen years after onset of eating disorder.** *J Clin Exp Neuropsychol* 2010, **32**(4):358–65. Epub 2009/10/27.
61. Rozenstein MH, Latzer Y, Stein D, Eviatar Z: **Perception of emotion and bilateral advantage in women with eating disorders, their healthy sisters, and nonrelated healthy controls.** *J Affect Disorder* 2011, **134**(1–3):386–95. Epub 2011/07/16.
62. Eshkevari E, Rieger E, Longo MR, Haggard P, Treasure J: **Increased plasticity of the bodily self in eating disorders.** *Psych Med* 2012, **42**(4):819–28. Epub 2011/10/25.
63. Hatch A, Madden S, Kohn MR, Clarke S, Touyz S, Gordon E, *et al*: **EEG in adolescent anorexia nervosa: impact of refeeding and weight gain.** *Int J Eating Disorders* 2011, **44**(1):65–75. Epub 2010/01/12.
64. McAdams CJ, Krawczyk DC: **Impaired neural processing of social attribution in anorexia nervosa.** *Psychia Res* 2011, **194**(1):54–63. Epub 2011/08/30.
65. Cowdrey FA, Harmer CJ, Park RJ, McCabe C: **Neural responses to emotional faces in women recovered from anorexia nervosa.** *Psychia Res* 2012, **201**(3):190–5. Epub 2012/04/03.
66. Powell J, Lewis PA, Roberts N, Garcia-Finana M, Dunbar RI: **Orbital prefrontal cortex volume predicts social network size: an imaging study of individual differences in humans.** *Proc Bio Sci/Royal Soc* 2012, **279**(1736): 2157–62. Epub 2012/02/03.
67. Dunbar R: **Psychology. Evolution of the social brain.** *Science* 2003, **302**(5648):1160–1. Epub 2003/11/15.
68. Freeberg TM, Dunbar RI, Ord TJ: **Social complexity as a proximate and ultimate factor in communicative complexity.** *Philos Trans R Soc Lond B Biol Sci London Series B, Biol Sci* 2012, **367**(1597):1785–801. Epub 2012/05/30.
69. Lawson EA, Donoho DA, Blum JI, Meenaghan EM, Misra M, Herzog DB, *et al*: **Decreased nocturnal oxytocin levels in anorexia nervosa are associated with low bone mineral density and fat mass.** *J Clin Psychia* 2011, **72**(11):1546–51. Epub 2011/09/10.
70. Demitrack MA, Lesem MD, Listwak SJ, Brandt HA, Jimerson DC, Gold PW: **CSF oxytocin in anorexia nervosa and bulimia nervosa: clinical and pathophysiologic considerations.** *Am J Psychia* 1990, **147**(7):882–6. Epub 1990/07/01.
71. Lawson EA, Holsen LM, Santin M, Meenaghan E, Eddy KT, Becker AE, *et al*: **Oxytocin secretion is associated with severity of disordered eating psychopathology and insular cortex hypoactivation in anorexia nervosa.** *J Clin Endocrinol Metab* 2012, **97**(10):E1898–908. Epub 2012/08/09.
72. Sternheim L, Startup H, Pretorius N, Johnson-Sabine E, Schmidt U, Channon S: **An experimental exploration of social problem solving and its associated processes in anorexia nervosa.** *Psychia Res* 2012, **200**(2–3):524–9. Epub 2012/07/20.
73. Zabala MJ, Macdonald P, Treasure J: **Appraisal of caregiving burden, expressed emotion and psychological distress in families of people with eating disorders: a systematic review.** *Eu Eating Disorders Rev: J Eating Disorders Assoc* 2009, **17**(5):338–49. Epub 2009/04/16.
74. Treasure J, Sepulveda AR, MacDonald P, Whitaker W, Lopez C, Zabala M, *et al*: **The assessment of the family of people with eating disorders.** *Eu Eating Disorders Rev: J Eating Disorders Assoc* 2008, **16**(4):247–55. Epub 2008/02/02.
75. Sepulveda AR, Kyriacou O, Treasure J: **Development and validation of the accommodation and enabling scale for eating disorders (AESED) for caregivers in eating disorders.** *BMC Health Services Res* 2009, **9**:171. Epub 2009/09/25.
76. Grover M, Naumann U, Mohammad-Dar L, Glennon D, Ringwood S, Eisler I, *et al*: **A randomized controlled trial of an Internet-based cognitive-behavioural skills package for carers of people with anorexia nervosa.** *Psych Med* 2011:1–11. Epub 2011/07/08.
77. Grover M, Williams C, Eisler I, Fairbairn P, McCloskey C, Smith G, *et al*: **An off-line pilot evaluation of a web-based systemic cognitive-behavioral**

intervention for carers of people with anorexia nervosa. *Int J Eating Disorders* 2011, **44**(8):708–15. Epub 2011/11/11.
78. Goddard E, Macdonald P, Sepulveda AR, Naumann U, Landau S, Schmidt U, *et al*: Cognitive interpersonal maintenance model of eating disorders: intervention for carers. *Brit J Psychia: J Men Sci* 2011, **199**(3):225–31. Epub 2011/07/06.
79. Raenker S, Hibbs R, Goddard E, Naumann U, Arcelus J, Ayton A, *et al*: Caregiving and coping in carers of people with anorexia nervosa admitted for intensive hospital care. *Int J Eating Disorders* 2012. Epub 2012/10/31.
80. Wade TD, Treasure J, Schmidt U: A case series evaluation of the Maudsley Model for treatment of adults with anorexia nervosa. *Eu Eating Disorders Rev: J Eating Disorders Assoc* 2011. Epub 2011/02/01.
81. Schmidt U, Oldershaw A, Jichi F, Sternheim L, Startup H, McIntosh V, *et al*: Out-patient psychological therapies for adults with anorexia nervosa: randomised controlled trial. *Brit J Psychiat: J Men Sci* 2012, **201**:392–9. Epub 2012/09/22.
82. MacLeod C, Mathews A: Cognitive bias modification approaches to anxiety. *Annu Rev Clin Psycho* 2012, **8**:189–217. Epub 2011/11/01.
83. Beard C, Sawyer AT, Hofmann SG: Efficacy of attention bias modification using threat and appetitive stimuli: a meta-analytic review. *Behav Ther* 2012, **43**(4):724–40. Epub 2012/10/11.
84. Meyer-Lindenberg A, Domes G, Kirsch P, Heinrichs M: Oxytocin and vasopressin in the human brain: social neuropeptides for translational medicine. *Nat Rev Neurosci* 2011, **12**(9):524–38. Epub 2011/08/20.
85. Van den Eynde F, Guillaume S, Broadbent H, Campbell IC, Schmidt U: Repetitive transcranial magnetic stimulation in anorexia nervosa: A pilot study. *Eu Psychiat: J Assoc Eu Psychiat* 2011. Epub 2011/09/02.

A systematic review of cognitive remediation therapy for anorexia nervosa – development, current state and implications for future research and clinical practice

Camilla Lindvall Dahlgren[1,2*] and Øyvind Rø[1,3]

Abstract

Objective: To systematically review studies of cognitive remediation therapy (CRT) for anorexia nervosa (AN), and to discuss findings with references to clinical practice and future research.

Method: The literature was reviewed using the PubMed, Web of Science and PsycINFO search terms "cognitive remediation therapy" AND "anorexia nervosa". Papers published online between 2005 and 2013 were selected on the basis of three inclusion criteria: 1) studies of any design focusing on CRT for AN, 2) papers that were written in English or had an available published English translation, and 3) papers published in peer reviewed journals.

Results: A total of 45 papers were identified of which 21 were recognized as being relevant for the review. Relevant papers were divided into three different categories 1) single case reports, 2) case series and 3) randomised controlled trials (RCTs). Single case studies and case series yielded strong evidence of feasibility and acceptability of CRT for AN despite great variety in sample compositions. Four RCTs demonstrate that CRT has the potential of enhancing the effectiveness of current treatments, reduce attrition, increase cognitive set-shifting abilities and quality of life, as well as reduce eating disorder psychopathology.

Discussion: The number of CRT studies published is growing rapidly, in particular RCTs. Further research is needed to define the primary aim of delivering CRT to patients with eating disorders, and to establish how to best measure the effect of the intervention. Moreover, researchers and clinicians should focus on identifying and assessing specific versus non-specific CRT contributions, and explore long-term effects of the intervention. It is imperative that adolescent RCTs are conducted to evaluate how CRT may be effective as a treatment for this young patient group.

Keywords: Cognitive remediation therapy, Anorexia nervosa, Review, Treatment, Neuropsychology, Eating disorders, Metacognition

Introduction

Anorexia nervosa (AN) is a multifaceted mental disorder characterized by pathological eating behaviours. It is a serious condition and in some cases, even life threatening [1] with significant psychiatric and physical co-morbidity, and poor quality of life [2,3]. Symptoms of the illness most commonly occur in early to late adolescence, and has a prevalence rate of 0.5-0.7% among adolescent females between 15 and 19 [4]. In the DSM-5 [5], AN is characterized by distorted body image and excessive dieting that leads to severe weight loss, with a pathological fear of becoming fat.

Although previous research in the field of eating disorders (EDs) has made important contributions to the understanding of AN, the evidence base for treatment efficacy in adult AN is scarce [6]. For younger patients, current research evidence suggests that a particular form

* Correspondence: camilla.lindvall@dahlgren.no
[1]Regional Department for Eating Disorders, Division of Mental Health and Addiction, Oslo University Hospital, Ullevål HF, Oslo, Norway
[2]Department of Psychiatry, Centre for Research on Eating Disorders at Oxford (CREDO), University of Oxford, Warneford Hospital, Oxford, UK
Full list of author information is available at the end of the article

of family based therapy, FBT [7], is the most efficient approach [8-10]. Despite numerous approaches currently being applied in the treatment of the disorder such as cognitive behavioural therapy (CBT), interpersonal therapy (IPT), cognitive analytic therapy (CAT), family based therapy (FBT) (for children and adolescents), nutritional counselling etc., existing randomised controlled trials (RCTs) are limited [11]. Also, those existing appear inconclusive as short vs. long-term investigations, sub group phenomena and current state of illness appear to influence treatment outcome, making it difficult to compare studies and predict long-term effects.

In recent years, there has been a substantial increase in papers investigating the impact of neuropsychology on eating disorder (ED) aetiology-, maintenance-, and recovery. Clinical neuropsychology is concerned with the applied science of brain-behaviour relationships, and in AN, the focus has been primarily to establish the extent to which weaknesses in cognitive flexibility (i.e. the inability to shift or change mental and behavioural strategies) and central coherence (i.e. the preoccupation with details at the cost of global/contextual processing) contribute to the development of the illness, its perseverance and the likelihood of recovery [12-16]. Early neuropsychological studies and clinical observations of adults with AN laid the groundwork for the development of cognitive remediation therapy (CRT), an intervention specifically tailored to remedy weaknesses in these two domains (i.e. cognitive flexibility and central coherence), and designed to encourage patients to reflect on their thinking styles. The CRT technique was originally conceptualized and developed from patients suffering from brain lesions [17], but over the last 50 years, the method and its application has been gradually adapted to suit individuals suffering from other health conditions as well. In psychiatry, CRT has been most commonly associated with the investigation of cognitive dysfunction in patients with schizophrenia, and dating back to the early 1990's, there is an extensive body of work describing positive outcomes of CRT for this patient group [18,19]. The approach has also been successful in treating other mental health conditions such as mood disorders [20] attention deficit hyperactivity disorder (ADHD) [21], alcohol dependence [22], geriatric depression [23] and obsessive compulsive disorder (OCD) [24].

CRT for AN is a relatively new treatment approach. For this patient group, the intervention has been delivered as an addition to treatment as usual, and focuses on the process of thinking (i.e. the how) rather than the content (i.e. the what). In contrast to traditional interventions that centre on increasing food intake and on addressing ED specific symptoms such as weight and shape concerns, CRT aims neither to address nor directly treat these. The focus is primarily to decrease rigidity (i.e. increase flexibility) and achieve a balance between local (detailed) and global (the bigger picture) information processing strategies.

The very first paper on CRT for AN was published in 2005 [25], and reports results from a single case study illustrating the use of CRT for an adult female inpatient refusing to participate in the core treatment approaches offered. The materials used were hand-picked from the set-shifting module in Delahunty & Morice's *"A training programme for the remediation of cognitive deficits in schizophrenia"* [26], and gradually thereafter, novel materials were developed and assembled in CRT manuals specifically tailored to remediate cognitive weaknesses in females with AN (e.g. [27]). Research on CRT for AN is evolving rapidly, and is currently transforming from feasibility and piloting trials into the realm of what is considered to be the gold standard when it comes to testing the effect of a specific treatment approach; RCTs. Alongside study design transformations, the aim of delivering CRT and contributions thought to be associated with the intervention also appear to have changed. CRT was initially hypothesized to improve thinking skills beneficial for every day living, and to prepare patients for therapeutic interventions focusing on thought, belief and emotion. However, during the course of its development and adaptation, exploration of potential intervention outcomes have expanded considerably, and now also include ED psychopathology, comorbidity, perfectionism, treatment attrition and comparisons to other neurocognitive interventions. As knowledge of the applicability of CRT for AN has accumulated during almost a decade, research and clinical work has now guided a small number of RCTs, and for the first time, researchers have been able to demonstrate the effect of the treatment.

Three papers have sought to describe the current evidence of CRT for AN, and its future directions [28-30]. The first of these was published seven years ago [28] (merely two years after the first CRT for AN paper) and lacks a current update of the field. The second paper [29] describes how CRT for AN has been developed and refined, and suggests future research directions, but lacks a systematic overview of studies published in this field. The most recent summary paper published in 2013 [30] also aims to provide the reader with current evidence and future research directions, in addition to presenting an overview of published studies reporting CRT for AN. However, merely nine studies are included in this overview, leaving out a total of 12 studies published in this field, four of which are recently published effect studies (i.e. RCTs). As the intervention itself, as well as the assessment of its efficacy has gone through major recent developments, the current paper aims to contribute to the field further by presenting a systematic overview of *all* studies of CRT for AN. Doing so, the authors wish to add to the field by delineating the interventions developmental trajectory in both adults and adolescents, its current state, and it's potency in future treatment of AN.

Review

The literature was reviewed using the PubMed, Web of Knowledge and PsycINFO search terms "cognitive remediation therapy" AND "anorexia nervosa". The PubMed search yielded 27 publications, Web of Science 23 publications and PsycINFO 25 publications, all published online between August 2005 and November 2013. Together, the three searches yielded 75 publications, which were cross-referenced. After duplicates had been omitted, 45 unique publications were identified. Publication titles and abstracts were screened initially, and eligibility was established by reading the full texts. A manual reference search was conducted (i.e. references lists in papers from the initial database search were examined) to explore additional papers of relevance. One additional paper was identified during this search [29]. On the basis of the inclusion criteria outlined below, 21 papers were identified as being relevant, and selected for review.

Inclusion criteria

1) Studies of any design focusing on cognitive remediation therapy and AN.
2) Articles that are written in English or has an available published English translation.
3) Articles that are published in peer reviewed journals.

Results

Excluded studies

All in all, 24 publications were excluded from the review. Two CRT studies were excluded as they were written in Polish [31] and French [32], and one additional CRT publication was omitted as it had been published as a meeting abstract rather than in an article format [33]. Nine studies were excluded as these did not focus specifically on CRT for AN [34-42], and six publications were excluded as these represented either books or book chapters [43-48] rather than peer reviewed papers. Three studies evaluating the combination of cognitive remediation therapy and emotional skills training (CREST) [49-51] were excluded from the review as the design of these studies did not allow for assessment of CRT specific contributions. Finally, three theoretical CRT papers lacking clinical data were omitted [28-30]. The search strategy used to identify and screen studies for review is presented in the PRISMA flow diagram (Figure 1).

Overview of included studies

The 21 reviewed studies were published online between August 2005 and November 2013, with sample sizes ranging from 1 to 46 participants, and ages ranging from 12–62. Eleven studies explore CRT in adult samples (ages 18–45), six studies explore CRT in adolescents (ages 12–19), and the remaining four studies samples mix adolescent and adult patients (ages 14–62). With the exception of seven male participants, all patients included in the studies (receiving CRT) were female (N = 355), and the vast majority of participants were diagnosed with AN. One study had included patients with a current diagnosis of AN plus recently recovered AN patients (N = non specified) [52], and another study had included both current AN (N = 17) patients as well as participants with an eating disorder not otherwise specified (EDNOS) diagnosis (N = 7) [53]. Three of the 21 publications were based on the same sample [54-56]. The authors are not aware of additional sample overlaps. One of the most recent studies explores transdiagnostic CRT without specifying ED diagnosis [57]. Out of the 21 studies reviewed, four reported results from RCTs, all which were published online in 2013 [57-60]. Participants in the included studies were currently enrolled in either in- or outpatient treatment for their ED, and all received CRT as a conjunctive intervention. Included studies varied widely, for example according to whether CRT was delivered individually, in groups or families, the number of sessions offered, the intensity of these and the materials used. Studies also varied according to the aim of the study and consequently, what outcome measures were applied. Three different types of CRT publications were identified:

1) Single case studies (n = 3).
2) Case series (n = 14).
3) RCTs (n = 4).

The main characteristics of the publications are presented in Table 1. Publications are stratified according to *publication type* and *chronological order*.

1) Single case studies

The three single case studies [25,61,62] represent the very beginning of the development of CRT for AN. All papers describe a single, adult female inpatient with longstanding AN, undergoing 10 sessions of individual CRT. The three papers illustrate how the CRT materials were adopted and adapted from the set-shifting module from Delahunty and Morice's work on patients with schizophrenia [26], and how this material became the corner stone in the development of the CRT materials that most clinicians and researchers use today. The earliest of the three papers [25] brings about the importance of bridging the gap between in-session task performance and its relevance to everyday undertakings, a crucial part of CRT, which has been adhered to in the majority of subsequent studies. In the most recent of these three single case studies [62], the concept of behavioural tasks (in subsequent studies often referred to as *homework*) is

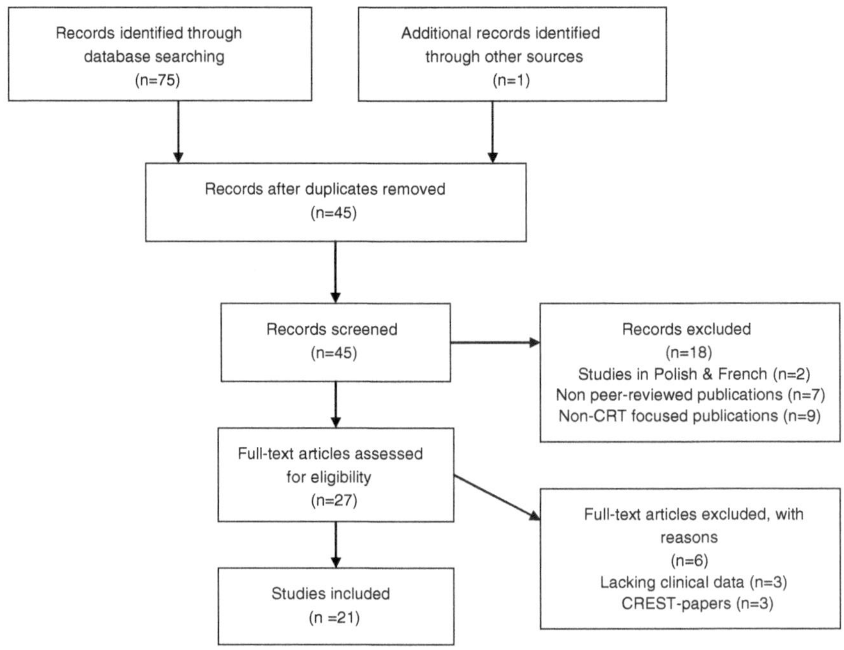

Figure 1 Search strategy used to identify and screen studies for review.

introduced as a part of the therapeutic work with the patient, aiming to facilitate the implementation of newly learned strategies to everyday life situations. This study is descriptive in it's nature, and focuses on patients' experiences with CRT. It delineates the potential of CRT in increasing the effectiveness of other interventions, and with regards to the development of a heightened awareness of the patients' thinking style. The two former papers [25,62] set out to investigate changes in neuropsychological functioning and clinical variables during the course of the intervention, and were identical in terms of outcome measures used. Results were inconclusive in that some performance measures had improved in one study, whereas they had not on the other study, and contrary, some measures did not improve in the first study, but did so in the latter.

2) Case series

Three different types of case series were identified: feasibility studies, studies focusing on pre and post CRT assessments, and studies that overlapped with regard to these two categories.

1. Feasibility studies

Six feasibility studies [55,63-67] were identified amongst the 21 papers. All studies investigated CRT for patients with AN, but the diversity of sample compositions e.g. sample size, age, in- and/or outpatients), intervention approaches (e.g. individual-, family- or group therapy, treatment intensity, intervention materials) and outcome measures (qualitative or quantitative, types of assessment instruments) rendered it difficult to compare studies and to generalize findings. Three papers reported results from patient feedback letters [65-67] with the two latter supporting the feasibility of CRT delivered in a group format, and the former when delivered individually. These three studies investigated feasibility for patients ranging widely in ages (13–54), strengthening the applicability of CRT across ages, and support the feasibility of the intervention at various stages of illness and developmental trajectories. The Wood et al. study [66] is the first to explore CRT for adolescents with AN, and it is also the first paper to present a detailed outline of the specific task(s) used each session. Results yielded evidence of feasibility and patient satisfaction, but also feedback on some of the drawbacks of delivering CRT in a group format (e.g. lack of relevance and unfavourable group dynamics). In 2013, the second paper exploring CRT for adolescents with AN was published. This time, the format of delivery had changed, and the 20 patients in the Dahlgren et al. study [55] received individually delivered CRT, tailored to meet each patient's specific needs. This was the first study to use materials developed specifically for children and adolescents [68]. The study published by Easter and Tchanturia [63] illustrates a novel approach to feasibility in its application of *therapists'* feedback letters to examine how CRT has been implemented in the daily life of the patients. It is pioneering

Table 1 Characteristics of included studies

SINGLE CASE STUDIES

Year author	Aim of study	N	Diagnosis	Age	Setting	Mode of delivery	No. of sessions	Intensity	Results
2005 Davies & Tchanturia	To illustrate how CRT can be used to stimulate mental activities and improve thinking skills.	1	AN	21	Inpatients	Individual	10	Two 3 weekly sessions + 2 twice weekly	Improvement in cognitive set-shifting.
2006 Tchanturia et al.	To demonstrate the potential benefits of CRT through a case-report.	1	AN	42	Inpatients	Individual	10	Once or twice weekly	The authors propose cognitive flexibility training as a pre-treatment intervention for treatment resistant inpatient cases.
2007 Pretorius & Tchanturia	To demonstrate how CRT has been adapted for AN through a case-report.	1	AN	31	Inpatients	Individual	10	Twice weekly	Increase in BMI, tasks were a bit repetitive but the patient was able to develop new flexible strategies for implementation in real-life settings.

CASE SERIES

Year author	Aim of study	N	Diagnosis	Age range (Mean)	Setting	Mode of delivery	No. of sessions	Intensity	Results
2007 Tchanturia et al.	Explore the effect of CRT in set-shifting and investigates in acceptability for AN patients.	4	AN	21-42	Inpatients	Individual	10	Not reported	Improved cognitive flexibility and positive feedback for CRT.
2008 Whitney et al.	To examine patients' experience of participating in CRT.	21	AN	17-54 (30.3)	Inpatients	Individual	10	Once or twice weekly	Positive that the intervention did not focus on food, helpful in reducing perfectionism and rigidity. More difficulty in tasks wanted, and help to implement newly learned skills.
2008 Tchanturia et al.	To explore neuropsychological task performance before and after CRT.	27	AN	(28.8)	Inpatients	Individual	10	Twice weekly	Improvements in cognitive performance on the Brixton & CatBat tasks. No sign improvements in other neuropsychological tasks. Significant decrease in depression.
2010 Genders & Tchanturia	To report CRT development and acceptability in a group format (2 male participants).	30	AN	14-62	Inpatients + Outpatients	Group	4	Once weekly	Statistically significant gains in self-reports of ability to change. CRT was found to be acceptable, useful and positive by both patient and group facilitators.
2010 Pitt et al.	To evaluate the benefit of CRT in terms of changes in self-reported perfectionism and patient feedback.	7	AN + Recovered AN	(29.5)	Outpatients	Individual	10	Once or twice weekly	Initially confusing but mentally stimulating. Increased awareness of ones own thinking style. Both higher and lower degrees of perfectionism post CRT.
2011 Wood et al.	To describe group CRT for adolescents.	9	AN	13-19	Inpatients	Group	10	Once and twice weekly	Patients found CRT fun and playful, helped develop a positive therapeutic relationship. Negative feedback involved tasks being boring, too easy tasks, repetitive, some negative group dynamics affected the group work.
2011 Easter & Tchanturia	To examine how CRT has been implemented in the daily life of the patients through therapist feedback letters.	26	AN	Adults	Inpatients	Not reported	10	Twice weekly	Feedback letters were positive and motivational, and highlighted challenges in metacognitive ability and in transferring in therapy skills to every day life for the patients.
2012 Abbate-Daga et al.	To measure the effect of CRT on cognitive flexibility.	20	AN	(22.5)	Outpatients	Individual	10	Once weekly	Improved neuropsychological performance. Significant improvement on impulse regulation, interoceptive awareness reflexive skills and awareness.

Table 1 Characteristics of included studies *(Continued)*

2012 Pretorius et al.	Evaluation of group CRT for adolescents with AN through self-reported flexibility and motivation.	30	AN + EDNOS	12-17 (15.6)	Outpatients	Group	4	Once weekly	No significant changes in flexibility and motivation to get better. Patient feedback: "interesting", "fun", "not too demanding", "helpful", but also "dull" and "repetitive". Patients wanted more variation in exercises.
2013 Zuchova et al.	To explore the feasibility and acceptability of group CRT for inpatients with AN.	34	AN	18-45	Inpatients	Group	10	Once a week	Group-based CRT could be well incorporated into the therapeutic program at the eating disorders unit, and was well received by the participants.
2013 Dahlgren et al. (a)	To assess the feasibility of CRT for children and adolescents with AN.	20	AN	13-18 (15.9)	Inpatients + Outpatients	Individual	7-12	Once or twice weekly	Results indicate feasibility for young patients with AN with regards to recruitment, materials, individual tailoring and delivery, and clinician feasibility.
2013 Dahlgren et al. (b)	To assess neuropsychological functioning pre and post CRT.	20	AN	13-18 (15.9)	Inpatients + Outpatients	Individual	7-12	Once or twice weekly	Significant changes in weight, depression, visio-spatial memory, global information processing and verbal fluency. Changes in weight had a significant effect on improvements in visio-spatial memory and verbal fluency.
2013 Dahlgren et al. (c)	To explore self-reports and parental ratings of executive function before and after CRT.	17	AN	13-18 (15.9)	Inpatients + Outpatients	Individual	7-12	Once or twice weekly	Decrease in patient BRIEF shift subscale post CRT. Parent reports revealed significant lower scores on shift-, emotional control- and working memory subscales, and on two composite indices.
2013 Lask & Roberts	To assess feasibility of CRT in family settings.	4	AN	14-19	Inpatients + Outpatients	Family	01/06/14	Varying from weekly to monthly	CRT is useful when applied in families, and authors suggest a subsequent formal evaluation of this mode of delivery.

RANDOMISED CONTROLLED TRIALS

Year author	Aim of study	N	Diagnosis	Age range (Mean)	Setting	Mode of delivery	No. of sessions	Intensity	Results
2013 Lock et al.	To evaluate the feasibility of using CRT to reduce attrition in RCT's for AN.	23*/ 23	AN	(22.7s)	Outpatients	Individual	8	8 sessions during 2 months	CRT is acceptable and feasible for use in RCTs. It may also reduce short-term attrition.
2013 Brockmeyer et al.	To investigate feasibility and efficacy of specifically tailored CRT, compared to NNT.	11*/ 14	AN	(23.6*/26.7)	Inpatients + Outpatients	Computer assisted & Individual	30	30 sessions over 3 weeks	Participants receiving CRT outperformed participants in the NNT condition in cognitive set-shifting. Both groups showed high treatment acceptance.
2013 Steinglass et al.	To evaluate AN-EXRP as an adjunctive strategy to improve eating behaviour during weight restoration.	15*/ 15	AN	16-45	Inpatients	Individual & Group	12	3 times a week over 4 weeks	AN-EXRP is associated with better caloric intake than CRT when assessed through laboratory meals.
2013 Dingemans et al.	To investigate the effectiveness of CRT in a randomised controlled trial comparing treatment as usual (TAU) and TAU plus CRT.	41*/ 41	ED	17-53	Mainly inpatients	Individual	10	10 sessions over 6 weeks	CRT plus TAU was superior in terms of ED-related quality of life and ED psychopathology. CRT appears to be promising in enhancing effectiveness of concurrent treatment.

Note. Results are presented descriptively due large discrepancies between studies, and for some papers, due to the lack of quantitative data.
* = Interventions details (i.e. mode of delivery, session details, intensity and intervention materials) refer to the CRT arm only.
AN = Anorexia Nervosa; *AN-EXRP* = Exposure and Response prevention for AN; *BMI* = Body Max Index; *CRT* = Cognitive Remediation Therapy; *ED* = Eating Disorder; *EDNOS* = Eating Disorder Not Otherwise Specified; *NNT* = Non-specific Neurocognitive Training; *RCT* = Randomised Controlled Trial.

and unique in its attempt to establish a more ecologically valid interpretation of how CRT affects the daily life of the patients. No subsequent studies have used this type of methodology, although many report using feedback letters. The most recent feasibility study explores the use of CRT when used in family settings [64] and reports clinical and observational data to illustrate its use in this novel mode of delivery. Results supported the acceptability for both patients and their caregivers, and the intervention appeared to increase motivation to change in the patients.

2. Studies assessing pre and post CRT functioning

Four studies investigate pre and post CRT functioning without using control groups [54,69-71], and illustrate how the use of a wide variety of outcome measures have been applied to investigate changes across the intervention span. Such investigations include ED psychopathology, comorbidity, impulse regulation, executive functions (including cognitive flexibility and decision-making), central coherence, and overall functioning. Similar in the four studies is that the patients appear to have received approximately the same number of sessions (i.e. 10). However, comparing the studies it is clear that contrasting features outnumber similarities in terms of age, treatment intensity, the CRT materials used and the choice of assessment instruments. Results also reveal how different aspects of the same measure have been used to evaluate changes post CRT. For example, both Tchanturia et al. [72] and Abbate-Daga et al. [59] found significant changes in Trail Making Test (TMT) [72] performance in adult patients with AN, whereas Dahlgren et al. [54] did not in adolescents with AN. However, results from a variety of TMT measures such as shifting time-, total completion time- and attention were reported in the different papers, rendering it difficult to compare results. Three studies [54,56,71] (of which the two latter are based on the same sample) report a decrease in depression post CRT, with one adolescent study [54] challenging the previously held notion that weight restoration alone does not significantly contribute to changes in neuropsychological functioning [25,71]. Further, the two studies published by Dahlgren et al. [54,70] address methodological issues previously ignored, such as test-retest effects and biases associated with the absence of proper controlling and corrections for multiple comparisons. In Dahlgren et al. [70], a novel approach to investigate pre and post CRT functioning is being used: the self-report measure "Behavior Rating Inventory of Executive Function" (BRIEF) [73]. In this paper, the authors compare patient and parental reports of executive functioning (EF) before and after CRT. On a group level, conclusions point in the direction of scorings within the normal range, and yields results of substantial discrepancies between parent- and patient's ratings of executive functioning. On an individual level however, large within-group differences emerge.

3. Overlapping studies

We identified four studies with a distinct overlap with regards to feasibility and pre and post CRT assessments without control groups [52,53,74,75]. The least recent publication from 2007 [74], although using a very small sample (N = 4), represents the transition from the single case study format, to a novel study design where larger groups of patients are included, and where authors set out to investigate both feasibility and neuropsychological performance before and after the CRT. Observed significant changes in set-shifting and patient feedback from this study was used to further develop CRT for patients with AN. Also, results from this study led to the refining of materials, and the inclusion of behavioural task in the updated [in-house] manual produced a few years later [Tchanturia & Davies: Cognitive Remediation Programme for Anorexia Nervosa: A Manual for Practitioners, Unpublished]. Group CRT was first described and evaluated in the study by Genders & Tchanturia [74] and similar to the Tchanturia et al.'s work from 2007, this study also sought to combine knowledge of feasibility and changes post CRT. Results supported acceptability for both patients and group facilitators, and heightened rates of self-reported ability to change were reported by the patients. No significant changes in cognitive flexibility or self-esteem were reported. When the second paper on group-CRT was published in 2012 [53] tasks had been adapted from the Genders & Tchanturia study mentioned above, but to accommodate the patients who were already engaged in an intense six-week programme, no more than four sessions were offered. Again, similar to the previous group CRT study, results supported the acceptability of the intervention, but did not support significant changes in self-reported flexibility. In 2010, Pitt et al. [52] made an important addition to the field in not only by exploring the feasibility through patient feedback, but by introducing a novel CRT outcome measure; perfectionism. As the first of its kind, this study provided data based solely on outpatients assessments. Similar to the data reported in Tchanturia et al. in 2007 [75], self-reported flexibility was significantly higher post CRT. In terms of perfectionism, results could not be calculated statistically due to the small sample (N = 7), and trends were inconclusive as both increases and decreases in scores were observed.

3) RCTs

The four most recent studies on CRT for AN are all RCTs in adults, and represent a giant leap from that of feasibility trials and case studies in terms of its potency of measuring intervention effects. The first of these studies [59] explores the role of CRT in reducing attrition in RCTs for AN. In this study, 46 patients with AN were randomised to receive either eight sessions of CRT or CBT over a period of two months. Following these initial eight sessions, both groups received 16 CBT sessions over a period of four months. For patients receiving CRT, results revealed lower dropout rates compared to the CBT group (13 and 33% respectively), as well as significant changes in set-shifting and central coherence at the end of the intervention. However, dropout rates were obtained through data collected at the main outcome point (session eight), after which the rate of attrition increased in the CRT group and eventually, rose to a level matching that of the CBT patient group. Also, no significant differences between CRT and CBT groups in outcome measures such as weight or ED psychopathology were observed at the end of treatment. In addition, results indicate that CRT has an effect on specific neurocognitive functions, but shows no superiority in terms of improving ED symptomatology compared to CBT. Somewhat later in 2013, Brockmeyer et al. [58] introduced a novel approach to CRT; face-to-face sessions *plus* computer assisted homework. Data from 25 treatment completers, 11 receiving CRT focusing specifically on cognitive flexibility, and 14 receiving non-specific neurocognitive therapy (NNT), was analysed. Similar to the study conducted by Lock and colleagues [59], no significant difference in treatment adherence was observed. However, in line with Lock et al.'s initial RCT [59], Brockmeyer et al. [58] also found changes in cognitive flexibility being significantly higher in the group receiving CRT, than in the control group (i.e. NNT). In November 2013, two additional RCTs were published (online) [57,60]. The first, a small study conducted by Steinglass and colleagues [60], sought to evaluate the effect of Exposure and Response Prevention for AN (AN-EXRP) on eating behaviour during weight restoration, by comparing it to CRT. Data from 15 inpatient treatment completers was analysed, and yielded evidence of superior caloric intake in the AN-EXRP arm compared to CRT, with improvements that were significantly associated with reduced eating related anxiety. The most recent RCT [57] is also the largest with 82 patients receiving either treatment as usual (TAU) (N = 41) or CRT plus TAU (N = 41). It is also the first transdiagnostic CRT study, exploring the effect of the intervention in a sample of ED patients without reporting specific ED subtypes. Results revealed that patients in the CRT plus TAU arm reported higher levels of ED-related quality of life at the end of treatment than those who received TAU alone, and also, patients with poor baseline set-shifting abilities benefited more from CRT than those performing within the norms a this time point. Dropout rates in the two groups were nearly identical at 6-month follow up (approximately 20%).

Discussion

To our knowledge, this is the first paper reviewing the whole literature for CRT for AN, and the first paper delineating its developmental trajectory from single case studies to RCTs. Because of the preliminary nature of case reports and case series, and the great variety amongst them, it is difficult to compare and generalize results. Methodological challenges such as short test-retest spans and its associated risk of learning effects, the use of identical pre and post CRT assessment instruments and the lack of control group renders it impossible to conclude whether observed changes (or the lack of these) are direct results of the intervention itself, or associated with other factors such as changes in comorbidity, ED psychopathology, or weight. However, results from these studies suggest that individual CRT appears to be associated with lower dropout rates than group CRT, and has the potential of creating a positive patient-therapist alliance [76]. Further, group therapy appears to appeal to patients in increasing awareness of shared cognitive styles, but has also been reported fostering negative group dynamics, and tasks assigned during the therapy is not always perceived as relevant [66]. At present, there is only one report of family CRT [64], and although it appears as family CRT strengthens the understanding of how cognitive styles affect family dynamics, improves communication and cooperation during treatment, one must stress that family CRT should not replace existing treatments, but rather be seen as a conjunct to ordinary treatment engagements. Overall, single case studies and case series presented in this paper support the feasibility of CRT across ages, illness severity, current treatment engagements and when delivered in a number of different formats.

As evident from Table 1, the mode of CRT delivery is changing rapidly, and as new modalities are described, tested and evaluated, it is crucial to attempt comparing results so as to understand the advantages and disadvantages of each approach. With the emergence of RCTs, the potential of measuring the effectiveness of CRT has increased dramatically, and so has the possibility of comparing results.

The four RCTs presented in this paper, although varying in terms of study design and aims, depicts how CRT is currently being implemented in a variety of settings, with patients suffering from various forms of EDs, and through different means of delivery. The first two studies [58,59] support its efficiency in improving specific neurocognitive functions, whereas the first [59] and last [57] RCT published yielded evidence of its potency in reducing attrition and enhancing the effectiveness of concurrent treatment. In terms of moderator analyses, Lock et al. [59] failed to find evidence of weight and comorbidity as moderators for treatment response, whereas Dingemans et al. [57] showed that patients with poor baseline set-shifting abilities benefited more from CRT than those scoring within the norms. The emergence of the novel mode of delivery described in Brockmeyer et al. [58] exemplifies how face-to-face treatment in combination with computer assisted sessions might intensify learning and awareness, and how conjunctive CRT might help empowering patients to practice new skills using novel technologies.

The potency of CRT with regards to improvements in ED psychopathology and comorbid psychiatric illnesses still remains uncertain, and larger RCTs are needed to further address this issue. Also, as the mode of delivery and study aims in the four RCTs differ substantially, interpretation of results should be viewed as specific to each study rather than general, and comparisons should take into account the observed variation in study designs, mode of treatment delivery, choice of outcome measures and patient characteristics.

To date, adolescent CRT case studies- and series have supported the feasibility and acceptability of the intervention, both when delivered individually [53,55] in groups [67] and in families [65]. However, as all current RCTs are oriented towards adult patients, we still know little about the intervention's potential in terms of efficacy in younger AN populations. Further, as many recent studies fail to detect neuropsychological impairment in adolescent AN patients [12,40,77-81], it might be timely to consider other components than neuropsychological performance when assessing the effect of CRT in this patient group, and to learn from recent results suggesting that CRT is more beneficent for those struggling with cognitive weaknesses than in those who perform within the norms [57]. For young AN patients, one might suggest revisiting one of the original aims of the intervention; preparation for subsequent treatment [25,61], but also to pay attention to results recently surfaced such as attrition reduction [59] and enhancing the effectiveness of concurrent treatments [57]. Further, as CRT aims to address thoughts and behaviours as they manifest in the patient's everyday life, novel measures such as metacognitive abilities, quality of life or every day coping strategies might also be useful in assessing outcomes associated with the intervention. Finally, as evident from the papers presented in this paper, there are considerable discrepancies with regard to the aim of delivering CRT to patients with EDs. Although it is clear that CRT is still in its developmental phase and has followed a logic course of methodology (from single case studies to RCTs), the field would benefit greatly from finding a common ground on which the aim of delivering the intervention is based, and subsequently, using similar outcome measures to assess global intervention effects.

Conclusion

The main conclusion of this review is that there is strong evidence of feasibility of CRT for AN across ages and illness severity. With the emergence of several recent RCTs, new evidence also suggest that that the intervention is effective in reducing attrition, enhancing the efficacy of concurrent treatment and improve cognitive set-shifting. To further strengthen our understanding of mechanisms of action in CRT, future studies should focus on (1) exploring the long-term effects of the treatment, (2) investigate the influence of moderators such as comorbidity (e.g. depression, anxiety and OCD), illness severity and duration of illness, personality, and other pre-treatment patient characteristics, (3) devising RCTs exploring the effectiveness of CRT for adolescents, using age appropriate instruments taking into account the heterogeneity in neuropsychological functioning in young individuals with AN (e.g. instruments assessing metacognitive abilities, self-awareness, motivation, ability and willingness to change, therapeutic alliance, quality of life and everyday functioning), (4) exploring of the applicability and effectiveness of transdiagnostic versions of CRT in larger samples, and finally, (5) the continuous investigation of family CRT as a conjunctive treatment for young girls with AN.

Abbreviations

ADHD: Attention deficit hyperactivity disorder; AN: Anorexia nervosa; AN-EXRP: Exposure and response prevention for AN; BMI: Body mass index; BRIEF: Behavior rating inventory of executive function; CAT: Cognitive analytic therapy; CBT: Cognitive behavioral therapy; CREST: Cognitive remediation therapy and emotional skills training; CRT: Cognitive remediation therapy; DSM-5: The diagnostic and statistic manual of mental Disorders Fifth Edition; ED: Eating disorder; EF: Executive function; EDNOS: Eating disorder not otherwise specified; FBT: Family based therapy; IPT: Interpersonal therapy; NNT: Non-specific neurocognitive therapy; OCD: Obsessive compulsive disorder; RCT: Randomised controlled trial; TAU: Treatment as usual; TMT: Trail making test.

Competing interests

The authors declare that they have no competing interests.

Authors' contributions

CLD drafted the manuscript, conducted the literature search, assembled and analysed all data and wrote the paper. ØR participated in the formulation of the aims of the study, in the interpretation of the main findings and in drafting the manuscript. Both authors read and approved the final manuscript.

Acknowledgements

The work on this paper has been supported by the Centre for Research on Eating Disorders at Oxford (CREDO), Oxford University, and by the Regional Department for Eating Disorder, Department of Mental Health and Addiction, Oslo University Hospital, Ullevål. The authors would also like to thank the reviewers for valuable comments.

Author details

[1]Regional Department for Eating Disorders, Division of Mental Health and Addiction, Oslo University Hospital, Ullevål HF, Oslo, Norway. [2]Department of Psychiatry, Centre for Research on Eating Disorders at Oxford (CREDO), University of Oxford, Warneford Hospital, Oxford, UK. [3]Division of Mental Health and Addiction, Institute of Clinical Medicine, University of Oslo, Oslo, Norway.

References

1. Arcelus J, Mitchell AJ, Wales J, Nielsen S: **Mortality rates in patients with anorexia nervosa and other eating disorders. a meta-analysis of 36 studies.** *Arch Gen Psychiatry* 2011, **68**(7):724–731.
2. Halvorsen I, Heyerdahl S: **Girls with anorexia nervosa as young adults: personality, self-esteem, and life satisfaction.** *Int J Eat Disord* 2006, **39**(4):285–293.

3. Keilen M, Treasure T, Schmidt U, Treasure J: **Quality of life measurements in eating disorders, angina, and transplant candidates: are they comparable?** *J R Soc Med* 1994, **87**(8):441–444.
4. Hoek HW, van Hoeken D: **Review of the prevalence and incidence of eating disorders.** *Int J Eat Disord* 2003, **34**(4):383–396.
5. American Psychological Association: *Diagnostic and Statistical Manual of Mental Disorders.* 5th edition. Arlington VA: American Psychiatric Association; 2013.
6. Fairburn CG: **Evidence-based treatment for anorexia nervosa.** *Int J Eat Disord* 2005, **37**(Suppl):S26–S30.
7. Lock J, Le Grange D, Agras WS, Dare C: *Treatment manual for anorexia nervosa: A family-based approach.* New York: Guilford Press; 2001.
8. Couturier J, Kimber M, Szatmari P: **Efficacy of family-based treatment for adolescents with eating disorders: a systematic review and meta-analysis.** *Int J Eat Disord* 2013, **46**(1):3–11.
9. Lock J, Le Grange D, Agras WS, Moye A, Bryson SW, Jo B: **Randomized clinical trial comparing family-based treatment with adolescent-focused individual therapy for adolescents with anorexia nervosa.** *Arch Gen Psychiatry* 2010, **67**(10):1025–1032.
10. National Institute for Health and Clinical Excellence (NICE): *Core interventions for the treatment and management of anorexia nervosa, bulimia nervosa and related eating disorders.* London UK: Abba Litho Sales Limited; 2004.
11. Gardner J, Wilkinson P: **Is family therapy the most effective treatment for anorexia nervosa?** *Psychiatr Danubina* 2011, **23**(Suppl 1):S175–S177.
12. Bühren K, Mainz V, Herpertz-Dahlmann B, Schafer K, Kahraman-Lanzerath B, Lente C, Konrad K: **Cognitive flexibility in juvenile anorexia nervosa patients before and after weight recovery.** *J Neural Transm* 2012, **119**(9):1047–1057.
13. Danner UN, Sanders N, Smeets PA, van Meer F, Adan RA, Hoek HW, van Elburg AA: **Neuropsychological weaknesses in anorexia nervosa: set-shifting, central coherence, and decision making in currently ill and recovered women.** *Int J Eat Disord* 2012, **45**(5):685–694.
14. Kanakam N, Treasure J: **A review of cognitive neuropsychiatry in the taxonomy of eating disorders: state, trait, or genetic?** *Cogn Neuropsychiatry* 2013, **18**(1–2):83–114.
15. Tchanturia K, Harrison A, Davies H, Roberts ME, Oldershaw A, Nakazato M, Stahl D, Morris R, Schmidt U, Treasure J: **Cognitive flexibility and clinical severity in eating disorders.** *PLoS One* 2011, **6**(6):e20462.
16. Tenconi E, Santonastaso P, Degortes D, Bosello R, Titton F, Mapelli D, Favaro A: **Set-shifting abilities, central coherence, and handedness in anorexia nervosa patients, their unaffected siblings and healthy controls: exploring putative endophenotypes.** *World J Biol Psychiatry* 2010, **11**(6):813–823.
17. Luria AR: *The Man with a Shattered World: The History of a Brain Wound.* Cambridge MA: Harvard University Press; 1972.
18. Kurtz MM: **Cognitive remediation for schizophrenia: current status, biological correlates and predictors of response.** *Expert Rev Neurother* 2012, **12**(7):813–821.
19. Wykes T, Spaulding WD: **Thinking about the future cognitive remediation therapy–what works and could we do better?** *Schizophr Bull* 2011, **37**(Suppl 2):S80–S90.
20. Bowie CR, Gupta M, Holshausen K: **Cognitive remediation therapy for mood disorders: rationale, early evidence, and future directions.** *Can J Psychiatry* 2013, **58**(6):319–325.
21. Stevenson CS, Whitmont S, Bornholt L, Livesey D, Stevenson RJ: **A cognitive remediation programme for adults with attention deficit hyperactivity disorder.** *Aust New Zeal J Psychiatr* 2002, **36**(5):610–616.
22. Rupp CI, Kemmler G, Kurz M, Hinterhuber H, Fleischhacker WW: **Cognitive remediation therapy during treatment for alcohol dependence.** *J Stud Alcohol Drugs* 2012, **73**(4):625–634.
23. Morimoto SS, Wexler BE, Alexopoulos GS: **Neuroplasticity-based computerized cognitive remediation for geriatric depression.** *Int J Geriatr Psychiatry* 2012, **27**(12):1239–1247.
24. Buhlmann U, Deckersbach T, Engelhard I, Cook LM, Rauch SL, Kathmann N, Wilhelm S, Savage CR: **Cognitive retraining for organizational impairment in obsessive-compulsive disorder.** *Psychiatry Res* 2006, **144**(2–3):109–116.
25. Davies H, Tchanturia K: **Cognitive remediation therapy as an intervention for acute anorexia nervosa: a case report.** *Eur Eat Disord Rev* 2005, **13**:311–316.
26. Delahunty A, Morice R: *A training programme for the remediation of cognitive deficits in schizophrenia.* Albury NSW: Department of Health; 1993.
27. Tchanturia K, Davies H, Reeder C, Wykes T: *Cognitive Remediation Programme for Anorexia Nervosa: A Manual for Practitioners.* London UK: Institute of Psychiatry; 2010. http://www.katetchanturia.com.
28. Baldock E, Tchanturia K: **Translating laboratory research into practice: foundations, functions and future of cognitive remediation therapy for anorexia nervosa.** *Therapy* 2007, **4**(3):285–292.
29. Tchanturia K, Lock J: **Cognitive remediation therapy for eating disorders: development, refinement and future directions.** *Curr Top Behav Neurosci* 2011, **6**:269–287.
30. Tchanturia K, Lloyd S, Kang K: **Cognitive remediation therapy for anorexia nervosa: current evidence and future research directions.** *Int J Eat Disord* 2013, **46**(5):492–495.
31. Cwojdzinska A, Markowska-Regulska K, Rybakowski F: **Cognitive remediation therapy in adolescent anorexia nervosa - case report.** *Psychiatr Pol* 2009, **43**(1):115–124.
32. Asch M, Esteves J, De Hautecloque D, Bargiacchi A, Le Heuzey MF, Mouren MC, Doyen C: **Cognitive remediation therapy for children and adolescents with anorexia nervosa in France: an exploratory study.** *Encéphale* 2014, **40**(3):240–6.
33. Vorgaft I, Bercovich S: **Cognitive remediation therapy for patients with anorexia nervosa.** *Isr J Psychiatry Relat Sci* 2012, **49**(1):19–19.
34. Fagundo AB, Santamaria JJ, Forcano L, Giner-Bartolome C, Jimenez-Murcia S, Sanchez I, Granero R, Ben-Moussa M, Magnenat-Thalmann N, Konstantas D, Lam T, Lucas M, Nielsen J, Bults RG, Tarrega S, Menchon JM, de la Torre R, Cardi V, Treasure J, Fernandez-Aranda F: **Video game therapy for emotional regulation and impulsivity control in a series of treated cases with bulimia nervosa.** *Eur Eat Disord Rev* 2013, **21**(6):493–499.
35. Hay PJ, Touyz S, Sud R: **Treatment for severe and enduring anorexia nervosa: a review.** *Aust New Zeal J Psychiatr* 2012, **46**(12):1136–44.
36. Nunn K, Frampton I, Fuglset TS, Torzsok-Sonnevend M, Lask B: **Anorexia nervosa and the insula.** *Med Hypotheses* 2011, **76**(3):353–357.
37. Safer DL, Chen EY: **Anorexia nervosa as a disorder of emotion dysregulation: theory, evidence, and treatment implications.** *Clin Psychol Sci Pract* 2011, **18**(3):203–207.
38. Guardia D, Luyat M, Cottecin O: **Anorexia nervosa, a body shape's story.** *Correspondances en Metabolismes Horm Diab et Nutr* 2011, **15**(9–10):316–320.
39. Martinez G, Cook-Darzens S, Chaste P, Mouren MC, Doyen C: **Anorexia nervosa in the light of neurocognitive functioning: new theoretical and therapeutic perspectives.** *Encéphale* 2014, **40**(2):160–167.
40. Lang K, Stahl D, Espie J, Treasure J, Tchanturia K: **Set shifting in children and adolescents with anorexia nervosa: an exploratory systematic review and meta-analysis.** *Int J Eat Disord* 2014, **47**(4):394–399.
41. Zuchova S, Kubena AA, Erler T, Papezova H: **Neuropsychological variables and clinical status in anorexia nervosa: relationship between visuospatial memory and central coherence and eating disorder symptom severity.** *Eat Weight Disord* 2013, **18**(4):421–428.
42. Tchanturia K, Smith E, Weineck F, Fidanboylu E, Kern N, Treasure J, Baron Cohen S: **Exploring autistic traits in anorexia: a clinical study.** *Mol Autism* 2013, **4**(1):44.
43. Lopez C, Davies H, Tchanturia K: **Neuropsychological inefficiences in anorexia nervosa targeted in clinical practice: The development of a module of cognitive remediation therapy.** In *Eating and its disorders.* Edited by Fox J, Goss K. UK: Wiley-Blackwell; 2012:185–197.
44. Adan RA, Kaye W: *Behavioural Neurobiology of Eating Disorders.* New York US: Springer-Verlag Publishing; 2011.
45. Grilo CM, Mitchell JE: *The Treatment of Eating Disorders - A Clinical Handbook.* New York US: Guilford Press; 2010.
46. Tchanturia K, Hambrook D: **Cognitive remediation therapy for anorexia nervosa.** In *The Treatment of Eating Disorders.* Edited by Grilo CM, Mitchell JE. New York US: Guilford Press; 2010.
47. Owen I, Dahlgren CL, Lask B: **Cognitive Remediation Therapy.** In *Eating Disorders in Childhood and Adolescence.* 4th edition. Edited by Lask B, Bryant-Waugh R. New York US: Routledge/Taylor & Francis Group; 2013:301–318.
48. Fox J, Goss K: *Eating and its disorders.* East Sussex UK: John Wile and Sons Ltd.; 2012.
49. Davies H, Fox J, Naumann U, Treasure J, Schmidt U, Tchanturia K: **Cognitive remediation and emotion skills training for anorexia nervosa: an observational study using neuropsychological outcomes.** *Eur Eat Disord Rev* 2012, **20**(3):211–217.
50. Money C, Genders R, Treasure J, Schmidt U, Tchanturia K: **A brief emotion focused intervention for inpatients with anorexia nervosa: a qualitative study.** *J Health Psychol* 2011, **16**(6):947–958.

51. Tchanturia K, Doris E, Fleming C: **Effectiveness of Cognitive Remediation and Emotion Skills Training (CREST) for anorexia nervosa in group format: a naturalistic pilot study.** *Eur Eat Disord Rev* 2014, **22**(3):200–205.
52. Pitt S, Lewis R, Morgan S, Woodward D: **Cognitive remediation therapy in an outpatient setting: a case series.** *Eat Weight Disord* 2010, **15**(4):281–286.
53. Pretorius N, Dimmer M, Power E, Eisler I, Simic M, Tchanturia K: **Evaluation of a cognitive remediation therapy group for adolescents with anorexia nervosa: pilot study.** *Eur Eat Disord Rev* 2012, **20**(4):321–325.
54. Dahlgren CL, Lask B, Landrø NI, Rø Ø: **Neuropsychological functioning in adolescents with anorexia nervosa before and after cognitive remediation therapy: a feasibility trial.** *Int J Eat Disord* 2013, **46**(6):576–581.
55. Dahlgren CL, Lask B, Landrø NI, Rø Ø: **Developing and evaluating cognitive remediation therapy (CRT) for adolescents with anorexia nervosa: a feasibility study.** *Clin Child Psychol Psychiatry* 2014, **19**(3):476–487.
56. Dahlgren CL, Lask B, Landrø NI, Rø Ø: **Patient and parental self-reports of executive functioning in a sample of young females with anorexia nervosa before and after cognitive remediation therapy.** *Eur Eat Disord Rev* 2013, **22**(1):45–52.
57. Dingemans AE, Danner UN, Donker JM, Aardoom JJ, van Meer F, Tobias K, van Elburg AA, van Furth EF: **The effectiveness of cognitive remediation therapy in patients with a severe or enduring eating disorder: a randomized controlled trial.** *Psychother Psychosom* 2014, **83**(1):29–36.
58. Brockmeyer T, Ingenerf K, Walther S, Wild B, Hartmann M, Herzog W, Bents H, Friederich HC: **Training cognitive flexibility in patients with anorexia nervosa: a pilot randomized controlled trial of cognitive remediation therapy.** *Int J Eat Disord* 2013, **47**(1):24–31.
59. Lock J, Agras WS, Fitzpatrick KK, Bryson SW, Jo B, Tchanturia K: **Is outpatient cognitive remediation therapy feasible to use in randomized clinical trials for anorexia nervosa?** *Int J Eat Disord* 2013, **46**(6):567–575.
60. Steinglass JE, Albano AM, Simpson HB, Wang Y, Zou J, Attia E, Walsh TB: **Confronting fear using exposure and response prevention for anorexia nervosa: a randomized controlled pilot study.** *Int J Eat Disord* 2013, **47**(2):174–180.
61. Pretorius N, Tchanturia K: **Anorexia nervosa: how people think and how we address it in cognitive remediation therapy.** *Therapy* 2007, **4**(4):423–432.
62. Tchanturia K, Whitney J, Treasure J: **Can cognitive exercises help treat anorexia nervosa?** *Eat Weight Disord* 2006, **11**(4):e112–e116.
63. Easter A, Tchanturia K: **Therapists' experiences of cognitive remediation therapy for anorexia nervosa: implications for working with adolescents.** *Clin Child Psychol Psychiatry* 2011, **16**(2):233–246.
64. Lask B, Roberts A: **Family cognitive remediation therapy for anorexia nervosa.** *Clin Child Psychol Psychiatr* 2013, [Epub ahead of print]. doi:10.1177/1359104513504313.
65. Whitney J, Easter A, Tchanturia K: **Service users' feedback on cognitive training in the treatment of anorexia nervosa: a qualitative study.** *Int J Eat Disord* 2008, **41**(6):542–550.
66. Wood L, Al-Khairulla H, Lask B: **Group cognitive remediation therapy for adolescents with anorexia nervosa.** *Clin Child Psychol Psychiatry* 2011, **16**(2):225–231.
67. Zuchova S, Erler T, Papezova H: **Group cognitive remediation therapy for adult anorexia nervosa inpatients: first experiences.** *Eat Weight Disord* 2013, **18**(3):269–273.
68. Lindvall C, Owen I, Lask B: *The CRT Resource Pack for Children and Adolescents with Anorexia Nervosa.* Oslo Norway: Oslo University Hospital, Ullevål HF; 2010. http://www.rasp.no.
69. Abbate-Daga G, Buzzichelli S, Marzola E, Amianto F, Fassino S: **Effectiveness of cognitive remediation therapy (CRT) in anorexia nervosa: a case series.** *J Clin Exp Neuropsychol* 2012, **34**(10):1009–1015.
70. Dahlgren CL, Lask B, Landro NI, Rø Ø: **Patient and parental self-reports of executive functioning in a sample of young female adolescents with anorexia nervosa before and after cognitive remediation therapy.** *European Eating Disorders Review* 2014, **22**(1):45–52.
71. Tchanturia K, Davies H, Lopez C, Schmidt U, Treasure J, Wykes T: **Neuropsychological task performance before and after cognitive remediation in anorexia nervosa: a pilot case-series.** *Psychol Med* 2008, **38**(9):1371–1373.
72. Delis D, Kaplan E, Kramer J: *Delis Kaplan Executive Function System (D-KEFS) - Technical Manual.* San Antonio TX: The Psychological Corporation; 2001.
73. Gioia GA, Isquith PK, Guy SC, Kenworthy L: *Behavior Rating Inventory of Executive Function: Professional Manual.* USA: Psychological Assessment Resources Inc.; 2000.
74. Genders R, Tchanturia K: **Cognitive remediation therapy (CRT) for anorexia in group format: a pilot study.** *Eat Weight Disord* 2010, **15**(4):e234–e239.
75. Tchanturia K, Davies H, Campbell IC: **Cognitive remediation therapy for patients with anorexia nervosa: preliminary findings.** *Ann Gen Psychiatr* 2007, **6**(14):1–16.
76. Dahlgren CL: *Cognitive Remediation Therapy for Young Female Adolescents with Anorexia Nervosa - Assessing the Feasibility of a Novel Eating Disorder Intervention*, PhD Thesis. Oslo, Norway: University of Oslo, Faculty of Social Sciences; 2014.
77. Fitzpatrick KK, Darcy A, Colborn D, Gudorf C, Lock J: **Set-shifting among adolescents with anorexia nervosa.** *Int J Eat Disord* 2012, **45**(7):909–912.
78. Rose M, Frampton I, Lask B: **A case series investigating distinct neuropsychological profiles in children and adolescents with anorexia nervosa.** *Eur Eat Disord Rev* 2012, **20**(1):32–38.
79. Rose M, Frampton I, Lask B: **Central coherence, organizational strategy, and visuospatial memory in Children and adolescents with Anorexia Nervosa.** *Appl Neuropsychol Child* 2013, [Epub ahead of print]. doi:10.1080/21622965.2013.775064.
80. Shott ME, Filoteo JV, Bhatnagar KA, Peak NJ, Hagman JO, Rockwell R, Kaye WH, Frank GK: **Cognitive set-shifting in anorexia nervosa.** *Eur Eat Disord Rev* 2012, **20**(5):343–349.
81. Stedal K, Frampton I, Landro NI, Lask B: **An examination of the ravello profile - a neuropsychological test battery for anorexia nervosa.** *Eur Eat Disord Rev* 2012, **20**(3):175–181.

8

The impact of indicated prevention and early intervention on co-morbid eating disorder and depressive symptoms: a systematic review

Rachel F Rodgers[1,2,3] and Susan J Paxton[3*]

Abstract

Background: Depressive and eating disorder symptoms are highly comorbid. To date, however, little is known regarding the efficacy of existing programs in decreasing concurrent eating disorder and depressive symptoms.

Methods: We conducted a systematic review of selective and indicated controlled prevention and early intervention programs that assessed both eating disorder and depressive symptoms.

Results: We identified a total of 26 studies. The large majority of identified interventions (92%) were successful in decreasing eating disorder symptoms. However fewer than half (42%) were successful in decreasing both eating disorder and depressive symptoms. Intervention and participant characteristics did not predict success in decreasing depressive symptoms.

Conclusions: Indicated prevention and early intervention programs targeting eating disorder symptoms are limited in their success in decreasing concurrent depressive symptoms. Further efforts to develop more efficient interventions that are successful in decreasing both eating disorder and depressive symptoms are warranted.

Keywords: Eating disorders, Depression, Prevention, Early intervention, Systematic review

Review

Eating disorders and depressive disorders have revealed strong associations, and their relationships contribute to the complexity, burden, and treatment resistance of these disorders [1]. In view of these factors, understanding the effects of prevention and early intervention efforts on both eating disorder and depressive symptoms is an important concern, and would help inform intervention. However, to date, little attention has been paid to the success of interventions in decreasing both of these concerns. The aim of the present study was therefore to conduct a systematic review of indicated prevention and early intervention programs that assessed both eating disorder and depressive symptoms in order to clarify the efficacy of these programs in decreasing both types of symptomatology.

The lifetime comorbidity between eating disorders and major depressive disorders is high with estimates of 40% for Anorexia Nervosa and 50% for Bulimia Nervosa [2]. Importantly, in relation to eating disorders, comorbid depressive symptoms have been found to negatively affect the successfulness of early intervention efforts. Depressive symptoms have been found to predict attrition in self-help programs for binge eating disorder [3], and to predict drop-out from Internet interventions that have become more numerous in recent years [4]. Similarly, depressive symptoms have been found to predict poorer prognosis in self-help programs for eating disorders [3].

Several types of relationships have been hypothesized and described between eating disorder and depressive symptoms, namely that 1) eating disorder and depressive symptoms may develop simultaneously; 2) eating disorder symptoms may be a risk factor for depressive symptoms; 3) depressive symptoms may be a risk factor for eating disorder symptoms. While all of these models have received empirical support [5-7], compelling evidence from twin studies has revealed the importance of shared genetic factors in the development of comorbid eating disorder and depressive symptoms [8,9]. In view of this, some authors have argued

* Correspondence: susan.paxton@latrobe.edu.au
[3]La Trobe University, Melbourne, Australia
Full list of author information is available at the end of the article

that the evidence to date provides greatest support for a comorbidity model in which eating disorders and depression stem from both common and specific etiological factors [10].

A number of theoretical models have proposed frameworks that account for these shared and specific risk factors including biological, cognitive, emotional-regulation, and feminist models. Biological models emphasize the importance of shared genetically transmitted biological factors, as described above, and in particular the importance of dysregulation of serotonergic pathways that have an impact on both mood and eating behaviors [11]. Cognitive models highlight the role of common cognitive distortions that play a role in the development of both depressive and eating disorder symptoms through a heightened focus on negative information [12-14]. Emotion-regulation models have revealed how maladaptive strategies for regulating emotions may contribute to both depressive and eating disorders symptoms [15]. Finally, feminist models of the comorbidity between depressive and eating disorder symptoms have highlighted the gendered aspects of these concerns and viewed both as products of the restricted roles accessible to women in Western society and the objectifying male gaze [16-18].

Despite the high rates of comorbidity and the number of theoretical frameworks accounting for this co-occurrence, to date little is known regarding the common course of eating disorder and depressive symptoms within interventions for high-risk individuals or early intervention programs. Previous work exploring the effect of prevention interventions for eating disorders on negative affect (which includes depressive symptoms but also more serious forms of negative affect) revealed that programs targeting individuals at high risk of eating disorders were more successful in decreasing negative affect [19]. Furthermore, programs including participants over the age of 15, in interactive formats, and including psychoeducational and cognitive dissonance content, produced the greatest decreases in negative affect [19]. While these findings are useful, they may not be transposable to depressive symptoms in interventions for symptomatic individuals as negative affect has not been found to affect prevention intervention attrition [20,21]. Increasing our understanding of intervention effects on comorbid eating disorder and depressive symptoms is crucial as it has important clinical implications. In addition, this knowledge would convey important information regarding treatment efficiency and costs. Finally, strong theoretical bases exist for hypothesizing common underlying mechanisms accounting for eating disorder and depressive symptoms. However, a finding that interventions targeting these mechanisms (e.g., cognitive and emotional factors) were not successful in decreasing both types of symptomatology would point to a disconnect between theory and practice, and suggest a need for the theoretical accounts of the eating disorder/depression comorbidity to be revisited.

The aim of the present study was, therefore, to conduct a systematic review of interventions for high risk (indicated prevention) and symptomatic individuals (early intervention) that included both eating disorder and depression outcomes. Furthermore, consistent with previous findings [19], we expected that interventions that targeted individuals with higher initial levels of eating disorders and depressive symptoms would be most successful in decreasing both of these concerns. In addition, we hypothesized that interventions including a greater number of sessions, among younger participants (which might represent a shorter duration of symptoms), with content targeting negative thoughts and feelings would be most successful. Finally, as cognitive-behavioural therapy is widely recognized as one of the first line recommended treatments for depressive symptoms particularly among young people [22], we hypothesized that interventions implementing CBT strategies would be most successful in decreasing depressive symptoms.

Methods

This review was conducted in accordance to the PRISMA guidelines for systematic reviews [23]. The flow of information through different phases of the systematic review is shown in Figure 1.

Data sources

The databases PsychInfo, ScienceDirect and Scopus were searched for studies and dissertations published between January 1984 and September 2013. Two searches were conducted in each database, first a title search, second a keyword search. The searches included combinations of words describing eating concerns (eating AND disorder or disordered or disorders or pathology or disturbance or disturbed), body image concerns (body image or dissatisfaction or shape or appearance), depressive symptoms (depression or depressive or negative affect) and controlled interventions (prevention or intervention or evaluation or program or self-help AND control or controlled). In addition, studies included in previous reviews of the efficacy of interventions aiming to reduce eating concerns as well as the reference sections of relevant articles were scanned for additional potentially eligible studies.

Study selection

The resulting list of studies was inspected by one author to identify those meeting the following criteria:

(1) Peer-reviewed published work.
(2) Controlled intervention design, compared to an active or minimally active condition such as treatment as usual, or psychoeducation (randomised or not).

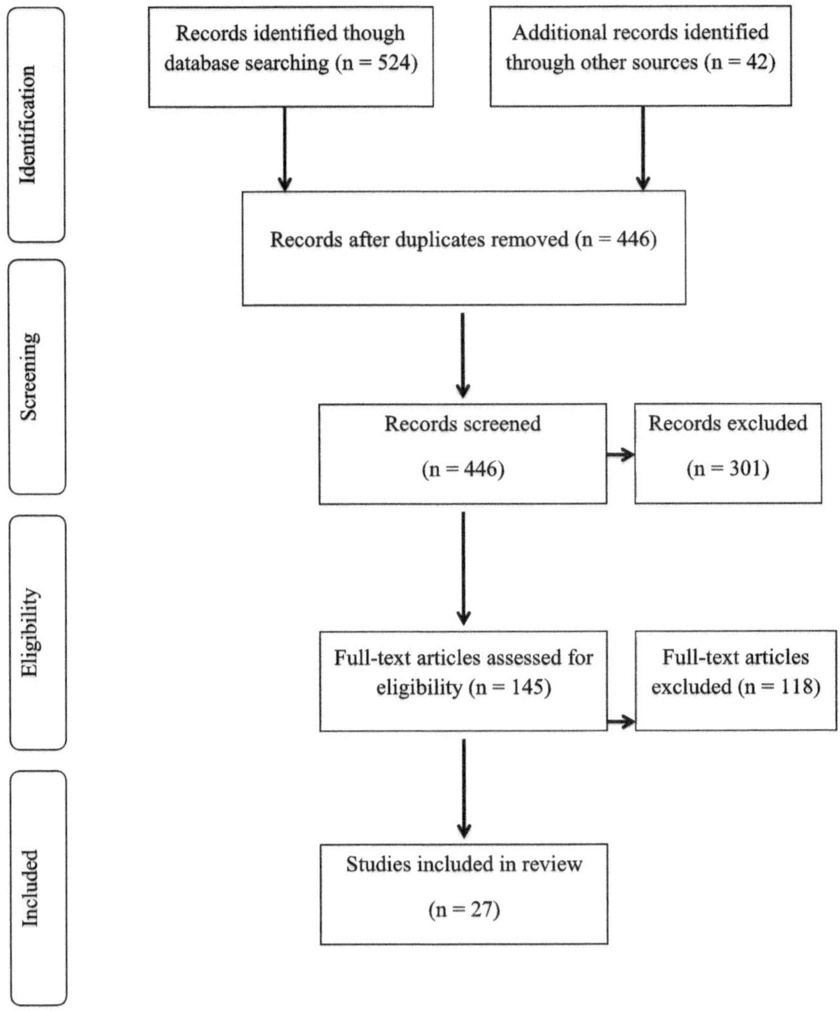

Figure 1 Systematic literature review flow diagram. Flow of information through the different phases of the systematic review.

(3) Indicated interventions defined as interventions aimed at individuals who were identified as having minimal detectable signs or symptoms of an eating but did not meet diagnostic criteria [24]. In our review we included interventions that included participants who had been screened for symptoms as well as interventions allowing participants to self-select as having high levels of concern. In addition, we included self-help and guided self-help interventions as representing the lowest intensity treatment in a stepped care model [25].

(4) The concurrent assessment of both disordered eating and depressive symptoms at baseline and post-intervention, using psychometrically established measures for assessing both eating concerns and depressive symptoms.

Data extraction

Data from the reviewed studies were extracted by one author (RR). The data extraction sheet listed the following categories designed to describe and compare the studies mean age, gender, country, inclusion criteria for the study, type of intervention, mode of delivery, depression and eating disorder symptom measure, effects of intervention at post-test and follow-up, baseline depression level, number of intervention sessions, and presence of content targeting negative thoughts and emotions.

Data analyses

Depression scores were transformed into percentile ranks using norms from the general population [26,27]. Chi-square tests were conducted to explore the effect of initial ED levels operationalized by recruitment criteria (self-selected versus screened), CBT strategies, content targeting negative thoughts and feelings, and face-to-face delivery on successfully decreasing depressive symptoms, and successfully decreasing both depressive and eating disorder symptoms. Independent t-tests were conducted to test the effect of mean age, number of sessions, and initial levels of depressive symptoms (percentile ranks) on successfully decreasing depressive symptoms, and successfully decreasing both depressive and eating disorder symptoms. All analyses were conducted using SPSS 22.

Results

Our review identified 26 studies corresponding to our inclusion criteria (Table 1). Of the 26, 13 studies (50%) were conducted in the U.S, 7 in Europe (27%), 4 (15%) in Australia, and 2 in Canada (8%). The age of participants ranged from 14.4 to 46.5 years old. Nineteen of the studies (73%) used the Beck Depression Inventory [28] as a measure of depressive symptoms, 3 (11%) used the Center for Epidemiology Depression Scale [29], 1 (4%) used the Montgomery-Asberg Depression Rating Scale, 1 (4%) used the Schedule for Affective Disorders and Schizophrenia for School-Age Children [30], 1 (4.33%) used the Kessler Distress Scale [31] and 1 (4%) used the Hospital Anxiety and Depression Scale [32].

Effect of interventions on eating disorder and depressive symptoms

Of the 27 studies, 24 (92%) revealed a statistically significant decrease in eating disorder symptoms while 12 (46%) revealed a statistically significant decrease in depressive symptoms. Eleven studies (42%) significantly decreased both depressive and eating disorder symptoms.

None of our hypothesized moderators of program success on depressive symptoms were supported. Programs with content targeting negative emotions or negative cognitions were not more likely to decrease depressive symptoms. Similarly, programs implementing CBT techniques were not more likely to decrease depressive symptoms. Furthermore, initial levels of depressive or eating disorder symptoms, age, and number of sessions also revealed no association with intervention efficacy in decreasing depressive symptoms (Table 2).

Similarly, none of the hypothesized moderators were able to distinguish between programs that successfully decreased both depressive and eating disorder symptoms, and those that were successful in decreasing only one, or none (Table 2). However, there was a trend for number of sessions, $t(24) = 1.75$, $p = 0.092$, with interventions with fewer sessions tending to be more likely to conjointly decrease eating disorder and depressive symptoms.

Discussion

The aim of the present study was to review the efficacy of indicated prevention and early interventions programs in decreasing concurrent depressive and eating disorder symptoms. Overall, the findings revealed that while the majority of interventions were successful in achieving decreases in eating disorder symptoms, fewer than half of the interventions identified were successful in decreasing both eating disorder and depressive symptoms. These results suggest that existing interventions may be limited in their overall impact and their long-term effects as remaining depressive symptoms could increase the likelihood of later recrudescence in eating disorder symptomatology [1]. Furthermore, these findings highlight the need for increased attention to comorbid depressive symptoms in intervention development and evaluation.

The findings from our review reveal that while 92% of the interventions resulted in significant decreases in eating disorder symptoms, only 42% were successfully in decreasing concurrent depressive and eating disorder symptoms. An important consideration lies in the fact that all of the interventions identified were primarily designed to target eating disorder symptoms, thus publication bias might have affected these ratios and made it more unlikely for our review to identify interventions successful only in decreasing depressive symptoms. Nevertheless, despite the seemingly widespread recognition of the important role of depressive symptoms in eating disorder pathology, illustrated by the frequent inclusion of depressive symptoms as a secondary outcome and the consideration of the effects of eating disorder interventions on depressive symptoms or negative affect in meta-analyses of eating disorder prevention interventions [19], our findings suggest that eating disorder interventions reveal a limited capacity to decrease depressive symptoms. Interestingly, while their importance as a secondary outcome is recognized, the failure to impact depressive symptoms seems to have received little attention. One potential explanation could be a lack of clarity in the conceptualization of depressive symptoms within intervention evaluation. Depressive symptomatology might be assessed as a control factor that could moderate intervention effects, and consequently the lack of intervention effects on this dimension would not be interpreted as a limitation of the intervention success. However, the studies included in the present review assessed for change in depressive symptoms, and frequently referred to it as a secondary outcome, suggesting that the intervention had been hypothesized to positively impact depressive symptoms.

The limited success of the interventions included in this review in decreasing depressive symptoms given their general success in decreasing eating disorder symptoms, suggests that, consistent with theories of comorbidity in a subset of individuals at least, depressive symptoms may not be secondary to eating disorder symptomatology [10]. Some

Table 1 Characteristics of studies included in the systematic review

Study	N intervention; N control; Gender	Mean age	Country	Inclusion criteria	Intervention; number of sessions	Depression assessment instrument	*p* -post	*p* – follow up	Eating disorder symptoms	*p* -post	*p* – follow up
Alloway [33]	N intervention =8; N control = 6; F	32	Canada	Diabetes	Psycho-education; 6 sessions	Beck depression inventory	ns	ns		ns	ns
				EDI ≥40					EDI		
				EAT ≥17					EDI		
Banasiak [34]	N intervention =54; N control =55; F	45	Australia	meeting full or modified criteria for BN	Guided self-help vs TAU; 8 sessions	Beck depression inventory	*	N/A	EDE-Q	*	N/A
									EDI	*	N/A
Bearman [35]	N intervention =38; N control =35; F	18.9	USA	Self-selected undergrads	CBT vs control; 4 sessions	Beck depression inventory	*	ns	BPS	*	*
									DRES	*	*
									EDE-Q	*	ns
Carrard [36]	N intervention =37; N control =37; F	36	Switzerland	1 OBE a week for the past 3 months, meeting BED	Internet CBT vs control; 11 sessions	Beck depression inventory	ns	N/A	EDE-Q	*	N/A
									EDI	*	N/A
									TFEQ	*	N/A
Carrard [37]	N intervention =22; N control =20; F	42	Switzerland	BED patients 30 < BMI < 50	Internet CBT vs control; 11 sessions	Beck depression inventory	*	ns	EDE-Q	ns	ns
									TFEQ	ns	ns
Carter [38]	N intervention =28/28; N control =29; F	27	USA	BN	CBT self-help vs nonspecific self-help vs control; 8 sessions	Beck depression inventory	ns	N/A	OBE	*	N/A
									EDE-Q	ns	N/A
Fichter [39]	N intervention =68; N control =61; F	25	Germany	AN-B/P patients	Self-help vs waitlist; 6 sessions	Beck depression inventory	ns	N/A	EDI	ns	N/A
									SIAB-EX	*	N/A
Grilo [40]	N intervention =38/37; N control =15; M & F	46.5	USA	BED	CBT vs behavioural weight-loss vs control; 12 sessions	Beck depression inventory	ns	N/A	EDE-Q	*	N/A
									TFEQ	*	N/A
Grilo [41]	N intervention =24; N control =24; M & F	45.8	USA	Obese with BED	Self-help CBT vs TAU; 8 sessions	Beck depression inventory	ns	N/A	EDE-Q	*	N/A
Heinicke [42]	N intervention =36; N control =37; F	14.4	Australia	Self-selected for body image or eating concerns	CBT vs WT; 6 sessions	Beck depression inventory	*	*	BSQ	*	*
									DEBQ	*	*
									EWLB	*	*
									EDI	*	*
									SATAQ	*	*
Jacobi [43]	N intervention =51; N control =52; F	22.3	Germany	> 42 WCS	Internet CBT vs control; 8 sessions	Beck depression inventory	d = .14	d = .15	EDE-Q	d = .23-.35	d = .41-.62
									EDI	d = .08-.32	d = .35-.54
Ljotsson [44]	N intervention =35; N control =36; M & F	34	Sweden	MADRS score <30 BED or BN full or sub-threshold	Self-help CBT vs control; 12 sessions	Montgome-ry asberg depression rating scale	*	*	EDE-Q	*	*
									EDI	*	*
									BSQ	*	*

Table 1 Characteristics of studies included in the systematic review *(Continued)*

McLean [45]	N intervention =32; N control =3629 F	43.92	Australia	BSQ ≥90 or EDE-Q WSC ≥3.5	CBT vs control; 8 sessions	KDS	ns	*	BSQ	*	*
									EDEQ	*	*
									BIAQ	*	*
									SATAQ	*	*
									DEBQ	*	*
Mitchell [46]	N intervention =30/33; N control =30; F		USA	Self-selected	CD vs yoga vs control; 6 sessions	CES-D	ns	N/A	EDDS	* (CD)	N/A
									BES	ns	N/A
									EDI	* (CD)	N/A
									IBSS	ns	N/A
									TFEQ	ns	N/A
									BSQ	ns	N/A
O'Brien [47]	N intervention =13; N control =11; F	22.2	Canada	EDI > 10, skipping 2 meals a week	Control vs psycho-education; 8 sessions	Beck depression inventory	ns	ns	BULIT	*	*
									BSQ	*	ns
									EAT	*	*
									FFS	*	ns
Paxton [48]	N intervention =42/37; N control =37; F	25	Australia	BSQ >100, or BSQ =90-99 AND BULIT-R >104	CBT vs internet CBT vs waitlist; 8 sessions	Beck depression inventory	*	N/A	BSQ	*	N/A
									BULIT	*	N/A
									DEBQ	*	N/A
									BIAQ	*	N/A
									SATAQ	*	N/A
Robinson [49]	N intervention =36/34; N control =27; M & F	28	UK	BN, BED or EDNOS	eCBT vs writing vs waitlist; 24 sessions	Beck depression inventory	ns	N/A	QEDD	*	N/A
									BITE	ns	N/A
Sánchez [50]	N intervention =38; N control =38; F	23.9	UK	BN or EDNOS	iCBT vs waitlist; 8 sessions	Hospital anxiety and depression scale	N/A	*	EDE-Q	N/A	*
Stice [51]	N intervention =203; N control =205; F	21.6	USA	Self-selected and phone screened	CD vs education brochure; 4 sessions	Beck depression inventory	*	*	EDDI	*	*
									DRES	*	*
									BPS	*	*
Stice [52]	N intervention =25; N control =70; F	21.3	USA	Self-selected into eating disorders seminar	Psycho-education vs control; 28 sessions	Beck depression inventory	ns	ns	IBSS	*	*
									BPS	*	*
									DRES	*	*
									EDDS	*	*
Stice [53]	N intervention =139; N control =167; F	15.7	USA	Self-selected	CD vs control; 4 sessions	CES-D	ns	ns	IBSS	*	ns
									BPS	*	*

Table 1 Characteristics of studies included in the systematic review *(Continued)*

									DRES	*	*
									EDDI	*	*
Stice [54]	N intervention =39/19; N control =29/20; F	21.6	USA	Self-selected	CD vs ECD vs psycho-education; 4 sessions	Beck depression inventory	*	N/A	IBSS	*	N/A
									BPS	*	N/A
									DRES	*	N/A
									EDDI		N/A
Stice [55]	N intervention =198; N control =200; F	18.4	USA	Self-selected	HW vs psycho-education; 4 sessions	K-SADS	ns	ns	BDS	*	ns
									DRES	*	*
									EDDI	*	ns
Stice [56]	N intervention =55/44; N control =75; F	20.9	USA	Self-selected	CD vs Peer CD vs educational brochure; 4 sessions	Beck depression inventory	*		IBSS	*	*
									BPS	*	*
									DRES	*	*
									EDDI	*	*
Striegel [57]	N intervention =59; N control =64; M & F	37.2	USA	binge eating on average at least twice a week but missed more than one criterion for BN or BED	Guided self-help vs TAU; 8 sessions	Beck depression inventory	*	*	EDE-Q	*	*
Taylor [58]	N intervention =206; N control =215; F	20.8	USA	WCS >50	ECBT vs waitlist; 8 sessions	CES-D	ns	ns (.07)	WCS	*	*
									EDI	*	*

Note: BED = Binge Eating Disorder; BES = Binge Eating Scale [59]; BIAQ = Body Image Avoidance Questionnaire [60]; BITE = Bulimia Investigatory Test Edinburgh [61]; BN = Bulimia nervosa; BPS = Satisfaction and Dissatisfaction with Body Parts Scale [62]; BPSS = BSQ = Body Shape Questionnaire [63]; BULIT = Bulimia Test Revised [64]; Beck Depression Inventory [28]; CBT = Cognitive Behavioural Therapy; CES-D = The Center for Epidemiologic Studies Depression Scale [29]; DRES = Dutch Restrained Eating Scale [65]; EAT = Eating Attitudes Test [66]; EDDI = Eating Disorder Diagnostic Interview [53]; EDDS = Eating Disorder Diagnostic Scale [67]; EDE-Q = Eating Disorder Examination Questionnaire [68]; EDI = Eating Disorders Inventory [69]; EDNOS = Eating Disorder Not otherwise Specified; EWLB = Extreme Weight Loss Behaviors; IBSS = Ideal Body Stereotype Scale [70]; FFS = Forbidden Food Survey [71]; Hospital Anxiety and Depression Scale [32]; KDS = Kessler Distress Scale [31]; K-SADS Schedule for Affective Disorders and Schizophrenia for School-Age Children [30]; MADRS = Montgomery Asberg Depression Rating Scale [72]; OBE = Objective Binge Episodes; SATAQ = Sociocultural Attitudes Towards Appearance Questionnaire [73]; SIAB-EX = Structured Inventory for Anorexic and Bulimic Disorders [74]; TAU = treatment as usual; TFEQ = Three Factor Eating Questionnaire [75]; WCS = Weight and Shape Concerns Scale [76].

*p<.05 or lower, ns = non-significant, that is p > .05.

Table 2 Characteristics of studies according to their success in decreasing depressive symptoms

	Range	Decreases in depressive symptoms[a]		Decreases in both depressive and eating disorder symptoms[b]	
		Significant decrease (12 studies)	No significant decrease (15 studies)	Significant decrease (11 studies)	No significant decrease (16 studies)
Participant age [mean years, (SD)]	14.4-46.5	27.2 (9.8)	28.7 (10.5)	25.4 (8.8)	33.3 (10.7)
Number of sessions[mean (SD)]	4-28	7.1 (2.7)	10.1 (7.1)	6.7 (2.4)	10.4 (7.1)
Initial depressive symptoms percentile rank [mean rank(SD)][c]	55-99	88.1 (6.9)	85.4 (13.4)	87.1 (7.8)	86.3 (13.1)
Use of a screening cut-off score , N (%)		7 (58%)	10 (67%)	6 (55%)	11 (69%)
Face to face format, N (%)		8 (67%)	10 (67%)	9 (82%)	9 (56%)
CBT theoretical framework, N (%)		9 (75%)	8 (53%)	8 (73%)	9 (56%)
Content targeting negative emotions and cognitions, N (%)		9 (75%)	10 (37%)	9 (82%)	10 (62%)

[a]For the 12 studies that found significant decreases in depressive symptoms, and the 15 that found no significant decrease, the mean age of participants, the mean depressive symptoms percentile rank at baseline, and the number of studies using a cut-off score, face-to face format, CBT framework, and content targeting emotions and cognitions are presented.

[b]The same information as in column [a]is provided for the 11 studies that found significant decreases in both depressive and eating disorder symptoms, and the 16 that did not.

[c]Higher rank indicates that the participants in the study reported higher initial levels of depression.

authors have suggested that individuals suffering from eating disorder symptoms may experience depressive symptoms due to the burden of the illness [5]. However, the finding that the improvement of eating disorder symptomatology was not robustly associated with improvement in depressive symptoms, suggests this may not be the only mechanism accounting for the comorbidity and supports theories highlighting common etiological factors [10].

Overall, our proposed moderating factors were not predictive of success in decreasing depressive symptoms. One potential explanation for this failure is that we lacked statistical power due to using dichotomous variables as outcomes and for many moderators, or that the continuous variables assessed lacked variability. However, it might also be that variables other than those assessed in these studies, predict intervention effects on depressive symptoms. Our finding did reveal a trend-level finding regarding number of sessions, with shorter interventions revealing a higher likelihood of decreasing both eating disorder and depressive symptoms. This finding is consistent with those of meta-analytic reviews of interventions targeting depressive symptoms among children and adolescents [77]. These authors hypothesized that engagement may be higher with shorter programs, accounting for the stronger effects.

Our study was limited by some aspects of the available data. We used participant recruitment criteria (self-selected versus screened) as a proxy for eating disorder severity in part due to the wide variability in eating disorder instruments used and the lack of available normative data for some of those instruments. Using a more sensitive measure of eating disorder severity might have produced different results. Furthermore, while some studies provided rates of diagnosable depression in their sample of baseline, rates of depression at post-test were not available, precluding examination of decreases in diagnosable depression.

Nevertheless, these findings reveal the gap in knowledge and practice regarding the treatment of concurrent eating disorder and depressive symptoms and suggest some directions for future work:

(1) Increasing our understanding of the course of depressive symptoms in relation to eating disorder symptoms during interventions might help clarify the mechanism of change in depressive symptoms and identify individuals benefiting less from the intervention effects on depressive symptoms.

(2) Exploring participants' experience of the causes of depressive symptoms, in particular as related or unrelated to their eating disorder symptoms, would contribute to increasing our understanding of the partial success of eating disorder interventions in decreasing concurrent eating disorder and depressive symptoms.

(3) The development and evaluation of depression-specific modules in eating disorder interventions would provide evidence of increased efficacy in decreasing depressive symptoms.

(4) Including measures of eating disorder symptoms in interventions primarily targeting depressive symptoms could further inform interventions for these comorbid concerns, and contribute to greater treatment efficiency.

Conclusions

Eating disorder and depressive symptoms are frequently comorbid and, in recognition of this, eating disorder interventions have often assessed depressive symptoms. The effect indicated prevention and early intervention programs on depressive symptoms is somewhat limited, however, and the characteristics of successful interventions are unclear. Further efforts are required to develop interventions that are successful in decreasing both eating disorder and depressive symptoms in order to increase treatment efficiency and the maintenance of therapeutic effects.

Competing interests

The authors declare that they have no competing interests.

Authors' contributions

RR conducted the literature search, data extraction and analysis, and prepared the manuscript. SP reviewed data extraction and interpretation, and contributed to writing of manuscript. Both authors read and approved the final manuscript.

Authors' information

Rachel F Rodgers this work was conducted as a Honorary Visiting Academic at La Trobe University.

Acknowledgements

The publication costs of this paper were supported by *beyondblue*. The authors are responsible for all content.

Author details

[1]Department of Counseling and Applied Educational Psychology, Northeastern University, Boston, USA. [2]Laboratoire de Stress Traumatique, Universite Paul Sabatier, Toulouse, France. [3]La Trobe University, Melbourne, Australia.

References

1. Berkman ND, Lohr KN, Bulik CM: **Outcomes of eating disorders: a systematic review of the literature.** *Int J Eat Disord* 2007, **40:**293–309.
2. Hudson JI, Hiripi E, Pope HG Jr, Kessler RC: **The prevalence and correlates of eating disorders in the National Comorbidity Survey Replication.** *Biol Psychiatry* 2007, **61:**348–358.
3. Masheb RM, Grilo CM: **Examination of predictors and moderators for self-help treatments of binge-eating disorder.** *J Consult Clin Psychol* 2008, **76**(5):900–904.
4. Von Brachel R, H√∂tzel K, Hirschfeld G, Rieger E, Schmidt U, Kosfelder J, Hechler T, Schulte D, Vocks S: **Internet-based motivation program for women with eating disorders: eating disorder pathology and depressive mood predict dropout.** *J Med Internet Res* 2014, **16:**e92.
5. Stice E, Hayward C, Cameron RP, Killen JD, Taylor CB: **Body-image and eating disturbances predict onset of depression among female adolescents: a longitudinal study.** *J Abnorm Psychol* 2000, **109:**438–444.
6. Stice E, Presnell K, Spangler D: **Risk factors for binge eating onset in adolescent girls: a 2-year prospective investigation.** *Health Psychol* 2002, **21:**131–138.
7. Presnell K, Stice E, Seidel A, Madeley MC: **Depression and eating pathology: prospective reciprocal relations in adolescents.** *Clin Psychol Psychother* 2009, **16:**357–365.
8. Wade TD, Bulik CM, Neale M, Kendler KS: **Anorexia nervosa and major depression: shared genetic and environmental risk factors.** *Am J Psychiatry* 2000, **157:**469–471.
9. Mangweth B, Hudson J, Pope H, Hausmann A, De Col C, Laird N, Beibl W, Tsuang M: **Family study of the aggregation of eating disorders and mood disorders.** *Psychol Med* 2003, **33:**1319–1323.
10. Bulik CM: **Anxiety, Depression, and Eating Disorders.** In *Eating Disorders and Obesity: A Comprehensive Handbook.* 2nd edition. Edited by Fairburn CG, Brownell KD. ; 2002:193–198.
11. Kaye W: **Neurobiology of anorexia and bulimia nervosa.** *Physiol Behav* 2008, **94:**121–135.
12. Cooper MJ: **Cognitive theory in anorexia nervosa and bulimia nervosa: progress, development and future directions.** *Clin Psychol Rev* 2005, **25:**511–531.
13. Benas JS, Gibb BE: **Weight-related teasing, dysfunctional cognitions, and symptoms of depression and eating disturbances.** *Cogn Ther Res* 2008, **32**(2):143–160.
14. Cooper MJ: **Beliefs and their relationship to eating attitudes and depressive symptoms in men.** *Eat Behav* 2006, **7:**423–426.
15. Aldao A, Nolen-Hoeksema S, Schweizer S: **Emotion-regulation strategies across psychopathology: a meta-analytic review.** *Clin Psychol Rev* 2010, **30:**217–237.
16. Fredrickson BL, Roberts TÄ: **Objectification theory.** *Psychol Women Q* 1997, **21:**173–206.
17. Tiggemann M, Kuring JK: **The role of body objectification in disordered eating and depressed mood.** *Br J Clin Psychol* 2004, **43:**299–311.
18. Gilbert S, Thompson JK: **Feminist explanations of the development of eating disorders: common themes, research findings, and methodological issues.** *Clin Psychol Sci Pract* 1996, **3:**183–202.
19. Stice E, Shaw H, Marti CN: **A meta-analytic review of eating disorder prevention programs: encouraging findings.** *Ann Rev Clin Psychol* 2007, **3:**207–231.
20. Stice E, Rohde P, Shaw H, Gau J: **An effectiveness trial of a selected dissonance-based eating disorder prevention program for female high school students: long-term effects.** *J Consult Clin Psychol* 2011, **79:**500–508.
21. Stice E, Ragan J: **A preliminary controlled evaluation of an eating disturbance psychoeducational intervention for college students.** *Int J Eat Disord* 2002, **31:**159–171.
22. Whitty P, Gilbody S: **NICE, but will they help people with depression? The new national institute for clinical excellence depression guidelines.** *Br J Psychiatry* 2005, **186:**177–178.
23. Moher D, Liberati A, Tetzlaff J, Altman DG: **Preferred reporting items for systematic reviews and meta-analyses: the PRISMA statement.** *PLoS Med* 2009, **6:**e1000097.
24. Medicine NRCalo: *Preventing Mental, Emotional, and Behavioral Disorders Among Young People: Progress and Possibilities.* Washington DC: The National Academic Press; 2009.
25. Wilson GT, Vitousek KM, Loeb KL: **Stepped care treatment for eating disorders.** *J Consult Clin Psychol* 2000, **68:**564–572.
26. Crawford J, Cayley C, Lovibond PF, Wilson PH, Hartley C: **Percentile norms and accompanying interval estimates from an Australian general adult population sample for self-report mood scales (BAI, BDI, CRSD, CES-D, DASS, DASS-21, STAI-X, STAI-Y, SRDS, and SRAS).** *Aust Psychol* 2011, **46:**3–14.
27. Slade T, Grove R, Burgess P: **Kessler psychological distress scale: normative data from the 2007 Australian national survey of mental health and wellbeing.** *Aust N Z J Psychiatry* 2011, **45:**308–316.
28. Beck AT, Ward C, Mendelson M: **Beck depression inventory (BDI).** *Arch Gen Psychiatry* 1961, **4:**561–571.
29. Radloff LS: **The CES-D scale a self-report depression scale for research in the general population.** *Appl Psychol Meas* 1977, **1:**385–401.
30. Kaufman J, Birmaher B, Brent D, Rao U, Flynn C, Moreci P, Williamson D, Ryan N: **Schedule for affective disorders and schizophrenia for school-age children-present and lifetime version (K-SADS-PL): initial reliability and validity data.** *J Am Acad Child Adolesc Psychiatry* 1997, **36:**980–988.
31. Kessler RC, Andrews G, Colpe LJ, Hiripi E, Mroczek DK, Normand S-LT, Walters EE, Zaslavsky AM: **Short screening scales to monitor population prevalences and trends in non-specific psychological distress.** *Psychol Med* 2002, **32:**959–976.
32. Zigmond AS, Snaith RP: **The hospital anxiety and depression scale.** *Acta Psychiatr Scand* 1983, **67:**361–370.
33. Alloway SC, Toth EL, McCargar LJ: **Effectiveness of a group psychoeducation program for the treatment of subclinical disordered eating in women with type 1 diabetes.** *Can J Diet Pract Res* 2000, **62:**188–192.
34. Banasiak SJ, Paxton SJ, Hay P: **Guided self-help for bulimia nervosa in primary care: a randomized controlled trial.** *Psychol Med* 2005, **35:**1283–1294.

35. Bearman SK, Stice E, Chase A: **Evaluation of an intervention targeting both depressive and bulimic pathology: a randomized prevention trial.** *Behav Ther* 2003, **34**:277–293.
36. Carrard I, Crépin C, Rouget P, Lam T, Golay A, Van der Linden M: **Randomised controlled trial of a guided self-help treatment on the internet for binge eating disorder.** *Behav Res Ther* 2011, **49**:482–491.
37. Carrard I, Crépin C, Rouget P, Lam T, van der Linden M, Alain Golay A: **Acceptance and efficacy of a guided Internet self-help treatment program for obese patients with binge eating disorder.** *Clin Pract Epidemiol Ment Health* 2011, **7**:8–18.
38. Carter JC, Olmsted MP, Kaplan AS, McCabe RE, Mills JS, Aimé A: **Self-help for bulimia nervosa: a randomized controlled trial.** *Am J Psychiatry* 2003, **160**:973–978.
39. Fichter M, Cebulla M, Quadflieg N, Naab S: **Guided self-help for binge eating/purging anorexia nervosa before inpatient treatment.** *Psychother Res* 2008, **18**:594–603.
40. Grilo CM, Masheb RM: **A randomized controlled comparison of guided self-help cognitive behavioral therapy and behavioral weight loss for binge eating disorder.** *Behav Res Ther* 2005, **43**:1509–1525.
41. Grilo CM, White MA, Gueorguieva R, Barnes RD, Masheb RM: **Self-help for binge eating disorder in primary care: a randomized controlled trial with ethnically and racially diverse obese patients.** *Behav Res Ther* 2013, **51**:855–861.
42. Heinicke BE, Paxton SJ, McLean SA, Wertheim EH: **Internet-delivered targeted group intervention for body dissatisfaction and disordered eating in adolescent girls: a randomized controlled trial.** *J Abnorm Child Psychol* 2007, **35**:379–391.
43. Jacobi C, Völker U, Trockel MT, Taylor CB: **Effects of an internet-based intervention for subthreshold eating disorders: a randomized controlled trial.** *Behav Res Ther* 2012, **50**:93–99.
44. Ljotsson B, Lundin C, Mitsell K, Carlbring P, Ramklint M, Ghaderi A: **Remote treatment of bulimia nervosa and binge eating disorder: a randomized trial of Internet-assisted cognitive behavioural therapy.** *Behav Res Ther* 2007, **45**:649–661.
45. McLean SA, Paxton SJ, Wertheim EH: **A body image and disordered eating intervention for women in midlife: a randomized controlled trial.** *J Consult Clin Psychol* 2011, **79**:751–758.
46. Mitchell KS, Mazzeo SE, Rausch SM, Cooke KL: **Innovative interventions for disordered eating: evaluating dissonance-based and yoga interventions.** *Int J Eat Disord* 2007, **40**:120–128.
47. O'Brien KM, LeBow MD: **Reducing maladaptive weight management practices: developing a psychoeducational intervention program.** *Eat Behav* 2007, **8**:195–210.
48. Paxton SJ, McLean SA, Gollings EK, Faulkner C, Wertheim EH: **Comparison of face-to-face and internet interventions for body image and eating problems in adult women: an RCT.** *Int J Eat Disord* 2007, **40**:692–704.
49. Robinson P, Serfaty M: **Getting better byte by byte: a pilot randomised controlled trial of email therapy for bulimia nervosa and binge eating disorder.** *Eur Eat Disord Rev* 2008, **16**:84–93.
50. Sánchez-Ortiz V, Munro C, Stahl D, House J, Startup H, Treasure J, Williams C, Schmidt U: **A randomized controlled trial of internet-based cognitive-behavioural therapy for bulimia nervosa or related disorders in a student population.** *Psychol Med* 2011, **41**:407–417.
51. Stice E, Butryn ML, Rohde P, Shaw H, Marti CN: **An effectiveness trial of a new enhanced dissonance eating disorder prevention program among female college students.** *Behav Res Ther* 2013, **51**:862–871.
52. Stice E, Orjada K, Tristan J: **Trial of a psychoeducational eating disturbance intervention for college women: a replication and extension.** *Int J Eat Disord* 2006, **39**:233–239.
53. Stice E, Rohde P, Gau J, Shaw H: **An effectiveness trial of a dissonance-based eating disorder prevention program for high-risk adolescents girls.** *J Consult Clin Psychol* 2009, **77**:825–834.
54. Stice E, Rohde P, Durant S, Shaw H: **A preliminary trial of a prototype internet dissonance-based eating disorder prevention program for young women with body image concerns.** *J Consult Clin Psychol* 2012, **80**:907–916.
55. Stice E, Rohde P, Shaw H, Marti CN: **Efficacy trial of a selective prevention program targeting both eating disorder symptoms and unhealthy weight gain among female college students.** *J Consult Clin Psychol* 2012, **80**:164–170.
56. Stice E, Rohde P, Durant S, Shaw H, Wade E: **Effectiveness of peer-led dissonance-based eating disorder prevention groups: results from two randomized pilot trials.** *Behav Res Ther* 2013, **51**:197–206.
57. Striegel-Moore RH, Wilson GT, DeBar L, Perrin N, Lynch F, Rosselli F, Kraemer HC: **Cognitive behavioral guided self-help for the treatment of recurrent binge eating.** *J Consult Clin Psychol* 2010, **78**:312–321.
58. Taylor CB, Bryson S, Luce KH, Cunning D, Doyle AC, Abascal LB, Rockwell R, Dev P, Winzelberg AJ, Wilfley DE: **Prevention of eating disorders in at-risk college-age women.** *Arch Gen Psychiatry* 2006, **63**:881–888.
59. Gormally J, Black S, Daston S, Rardin D: **The assessment of binge eating severity among obese persons.** *Addict Behav* 1982, **7**:47–55.
60. Rosen JC, Srebnik D, Saltzberg E, Wendt S: **Development of a body image avoidance questionnaire.** *Psychol Assess J Consult Clin Psychol* 1991, **3**:32–37.
61. Henderson M, Freeman CP: **A self-rating scale for bulimia. The'BITE'.** *Br J Psychiatry* 1987, **150**:18–24.
62. Berscheid E, Walster E, Bohrnstedt G: **The happy American body: a survey report.** *Psychol Today* 1973, **7**:119–131.
63. Cooper PJ, Taylor MJ, Cooper Z, Fairbum CG: **The development and validation of the body shape questionnaire.** *Int J Eat Disord* 1987, **6**:485–494.
64. Thelen MH, Farmer J, Wonderlich S, Smith M: **A revision of the bulimia test: the BULIT—R.** *Psychol Assess J Consult Clin Psychol* 1991, **3**:119–124.
65. Van Strien T, Frijters JE, Van Staveren WA, Defares PB, Deurenberg P: **The predictive validity of the Dutch restrained eating scale.** *Int J Eat Disord* 1986, **5**:747–755.
66. Garner DM, Garfinkel PE: **The eating attitudes test: an index of the symptoms of anorexia nervosa.** *Psychol Med* 1979, **9**:273–279.
67. Stice E, Telch CF, Rizvi SL: **Development and validation of the eating disorder diagnostic scale: a brief self-report measure of anorexia, bulimia, and binge-eating disorder.** *Psychol Assess* 2000, **12**:123–131.
68. Fairburn CG, Beglin SJ: **Assessment of eating disorders: interview or self-report questionnaire?** *Int J Eat Disord* 1994, **16**:363–370.
69. Garner DM, Olmstead MP, Polivy J: **Development and validation of a multidimensional eating disorder inventory for anorexia nervosa and bulimia.** *Int J Eat Disord* 1983, **2**:15–34.
70. Stice E, Schupak-Neuberg E, Shaw HE, Stein RI: **Relation of media exposure to eating disorder symptomatology: an examination of mediating mechanisms.** *J Abnorm Psychol* 1994, **103**:836–840.
71. Ruggiero L, Williamson D, Davis C, Schlundt DG, Carey MP: **Forbidden food survey: measure of bulimic's anticipated emotional reactions to specific foods.** *Addict Behav* 1988, **13**:267–274.
72. Svanborg P, Åsberg M: **A new self-rating scale for depression and anxiety states based on the comprehensive psychopathological rating scale.** *Acta Psychiatr Scand* 1994, **89**:21–28.
73. Thompson JK, van den Berg P, Roehrig M, Guarda AS, Heinberg LJ: **The sociocultural attitudes towards appearance scale-3 (SATAQ-3): development and validation.** *Int J Eat Disord* 2004, **35**:293–304.
74. Fichter MM, Herpertz S, Quadflieg N, Herpertz-Dahlmann B: **Structured interview for anorexic and bulimic disorders for DSM-IV and ICD-10: updated (third) revision.** *Int J Eat Disord* 1998, **24**:227–249.
75. Stunkard AJ, Messick S: **The three-factor eating questionnaire to measure dietary restraint, disinhibition and hunger.** *J Psychosom Res* 1985, **29**:71–83.
76. Jacobi C, Abascal L, Taylor CB: **Screening for eating disorders and high-risk behavior: caution.** *Int J Eat Disord* 2004, **36**:280–295.
77. Stice E, Shaw H, Bohon C, Marti CN, Rohde P: **A meta-analytic review of depression prevention programs for children and adolescents: factors that predict magnitude of intervention effects.** *J Consult Clin Psychol* 2009, **77**:486–503.

Loss of control eating with and without the undue influence of weight or shape on self-evaluation: evidence from an adolescent population

Carmel Harrison[1*], Jonathan Mond[1,2], Caroline Bentley[1], Kassandra Gratwick-Sarll[1], Elizabeth Rieger[1] and Bryan Rodgers[3]

Abstract

Background: The overvaluation of weight and/or shape ("overvaluation"), a diagnostic criterion for anorexia nervosa and bulimia nervosa, is increasingly supported for inclusion in the Diagnostic and Statistical Manual of Mental Disorders 5th Edition (DSM-5) criteria of binge eating disorder (BED). However, current evidence has been largely confined to adult populations. The current study aims to examine the status of overvaluation among adolescents with loss of control (LOC) eating recruited from a large, population-based sample.

Method: Subgroups of female adolescents – LOC eating with overvaluation (n = 30); LOC eating without overvaluation (n = 58); obese no LOC eating ("obese control") (n = 36); and "normal-weight control" (normal-weight, no LOC eating) (n = 439) – recruited from secondary schools within the Australian Capital Territory (ACT) were compared on measures of eating disorder psychopathology, general psychological distress and quality of life.

Results: Participants in the LOC eating with overvaluation subgroup reported significantly higher levels of eating disorder psychopathology than all other groups, while levels did not differ between participants in the LOC eating without overvaluation and obese control subgroups. On measures of distress and quality of life there were no significant differences between LOC eating with and without overvaluation subgroups. Both reported significantly greater distress and quality of life impairment than normal-weight controls. LOC eating with overvaluation participants had significantly higher levels of distress and quality of life impairment than obese controls, whereas scores on these measures did not differ between LOC eating without overvaluation and obese control subgroups.

Conclusion: The results suggest that the presence of overvaluation among adolescents with LOC eating indicates a more severe disorder in terms of eating disorder psychopathology, however may not indicate distress and disability as clearly as it does among adults with BED.

Keywords: Binge eating disorder, Loss of control eating, Diagnostic criteria, Overvaluation, Adolescents

* Correspondence: Carmel.Hill@anu.edu.au
[1]Research School of Psychology, Australian National University, Canberra, Australia
Full list of author information is available at the end of the article

Background

The overvaluation of weight and/or shape ("overvaluation") is described as a dysfunctional system of self-worth, such that the individual evaluates his or her self-worth based primarily or solely on their weight and/or shape [1]. Findings from both community and clinical samples in adults suggest that, among individuals with binge eating disorder (BED) or variants of BED, overvaluation indicates a significantly more severe disorder in terms of eating disorder symptomatology, comorbid psychopathology, and psychosocial impairment [2-5]. Conclusions from such findings suggest that overvaluation should be incorporated among Diagnostic and Statistical Manual of Mental Disorders 5th Edition (DSM-5) criteria for BED, either as a diagnostic specifier or a diagnostic criterion, inline with the other formal eating disorders anorexia nervosa and bulimia nervosa [6-8]. Concerns have been expressed that the absence of overvaluation in the diagnosis of BED may hinder both clinical practice and epidemiological research [9].

A conspicuous limitation of the existing literature however, is that it is almost entirely confined to adult populations [4,5,7]. Given that binge eating is common among children and adolescents, and given the need to develop classification schemes that take in to account eating disturbances across the lifespan, this is problematic [10]. Further, it is increasingly recognised that the DSM-5 definition of binge eating, which requires both consumption of an objectively large amount of food and loss of control over eating, may be problematic in children and adolescents, such that loss of control over eating – but not the amount of food consumed – is key in this population [11,12]. Hence, an alternative diagnostic criterion for BED in children and adolescents, in which the term loss of control (LOC) eating is used in preference to binge eating, has been suggested [11,12].

To our knowledge, only two studies have examined the status of overvaluation in young people with LOC eating [13,14]. Hilbert and Czaja found, in a community based study of children (aged 8–13 years), that overvaluation successfully identified children experiencing high recurrent LOC eating as a more severe presentation, in terms of eating disorder psychopathology, depressive symptoms and behavioural problems than all other groups [13]. Further, overvaluation aided in delineating eating defined as "normal", and LOC eating among children, thereby enhancing the specificity of classification [13]. Goldschmidt et al. compared overweight youth with LOC eating with ("moderate") and without ("minimal or no") overvaluation, along with comparison groups of overweight youth with no LOC eating with and without overvaluation, on measures of eating disorder psychopathology, behavioural problems and self-esteem [14]. Youth with LOC eating and overvaluation reported greater eating disorder symptomatology than all other groups, whereas youth with LOC eating without overvaluation were comparable to the overweight comparison group of no LOC eating, but reporting overvaluation. Further, youth reporting LOC eating with overvaluation experienced lower self-esteem than the overweight controls without overvaluation, whilst no other significant differences were found between groups on this measure. Both youth experiencing LOC eating with and without overvaluation reported significantly more behavioural problems than overweight controls regardless of overvaluation status. However, overvaluation did not distinguish between LOC eating subgroups on outcome measures of self-esteem and behavioural problems. The authors concluded that overvaluation failed to indicate a more severe symptomatology in adolescence [14].

One reason why anticipated differences may not have emerged in Goldschmidt et al.'s study, is that LOC eating was deemed to be present if participants reported one or more episodes of this behaviour in the past three months, as opposed to the DSM-5 binge frequency criterion for BED of one or more episodes per week [14]. Given the use of this relatively liberal criterion for "regular LOC eating", it is possible that LOC eating in Goldschmidt et al.'s study was not severe enough for differences between groups to emerge. The use of overweight – as opposed to obese – comparison groups could have further minimised group differences. Finally, Hilbert and Czaja's study included youth up to age 13 years, thus Goldschmidt et al.'s study is the only study to our knowledge, investigating overvaluation in BED and variants of BED within adolescents aged 13–18 years. Given recent interest in developing diagnostic criteria for eating disorders that are applicable across the lifespan [10], and observed differences between children and adults in terms of overeating behaviour [11,12], the lack of research addressing the status of overvaluation among adolescents with LOC eating is problematic.

The aim of the present study was, therefore, to examine the status of overvaluation in relation to LOC eating in an adolescent sample. Specifically, we sought to compare levels of eating disorder psychopathology, general psychological distress and impairment in psychosocial functioning, between four subgroups of female adolescents who: (1) reported LOC eating with overvaluation; (2) reported LOC eating without overvaluation; (3) were obese individuals without LOC eating (obese controls); and (4) were normal weight without LOC eating (normal-weight controls). In view of the paucity of existing evidence, our only hypothesis was that adolescents with LOC eating who overvalued their weight or shape would have significantly higher levels of eating disorder psychopathology than obese controls and normal-weight controls.

Method

Study design and recruitment of participants

Participants were recruited as part of the *ACT Schools Mental Health Literacy Survey*, a cross-sectional study examining eating-disordered behaviour among secondary school students attending schools within the Australian Capital Territory (ACT) region of Australia (population of approx. 370,000 in 2012), which includes the city of Canberra [15]. The recruitment procedures have been detailed previously [16]. In brief, participants were recruited from 12 ACT schools, which varied in terms of type (Government, Independent, and Catholic), location and numbers of students at the school. The study was presented as an opportunity for schools to promote "mental health literacy" and no remuneration was provided. Consent to participate was required from both students and their parents. The study design and methods were approved by the Australian National University Human Research Ethics Committee (2011/573), the ACT Department of Education and Training (2011/00468-8) and the Catholic Education Office (R106903).

All students in classes selected for participation who attended class on the day(s) assigned for data collection were invited to complete a printed, self-report questionnaire, in their classrooms, under the supervision of a teacher and one or more members of the research team. The questionnaire included measures of eating disorder symptoms, general psychological distress, quality of life and basic demographic information. Body mass index (BMI: kg/m^2) was calculated from self-reported height and weight [16]. Classification of weight status was based on the age-and-gender-specific BMI cut-points recommended by the Centers for Disease Control and Prevention (CDC) [17].

Completed questionnaires were received from 1749 students, a participation rate of 78.7% of all students invited to participate. Data for nine participants who were less than 12 years of age or greater than 18 years and a further 70 participants (4.0%) who were found to have unacceptably high levels of missing data or implausible data were excluded. The final sample therefore comprised of 1670 students aged 12–18 years. Of these, 1135 (68.0%) were female, 531 were male and 4 did not indicate their gender. The overrepresentation of female students, which reflected greater perceived relevance of the study material among the principals of all-girls schools and/or among the heads of faculties (e.g. psychology) in which female students were over-represented, was anticipated and was considered advantageous in addressing study aims that dictated relatively large numbers of participants with eating disorder symptoms [18]. The mean (SD) ages of male and female participants were, respectively, 14.85 (1.70) years and 15.51 (1.63) years. The sample comprised of 3.6% of all male secondary school students in the ACT in 2012 and 7.8% of all female secondary school students [19]. Reflecting the demographic profile of the ACT region, [20] the vast majority of participants were born in Australia (88.3%) and had English as a first language (90.4%).

Participants in the current study were the 1135 female adolescents. Male participants were excluded because the comparatively low prevalence of LOC eating among males precluded meaningful subgroups analysis. Although it would have been possible to combine male and female participants, this course was not taken because the goal of the current study was to extend prior research in women with BED and variants of BED to an adolescent population [7] and because, in the absence of any prior research on the status of overvaluation in males with BED or variants of BED, it was unclear how the inclusion of males might affect the findings.

Study measures

Eating Disorder Examination Questionnaire (EDE-Q)

The EDE-Q is a 36-item self-report measure that assesses the occurrence and frequency of eating disorder features during the past 28 days [21]. A global score is derived from 22 items assessing core attitudinal features, namely, dietary restraint, concerns about eating, weight concern and shape concern. Scores on these items range from "0" to "6", with higher scores indicating higher symptom levels [21]. Cronbach's alpha for the global score in the current study sample was 0.97.

Remaining items of the EDE-Q assess the occurrence and frequency of specific eating disorder behaviours, namely, binge eating and the use of self-induced vomiting, laxative misuse and excessive exercise, as a means of controlling weight or shape. For the current study, an additional item assessing the occurrence of subjective binge eating episodes, namely, episodes of perceived overeating in which a loss of control is experienced but the amount of food consumed is not unusually large, was included. The inclusion of this item permitted the assessment of LOC eating, this being defined as the occurrence of objective and/or subjective binge eating episodes [16]. As in previous studies [22,23], minor changes to the wording of some EDE-Q items were made in order to ensure the suitability of the instrument for use in an adolescent population.

Assessment of psychosocial functioning

Psychosocial functioning was assessed using measures of general psychological distress and quality of life as detailed below.

Kessler (10-item) psychological distress scale (K-10)

The K-10 is a 10-item measure of general psychological distress developed for use as a screening instrument in epidemiological studies of mental disorders and widely used for this purpose [24,25]. In Australia, it is also used as an outcome measure for individuals treated in community mental health services and for routine population health monitoring [26]. Participants are required to indicate the frequency or occurrence of 10 symptoms of anxiety or depression during the past four weeks. Responses are scored on a five-point, Likert-type scale ranging from "none of the time" ("1") to "all of the time" ("5"). Total scores therefore range from 10 to 50, with higher scores indicating higher levels of distress. The K-10 has very good psychometric properties and is suitable for use in both adult and adolescent populations [24,25,27,28]. Cronbach's alpha for participants in the current study sample was 0.91.

Pediatric quality of life inventory (15-item) (PedsQL™ 4.0 SF15)

The *PedsQL™ 4.0 SF15* is a 15-item, self-report, generic measure of quality of life developed specifically for use in paediatric populations [29,30]. Participants are asked how true each of a series of 15 statements were for them during the past four weeks, with items designed to address individuals' perceived functioning in each of four domains: physical health (5 items); emotional well-being (4 items); social functioning (3 items); and academic (school) functioning (3 items). Responses are scored on a five-point, Likert-type scale ranging from "never" ("0") to "always" ("4"), with higher scores indicating poorer perceived functioning in the domain concerned. In the current study, domain scores were calculated as mean scores of the specific items comprising each domain. The *PedsQL™ 4.0 SF15* has been found to be a reliable and valid measure of quality of life in young people, with psychometric properties comparable to those of the original (23-item) instrument [29,30]. Cronbach alphas in the current study sample ranged from 0.80 (physical health subscale) to 0.89 (total score).

Creation of study subgroups

Consistent with the study aims, four subgroups of participants were created: (1) LOC eating with overvaluation; (2) LOC eating without overvaluation; (3) obese no LOC eating (obese controls); and (4) normal-weight no LOC eating (normal-weight controls).

Given that LOC eating, regardless of the amount of food consumed, indicates eating disorder and general psychopathology in youth [11,12], the current study, inline with prior research [14], focused on LOC eating. Consistent with DSM-5 criteria for binge frequency [31], "LOC eating" was defined as at least weekly LOC episodes during the past four weeks. Further, and also consistent with the DSM-5 criteria for BED, inclusion in the LOC subgroups required that regular LOC eating occurred in the absence of the regular use of extreme weight-control behaviours. In the absence of any agreed-upon operational definition of "regular extreme weight-control behaviours", a conservative threshold, namely, twice per month, was employed in order to clearly distinguish participants in the LOC subgroups from individuals with a sub-threshold form of bulimia nervosa [32]. Thus, regular purging was defined as self-induced vomiting or misuse of laxatives or diuretics as a means of controlling weight or shape at least twice in the past 28 days. Regular extreme dietary restriction was defined, using an item of the EDE-Q, as going for long periods (8 or more waking hours) without eating anything at all as a means of controlling weight or shape more than 1–5 times in the past 28 days, and regular excessive exercise was defined as exercising in a "driven" or "compulsive" way as a means of controlling weight or shape at least twice in the past 28 days. These definitions have been used in previous, population-based studies of young women [7,33].

Participants with LOC eating were separated into those with and without overvaluation on the basis of responses to the two EDE-Q items that assess this construct, namely, "Over the past four weeks, how much has your *weight* influenced how you think about (judge) yourself as a person?" ("importance of weight") and "Over the past four weeks, how much has your *shape* influenced how you think about (judge) yourself as a person?" ("importance of shape"). Consistent with previous research employing the EDE-Q within community samples [4,5], participants who scored 5 or 6 on either (or both) of these items were considered to have overvaluation. Scores of this magnitude indicate that self-evaluation was influenced by their weight or shape either "markedly" (score of "6") or "more than moderately but less than markedly" ("5"). Items of the EDE-Q assessing overvaluation were omitted when comparing subgroups with respect to overall levels of eating disorder psychopathology as measured by the EDE-Q global score, thus creating a "revised" global score for the purpose of comparisons involving this outcome [7].

"Obese controls" were participants with a BMI above the 90th percentile for their age and sex [17] and who did not report any episodes of LOC eating during the past 28 days. "Normal-weight controls" were participants whose BMI was between the 5th and 85th percentile for their age and sex [17] and who reported no episodes of either LOC eating or extreme weight-control behaviours during the past 28 days. Participants who were underweight (BMI <5th percentile) were excluded from this subgroup. No attempt was made to exclude participants with overvaluation from the control groups since this would have detracted from the validity of comparisons between these groups and the LOC eating groups.

Of the 1,135 participants, 422 (37.2%) were classified as normal-weight controls, 36 (3.2%) were classified as obese controls, and 88 (7.8%) were classified as LOC eating. Among participants in the LOC eating subgroup, 30 (34.1%) overvalued their weight or shape while the remaining 58 participants (65.9%) did not have overvaluation.

Statistical analysis

One-way analysis of variance (ANOVA) was used to compare scores on measures of eating disorder psychopathology (EDE-Q revised global score), general psychological distress (K-10), and quality of life (*PedsQL™ 4.0 SF15*) between groups. Post-hoc tests were used to identify the source of any statistically significant F values. In view of the small subgroup sizes and small number of outcome variables, no adjustment for multiple comparisons was employed. A significance level of 0.05 was used for all tests and all analysis was conducted using the IBM SPSS statistical software package (version 20.0).

Results

As would be expected, differences between groups were observed with respect to BMI ($F_{(3,533)} = 156.65$, $p < .05$), whereas there were no differences between groups with respect to age, first language, country of birth, residential postcode or school type (all $p > .05$).

Results of the ANOVA appear in Table 1. As can be seen, significant differences between groups were observed for all outcome variables: EDE-Q (revised) global score ($F_{(3,542)} = 70.16$, $p < .05$), K-10 ($F_{(3,542)} = 15.70$, $p < .05$), and all subscales of the *PedsQL™ 4.0 SF15* ($F_{(3,541)} = 20.71$, $p < .05$). Post-hoc tests indicated that participants with LOC eating and overvaluation had higher EDE-Q global scores than women with LOC eating in the absence of overvaluation ($p < .05$), while scores on this measure did not differ between participants with LOC eating in the absence of overvaluation and obese controls ($p > .05$). Normal-weight participants had lower EDE-Q global scores than participants in all other groups ($p < .05$).

There were no significant differences between LOC eating with overvaluation and LOC eating without overvaluation subgroups with respect to levels of general psychological distress or on any of the *PedsQL™ 4.0 SF15* subscales (all $p > .05$) and both of these groups had higher levels of distress, and higher scores on each of the *PedsQL™ 4.0 SF15* subscales, than normal-weight controls (all $p < .05$). Participants in the LOC eating with overvaluation subgroup had higher levels of distress, and significantly greater impairment in emotional, social and academic functioning, than obese controls (all $p < .05$), whereas scores on these measures did not differ between LOC eating without overvaluation and obese control subgroups (all $p > .05$). However both LOC eating subgroups with and without overvaluation reported significantly greater impairment on the *PedsQL™ 4.0 SF15* total than the obese control subgroup ($p < .05$), whilst there were no differences between participants in either of the LOC eating subgroups and obese control participants on the physical health subscale of the *PedsQL™ 4.0 SF15* ($p > .05$).

Table 1 Mean (SD) scores on measures of eating disorder psychopathology (EDE-Q revised global score), general psychological distress (K-10), and quality of life (*PedsQL™ 4.0 SF15*) among study subgroups

	LOC eating with overvaluation of shape/ weight (1)	LOC eating without overvaluation of shape/ weight (2)	Obese controls (3)	Healthy controls (4)			Eta squared[i]	Post hoc
n	30	58	36	422				
	Mean (SD)	Mean (SD)	Mean (SD)	Mean (SD)	F	p		
Age	15.89 (1.37)	15.72 (1.72)	15.89 (1.56)	15.36 (1.70)	2.46	.062		
BMI	23.99 (4.89)	21.16 (3.46)	29.51 (3.83)	19.90 (2.21)	156.65	.000*		
	Mean (SE)	Mean (SE)	Mean (SE)	Mean (SE)	F	p		
EDE-Q revised global	3.31 (.20)	1.80 (.13)	1.80 (.20)	.94 (.05)	70.16	.000*	0.28	1 > 2,3 > 4
K10	27.23 (1.42)	24.40 (1.09)	20.64 (1.18)	19.73 (.34)	15.70	.000*	0.08	1, 2 > 4; 1 > 3
PedsQL™ 4.0 SF15 subscales								
Emotional well-being	3.00 (.12)	2.63 (.10)	2.23 (.13)	2.20 (.04)	12.39	.000*	0.06	1, 2 > 4; 1 > 3
Social functioning	2.31 (.18)	2.13 (.13)	1.81 (.15)	1.66 (.03)	12.51	.000*	0.06	1, 2 > 4; 1 > 3
Academic functioning	3.31 (.19)	3.01 (.12)	2.60 (.18)	2.56 (.04)	9.54	.000*	0.05	1, 2 > 4; 1 > 3
Physical health	2.10 (.15)	2.10 (.12)	1.80 (.13)	1.60 (.03)	13.02	.000*	0.07	1, 2 > 4,
PedsQL™ 4.0 SF15 Total	59.43 (2.51)	64.28 (2.09)	73.06 (2.69)	75.93 (.70)	20.71	.000*	0.10	1, 2 < 3, 4

*Significant p <0.05.
[i]eta squared effect size; 0.01 = small, 0.06 = medium, 0.14 = large [34].

Discussion

Summary of main findings

The current study compared subgroups of female adolescents with LOC eating, with and without overvaluation of weight and/or shape, on measures of eating disorder psychopathology, general psychological distress, and quality of life. Subgroups of obese participants reporting no LOC eating (obese controls) and adolescents of normal weight not experiencing LOC eating (normal-weight controls) were included for comparison purposes. Participants with LOC eating and overvaluation had significantly higher levels of eating disorder psychopathology than all other subgroups, whereas participants with LOC eating in the absence of overvaluation did not differ from obese controls with respect to levels of eating disorder psychopathology. There were no significant differences between LOC eating with overvaluation and LOC eating without overvaluation subgroups on any of the other measures. Participants with LOC eating and overvaluation had significantly higher levels of distress and impairment in emotional, social and academic functioning than obese controls, whereas no such differences were observed between LOC eating without overvaluation and obese controls.

Study implications

The finding that participants with LOC eating and overvaluation had significantly higher levels of eating disorder psychopathology than all other subgroups, when taken with the finding that participants in the LOC eating without overvaluation subgroup did not differ from obese controls in this regard, aligns with findings from previous research in adult [5-7] and adolescent populations [14]. Whilst overvaluation has been recognised as a distinct construct [6], high correlations between this construct and the broader construct of weight/shape concerns, as measured by the EDE-Q, exist [1,35]. The finding that the presence of overvaluation was associated with higher EDE-Q global scores, while notable, is not surprising, given significantly greater scores on the EDE-Q might reflect, in part, this association [35]. Nevertheless, the current findings in adolescents provides further evidence that overvaluation indicates disorder severity in terms of eating disorder psychopathology among individuals with BED and variants of BED [4,7]. Further, given that adolescents with LOC eating in the absence of overvaluation had comparable levels of eating disorder psychopathology to obese control participants, also in line with previous adult research [7], the current findings provide further evidence that LOC in the absence of overvaluation may not constitute a clinically significant pattern of behaviour.

Contrary to findings in both community and clinical samples of adult females with BED and variants of BED [4,7], but consistent with the findings of Goldschmidt and colleagues in adolescent females [14], no significant differences were observed between LOC eating subgroups on measures of psycho-social impairment, namely, general psychological distress and quality of life. However, there was evidence suggestive of such differences. Whereas participants with LOC eating and overvaluation had significantly higher levels of general psychological distress and impairment in social, psychological, and academic functioning than obese controls, there were no differences between participants with LOC eating in the absence of overvaluation and obese controls on any of these measures. These findings suggest that further investigation of the correlates of LOC eating with and without overvaluation in adolescents may be warranted.

At least two explanations for the lack of clear differences in levels of distress and disability between LOC eating subgroups among adolescents might be given, should this finding prove to be replicable. First, the concept of "overvaluation" may be more difficult for young people to grasp than for adults [10,14], making it more difficult to measure and differentiate between LOC eating with and without overvaluation. Second, evidence concerning the onset of overvaluation and its relationship to the onset of LOC eating and other eating disorder behaviours is lacking [36]. If overvaluation is associated with chronicity of overeating, then its influence on young people with LOC eating might only become apparent later in life. This interpretation would be consistent with the observation, in the current study and in Goldschmidt et al.'s study [14], that the presence of overvaluation among young people with LOC eating indicates greater severity in terms of eating disorder psychopathology but not in terms of distress and disability. Further population-based research, employing a prospective study design and, if possible, interview assessment of key constructs will be needed to elucidate these different possible interpretations.

Study limitations

At least four limitations of the current study methods should be noted. First, all variables were assessed using self-report measures. While self-report assessment of psycho-social functioning is unlikely to be problematic, limitations inherent in the self-report assessment of eating-disordered behaviour are well known [21,37,38]. In particular, the occurrence and/or frequency of binge eating may be overestimated when using self-report assessment and self-report assessment of loss of control over eating may be unreliable when the amount of food consumed is not unusually large [21,37,38]. Further, whereas high correlations between self-report and interview assessment of weight/shape concerns have been observed in several studies, little is known about the validity of self-report assessment of the more specific construct of overvaluation [21,37,38]. A study of young adult women supported the validity of self-report assessment of overvaluation, when compared with interview assessment [37], but evidence in adolescents is lacking [38]. It should also be noted that the EDE-Q assesses LOC eating and other behaviours over the past 28 days, as opposed to the 3-month duration specified in DSM-5 criteria for BED [31]. It is possible that different findings would have been observed had interview assessment and/or a 3-month time frame been employed.

Second, sample size for the LOC eating and obese control subgroups (n = 30, n = 58, n = 36) was relatively small. Hence, the failure to detect significant differences between these groups may reflect, in part, a lack of statistical power. The finding that there were significant differences between LOC eating with overvaluation and obese control participants on measures of distress and quality of life, but no such differences between LOC eating without overvaluation and obese control participants, is consistent with this interpretation.

Third, the cross-sectional design of the current study precludes any inferences as to the correlates of LOC eating with and without overvaluation over time. Research employing a prospective study design is needed to examine issues such as the utility of overvaluation in predicting outcomes among adolescents with LOC eating, and its temporal stability.

Finally, as in previous community-based studies, only females were included in the current study. Although very large sample sizes would be needed to examine the status of overvaluation among adolescent males with LOC eating in a community sample, research of this kind would be of interest given that LOC eating may be relatively common in boys [16].

Strengths of the current study include the recruitment of participants from a large, population-based sample, high participation rates, the inclusion of obese control and normal-weight control groups, and the inclusion of established measures of eating disorder psychopathology, general psychological distress and quality of life.

Conclusion

The results provide further evidence that the presence of overvaluation among adolescents with LOC eating indicates a more severe disorder in terms of eating disorder psychopathology, whereas overvaluation may not indicate distress and disability as clearly as it does among adults with BED and variants of BED.

Abbreviations

BED: Binge eating disorder; LOC eating: Loss of control eating; ACT: The Australian Capital Territory.

Competing interests

The authors declare that they have no competing interests.

Authors' contributions

JM and CH designed the study, CH, CB and KG carried out data collection. CH conducted the statistical analysis and drafted the manuscript. ER, JM and BR were consulted on the statistical analysis. All authors read and approved the final manuscript.

Author details

[1]Research School of Psychology, Australian National University, Canberra, Australia. [2]Department of Psychology, Macquarie University, Sydney, Australia. [3]Australian Demographic and Social Research Institute, Australian National University, Canberra, Australia.

References

1. Fairburn CG, Cooper Z, Shafran R: **Cognitive behaviour therapy for eating disorders: a "transdiagnostic" theory and treatment.** *Behav Res Ther* 2003, **41**:509–528.
2. Grilo CM, Hrabosky JI, White MA, Allison KC, Stunkard AJ, Masheb RM: **Overvaluation of shape and weight in binge eating disorder and overweight controls: refinement of a diagnostic construct.** *J Abnorm Psychol* 2008, **117**:414–419.
3. Grilo CM, Crosby RD, Masheb RM, White MA, Peterson CB, Wonderlich SA, Engel SG, Crow SJ, Mitchell JE: **Overvaluation of shape and weight in binge eating disorder, bulimia nervosa, and sub-threshold bulimia nervosa.** *Behav Res Ther* 2009, **47**:692–696.
4. Grilo CM, Masheb RM, White MA: **Significance of overvaluation of shape/weight in binge-eating disorder: comparative study with overweight and bulimia nervosa.** *Obesity (Silver Spring)* 2010, **18**:499–504.
5. Mond JM, Hay PJ, Rodgers B, Owen C: **Recurrent binge eating with and without the "undue influence of weight or shape on self-evaluation": implications for the diagnosis of binge eating disorder.** *Behav Res Ther* 2007, **45**:929–938.
6. Grilo CM: **Why no cognitive body image feature such as overvaluation of shape/weight in the binge eating disorder diagnosis?** *Int J Eat Disord* 2013, **46**:208–211.
7. Harrison C, Mond J, Rieger E, Hay P, Rodgers B: **Correlates of binge eating with and without overvaluation of weight or shape: further evidence from a general population sample of women.** *Adv Eat Disord Theory Res Pract* 2014. in press.
8. Mond JM: **Classification of bulimic-type eating disorders: from DSM-IV to DSM-5.** *J Eat Disord* 2013, **1**:33.
9. Mond J, Star A, Hay P: **Comorbidity and Related Considerations.** In *A Clinician's Guide to Binge Eating Disorder.* Edited by Alexander J, Goldschmidt A, Le Grange DA. New York: Routledge; 2013:66–77.
10. Workgroup for classification of eating disorders in children and adolescents (WCEDCA): **Classification of child and adolescent eating disturbances.** *Int J Eat Disord* 2007, **40**:S117–S122.
11. Goldschmidt AB, Jones M, Manwaring JL, Luce KH, Osborne MI, Cunning D, Taylor KL, Celio Doyle A, Wilfley DE, Taylor CB: **The clinical significance of loss of control over eating in overweight adolescents.** *Int J Eat Disord* 2008, **4**:153–158.
12. Morgan CM, Yanovski SZ, Nguyen TT, McDuffie J, Sebring NG, Jorge MR, Keil M, Yanovski JA: **Loss of control over eating, adiposity, and psychopathology in overweight children.** *Int J Eat Disord* 2002, **31**:430–441.
13. Hilbert A, Czaja J: **Binge eating in primary school children: towards a definition of clinical significance.** *Int J Eat Disord* 2009, **42**:235–243.
14. Goldschmidt A, Wilfley DE, Eddy KT, Boutelle K, Zucker N, Peterson CB, Celio-Doyle A, Le Grange D: **Overvaluation of shape and weight among overweight children and adolescents with loss of control eating.** *Behav Res Ther* 2011, **49**:682–688.
15. Australian Bureau of Statistics: *Population by Age and Sex, Regions of Australia, 2012. (cat. no. 3235.0).* Canberra: ACT: ABS; 2013.
16. Mond J, Hall A, Bentley C, Harrison C, Gratwick-Sarll K, Lewis V: **Eating-disordered behaviour in adolescent boys: eating disorder examination questionnaire norms.** *Int J Eat Disord* 2014, **47**:335–341.
17. Kuczmarski RJ, Ogden CL, Guo SS, Grummer-Strawn LM, Flegal KM, Mei Z, Wei R, Curtin LR, Roche AF, Johnson CL: **2000 CDC growth charts for the United States: Methods and development.** *Vital Health Stat* 2002, **246**:1–190.

18. Gratwick-Sarll K, Bentley C, Harrison C, Mond J: **Poor self-recognition of disordered eating among girls with bulimic-type eating disorders: cause for concern?** *Early Interv Psychiatry* 2014. in press.
19. Education and Training Directorate, ACT Government: *ACT School Census Feb 2012.* Canberra: ACT: ACT Government; 2012.
20. Australian Bureau of Statistics: *In fACT - Statistical Information on the ACT and Region, Feb 2011 (cat. no. 1308.8).* Canberra: ACT: ABS; 2011.
21. Fairburn CG, Beglin SJ: **Assessment of eating disorders: interview or self-report questionnaire?** *Int J Eat Disord* 1994, **16:**363–370.
22. Carter JC, Stewart DA, Fairburn CG: **Eating disorder examination questionnaire: norms for young adolescent girls.** *Behav Res Ther* 2001, **39:**625–632.
23. Mond JM, Marks P, Hay PJ, Rodgers B, Kelly C, Owen C, Paxton SJ: **Mental health literacy and eating-disordered behaviour: beliefs of adolescent girls concerning the treatment of and treatment-seeking for bulimia nervosa.** *J Youth Adolesc* 2007, **36:**753–762.
24. Andrews G, Slade T: **Interpreting scores on the kessler psychological distress scale (K10).** *Aust N Z J Public Health* 2001, **25:**494–497.
25. Kessler RC, Barker PR, Colpe LJ, Epstein JF, Gfroerer JC, Hiripi E, Howes MJ, Normand ST, Manderscheid RW, Walters EE, Zaslavsky AM: **Screening for serious mental illness in the general population.** *Arch Gen Psychiatry* 2003, **60:**184–189.
26. Australian Bureau of Statistics: *Information Paper: Use of the Kessler Psychological Distress Scale in ABS Health Surveys, Australia, 2007–08 (cat. no. 4817.0.55.001).* Canberra: ACT: ABS; 2012.
27. Huang JP, Xia W, Sun CH, Zhang HY, Wu LJ: **Psychological distress and its correlates in chinese adolescents.** *Aust N Z J Psychiatry* 2009, **43:**674–681.
28. Wake M, Canterford L, Patton GC, Hesketh K, Hardy P, Williams J, Waters E, Carlin JB: **Comorbidities of overweight/obesity experienced in adolescence: longitudinal study.** *Arch Dis Child* 2010, **95:**162–168.
29. Chan KS, Mangione-Smith R, Burwinkle TM, Rosen M, Varni JW: **Reliability and validity of the short-form generic core scales and asthma module.** *Med Care* 2005, **43:**256–265.
30. Varni JW, Burwinkle TM, Seid M, Skarr D: **The PedsQL 4.0 as a pediatric population health measure: feasibility, reliability, and validity.** *Ambul Pediatr* 2003, **3:**329–341.
31. American Psychiatric Association: *Diagnostic and Statistical Manual of Mental Disorders, 5th Edition (DSM-V).* Washington DC: American Psychiatric Association; 2013.
32. Cooper Z, Fairburn CG: **Refining the definition of binge eating disorder and nonpurging bulimia nervosa.** *Int J Eat Disord* 2003, **34:**S89–S95.
33. Mond JM, Hay PJ, Rodgers B, Owen C: **Eating disorder examination questionnaire (EDE-Q): norms for young adult women.** *Behav Res Ther* 2006, **44:**53–62.
34. Cohen JW: *Statistical Power Analysis for the Behavioral Sciences.* 2nd edition. Hillsdale, NJ: Lawrence Erlbaum Associates; 1988.
35. Hay PJ: **What is an eating disorder? Implications for current and future diagnostic criteria.** *Aust N Z J Psychiatry* 2013, **47:**208–211.
36. Walsh BT: **Eating disorders in DSM-5.** *Psychiatr Ann* 2012, **42:**399–400.
37. Mond JM, Hay PJ, Rodgers B, Owen C, Beumont PJV: **Validity of the eating disorder examination questionnaire (EDE-Q) in screening for eating disorders in community samples.** *Behav Res Ther* 2004, **42:**551–567.
38. Berg K, Peterson C, Frazier P, Crow S: **Psychometric evaluation of the eating disorder examination and eating disorder examination-questionnaire: a systematic review of the literature.** *Int J Eat Disord* 2012, **45:**428–438.

Eating disorder symptom trajectories in adolescence: effects of time, participant sex, and early adolescent depressive symptoms

Karina L Allen[1,2*], Ross D Crosby[3,4], Wendy H Oddy[1] and Susan M Byrne[2]

Abstract

Background: Adolescence is a period of developmental risk for eating disorders and eating disorder symptoms. This study aimed to describe the prevalence and trajectory of five core eating disorder behaviours (binge eating, purging, fasting, following strict dietary rules, and hard exercise for weight control) and a continuous index of dietary restraint and eating, weight and shape concerns, in a cohort of male and female adolescents followed from 14 to 20 years. It also aimed to determine the effect of early adolescent depressive symptoms on the prevalence and trajectory of these different eating disorder symptoms. Participants (N = 1,383; 49% male) were drawn from the Western Australian Pregnancy Cohort (Raine) Study, a prospective cohort study that has followed participants from pre-birth to age 20 years. An adapted version of the Eating Disorder Examination-Questionnaire was used to assess eating disorder symptoms at ages 14, 17 and 20 years. The Beck Depression Inventory for Youth was used to assess depressive symptoms at age 14. Longitudinal changes in the prevalence of eating disorder symptoms were tested using generalised estimating equations and linear mixed models.

Results: Symptom trajectories varied according to the eating disorder symptom studied, participant sex, and the presence of depressive symptoms in early adolescence. For males, eating disorder symptoms tended to be stable (for purging, fasting and hard exercise) or decreasing (for binge eating and global symptom scores) from 14 to 17 years, and then stable to 20 years. For females, fasting and global symptom scores increased from age 14 to peak in prevalence at age 17. Rates of binge eating in females were stable from age 14 to age 17 and increased significantly thereafter, whilst rates of purging and hard exercise increased from age 14 to age 17, and then remained elevated through to age 20. Depressive symptoms at age 14 impacted on eating disorder symptom trajectories in females, but not in males.

Conclusions: Prevention, screening and intervention initiatives for adolescent eating disorders need to be tailored to gender and age. Purging behaviour appears to be an important target for work with early to middle adolescent females.

Keywords: Eating disorders, Binge eating, Purging, Fasting, Dieting, Exercise, Adolescence, Trajectory, Raine study

* Correspondence: karina@ichr.uwa.edu.au
[1]Telethon Institute for Child Health Research, Centre for Child Health Research, The University of Western Australia, PO Box 855, West Perth, WA, Western Australia
[2]School of Psychology, The University of Western Australia, Crawley, Western Australia
Full list of author information is available at the end of the article

Background

Adolescence is regarded as a period of developmental risk for eating disorders [1,2] and eating disorder symptoms [3-5]. In general, eating disorder symptoms increase from 14–16 years in females [3,4], with peaks in binge eating onset at 16–17 years and purging onset at 17–18 years [1,6]. Few studies have considered the developmental trajectory of eating disorder symptoms in males, but available data suggest that boys may show reductions in eating pathology from early adolescence to mid adolescence, and then experience an increase in symptoms in late adolescence or early adulthood [3,5,7,8]. Eating disorder symptoms are associated with impairments in quality of life even when full criteria for an eating disorder are not met [9-11]. This makes it important that they are considered in research on the epidemiology and consequences of eating disorder psychopathology.

Studies have varied considerably in how eating disorder symptoms are conceptualised and assessed. Some research groups have used continuous questionnaire scores, which reflect a global index of cognitive and behavioural symptoms (such as dietary restraint and concerns about eating, weight and shape) and/or tendencies towards binge eating and purging (e.g., [3,7]). Others have assessed for discrete eating disorder behaviours, such as strict dieting, binge eating, or purging (e.g., [6,8]). In contrast to several large-scale cross-sectional projects [11,12], longitudinal studies in this area have not tended to assess for the full range of behaviours that may inform eating disorder diagnostic decisions, such as binge eating, purging, fasting and driven exercise in a single sample followed over time. An exception is in the study by Neumark-Sztainer et al. [5], where dieting, unhealthy weight control behaviours (defined as fasting, eating very little, using food substitutes, skipping meals or smoking cigarettes), extreme weight control behaviours (defined as diet pills, vomiting, laxatives or diuretics), and binge eating were assessed prospectively for male (n = 1030) and female (n = 1257) participants. Symptom trajectories varied according to the symptom in question, with marked increases being observed in the prevalence of extreme weight control behaviours across adolescence, but relative stability being observed in dieting behaviours [5]. Trajectories also varied for males and females, with symptom increases in middle adolescent females contrasting with symptom decreases in middle adolescent males. These findings highlight the importance of distinguishing between different symptom sets, and between male and female participants, when assessing eating disorder symptoms over time. To achieve this, longitudinal studies need to ensure that eating disorder assessment methods are broad enough to distinguish between different behaviours.

Eating disorders and eating disorder symptoms are strongly associated with other mental health difficulties, including depression, anxiety, substance misuse, and personality disorders [13-16]. These associations are particularly well documented for depression [14,16] and it has been established that depression and eating disorder symptoms show a bi-directional relationship, with each predicting increases in the other over time [17-19]. Most of this research has been conducted with females [17-20], but Sonneville and colleagues found significant associations between binge eating behaviour and later onset of depressive symptoms in male (n = 7843) and female (n = 9039) participants followed from adolescence to young adulthood in the Growing Up Today Study (GUTS) [8]. Conversely, Gardner and colleagues found that depression predicted increases in eating disorder symptoms in 6- to 14-year-old boys (n = 112) and girls (n = 104) over a 3-year period [21]. The dual-pathway model of bulimia nervosa (BN) also positions depressive symptoms as one pathway to binge eating and purging [22], and this model has been validated in male and female participants [23-25].

To date, studies on depression and eating pathology have tended to focus on binge eating and purging behaviours (e.g., [6,8]), or to use a global index of eating disorder symptoms (e.g., [17,19,26]). It is not clear whether depression also relates to other eating disorder symptoms, such as strict dietary restraint, purging without binge eating, or driven exercise for weight control. If depression predicts increases in some eating disorder symptoms but not others, it may be possible to tailor prevention programmes accordingly. Similarly, if these relationships differ across males and females, prevention efforts should be modified according to gender. The high prevalence of depressive symptoms in adolescence [27] makes delineation of these effects important, as results may facilitate targeted eating disorder screening, prevention and intervention work in adolescent populations.

Given the above, the current study had two aims:

1. To describe the prevalence and trajectory of five core eating disorder behaviours (binge eating, purging, fasting, following strict dietary rules, and hard exercise for weight control), and a continuous global index of eating pathology, in a cohort of male and female adolescents followed from 14 to 20 years.
2. To determine the effect of early adolescent depressive symptoms on the prevalence and trajectory of these different eating disorder symptoms over the 6-year time period, for males and females separately.

Methods

Design and participants

Participants were drawn from the Western Australian Pregnancy Cohort (Raine) Study, a prospective cohort study of 2,868 live birth babies followed to 20 years of age.

Full details regarding the Raine Study have been published previously [28,29]. In summary, 2,900 women were recruited from the antenatal booking clinics at King Edward Memorial Hospital for women (KEMH), the only public maternity hospital in Western Australia, between May 1989 and November 1991. Of the 2,900 women enrolled, 2,804 delivered live birth babies. Due to 64 multiple births, the initial cohort included 2,868 children. These children were assessed at birth and ages 1, 2, 3, 5, 8, 10, 14, 17 and 20 years.

This study focused on the 14, 17 and 20-year follow-ups, when detailed eating disorder data were collected. We used data from the earlier assessments to consider differences between participants included in this study and those lost to follow-up prior to adolescence. Eating disorder data were available for 1,598 participants at age 14 (56% of the original 2,868 births), 1,242 participants at age 17 (43%), and 1,243 participants at age 20 (43%). Analyses make use of participants with data at age 14 and at least one of the subsequent follow-ups, giving an effective sample size of 1,383 (49% male). This sample of 1,383 participants represents 48% of the original 2,868 births, 59% of the participants who were eligible for participation in the 14 through 20-year assessments (i.e., not deceased or lost to follow-up prior to age 14; N = 2,328), and 76% of the participants who completed at least one of the 14 through 20-year assessments (N = 1,878). Regarding attrition prior to age 14, 30 participants died in childhood (1% of the original 2,868 births), 162 were unable to be contacted (6%), and 348 had withdrawn (12%), resulting in a total possible sample of 2,328 adolescent participants (81%).

The mean age of the participants in this study was 14.01 years (SD = 0.19, range = 13.00–15.08) at the 14-year assessment, 16.92 years (SD = 0.24, range = 15.0–18.2) at the 17-year assessment, and 20.01 years (SD = 0.44, range = 19.00–22.08) at the 20-year assessment.

Procedure

Questionnaire packages were posted to adolescents at the 14, 17 and 20-year assessments, for at-home completion prior to a face-to-face assessment session. Height and weight were measured objectively during the face-to-face assessment.

All data collection occurred in accordance with Australian National Health and Medical Research Council Guidelines for Ethical Conduct in Human Research and was approved by the ethics committees of KEMH, Princess Margaret Hospital for Children, and the University of Western Australia.

Measures

Eating disorder symptoms at 14, 17 and 20 years

Eating disorder symptoms were assessed using 24 self-report items adapted from the Child Eating Disorder Examination (ChEDE) [30] and Eating Disorder Examination-Questionnaire (EDE-Q) [31]. These 24 items were self-report, as per the EDE-Q, but language was simplified or clarified when there was the possibility of confusion for 14-year-old adolescents. Response options were also simplified, so that the same four response options were used for all items: "not at all" (0); "some of the time (once per week / a few times a month)" (1); "a lot of the time (a few times a week)" (2); and "most of the time (every day or nearly every day)" (3). Questions referred to the previous month and the same items were used at all assessment points. Participants were asked to be conservative in their answers if they were unsure of the frequency of their behaviours. There is good evidence for the validity of self-report eating disorder assessment [31-36], including self-report assessment in adolescence [37].

Five categorical variables were computed to indicate the presence or absence of core eating disorder behaviours over the previous month: objective binge eating (eating an objectively large amount of food and feeling out of control of one's eating), purging (self-induced vomiting and/or laxative misuse), hard exercise specifically for weight control, fasting (not eating for 8 or more waking hours), and attempts to follow strict dietary rules. Behaviours were coded as present if they occurred at least "some of the time (once per week / a few times per month)". This frequency criterion is consistent with the requirements of DSM-5, which requires weekly binge eating / purging for diagnoses of bulimia nervosa and binge eating disorder [38]. A continuous, global index of eating disorder symptoms was also calculated by taking the mean of the items (n = 18) relating to dietary restraint and eating, weight and shape concern. Distinctions were not made between restraint and eating/weight/shape concerns, or between general weight and shape concerns and the over-evaluation of weight and shape, because of the high degree of correlation between these symptoms and their similar trajectories over time. Alpha coefficients for this global index were .90, .93 and .91, at the 14, 17 and 20-year assessments respectively.

Additional details on the eating disorder items have also been provided previously [29] and a copy of the questionnaire is provided in Appendix A.

Depressive symptoms at 14 years

Depressive symptoms at age 14 were assessed using the Beck Depression Inventory for Youth (BDI-Y) [39]. The BDI-Y is an adolescent adaptation of the adult Beck Depression Inventory-2 [40] and has excellent psychometric properties [39,41]. The possible score range is from 0 to 63. The alpha coefficient in this sample at age 14 was .97. Scores on the BDI-Y were stratified according to recommended cutpoints for the BDI-Y in early adolescence [39], to give a group with scores in the normal range (score ≤16) and a group with scores suggestive of at least mild depressive symptoms (score > 17).

Covariates

Family income and adolescent body mass index (BMI) were included as covariates in all analyses. Family income was reported by parents at the 14, 17 and 20-year assessments and dichotomised into low vs. medium-high income categories, where 'low' income included the lowest two Australian income quintiles and captured 15 - 20% of the sample at each assessment point. Adolescent height and weight measurements were taken by a trained researcher at each assessment point and used to calculate BMI according to the standard formula of weight (kg) / height $(m)^2$.

Parents also reported on family (e.g., family income, employment status, marital status), parent (e.g., parent physical and mental health) and child (e.g., child mental health) characteristics at the 5, 8 and 10-year assessments. These data were used in preliminary analyses comparing the current sample to Raine Study participants lost to follow-up.

Statistical analysis

All analyses were conducted in SPSS Statistics Version 19.

Preliminary analyses

Participants included in this study (n = 1,383) were compared to Raine Study participants lost to follow-up before adolescence (n = 961). Participants were compared on family, parent and psychosocial variables at ages 5, 8 and 10 years, using independent-samples *t*-tests (continuous variables) and Chi square tests (categorical variables). The same comparisons were conducted across participants included in this study and those who completed only one adolescent assessment (n = 495), and adolescent eating disorder symptoms were also compared across participants included in this study and those who took part in only one adolescent assessment.

After data screening, imputation techniques were used to impute missing eating disorder data for participants who completed two out of three adolescent assessments. Multiple imputation and EM estimation using maximum likelihood were both trialled, using established principles and techniques [42-44]. EM imputation was retained as providing the most appropriate imputation outcomes. Additional details are provided under Results, below.

Core analyses

Longitudinal changes in the prevalence of eating disorder behaviours were tested using generalised estimating equations (GEE) [45], which account for correlations within individuals over time. Initially, base models were run to determine if the prevalence of eating disorder symptoms varied significantly over time. Logistic binomial models were specified with a main effect of time, for each symptom. An independent working correlation model was used [46]. Subsequently, models were re-run to examine the predictive effects of 14-year depressive symptoms on changes in eating disorder symptoms over adolescence. These explanatory models were specified with a main effect of time, a main effect of 14-year depression status, and an interaction effect between time and depression. The categorical interaction term was created using three levels of time (1 = age 14, 2 = age 17, 3 = age 20) and two levels of depression (0 = no marked depression at age 14, 1 = pronounced depressive symptoms at age 14).

Longitudinal changes in global eating disorder symptoms scores were examined using linear mixed models. Again, a base model was specified to determine if scores varied significantly over time. Subsequently, time and 14-year depression status were specified as main effects, along with a time × depression interaction.

Models were adjusted for family income and adolescent BMI, and run separately for male and female participants.

Results

Preliminary analyses

Raine Study participants lost to follow-up before adolescence (n = 961) were significantly more likely to be from single-parent families at ages 5 (X^2 [1] = 17.13, $p < .001$), 8 (X^2 [1] = 23.29, $p < .001$), and 10 (X^2 [1] = 10.51, $p < .001$) years; were significantly less likely to have employed parents at ages 5 (X^2 [1] = 15.51, $p < .001$), 8 (X^2 [1] = 13.96, $p < .001$), and 10 (X^2 [1] = 24.19, $p < .001$) years; had significantly lower family incomes at ages 5 (t [1724] = 5.10, $p < .001$), 8 (t [1636] = 5.38, $p < .001$), and 10 (t [1578] = 4.67, $p < .001$) years; and had significantly higher CBCL Externalising Problem scores at ages 5 (t [1738] = 2.76, $p = .007$), 8 (t [1656] = 4.22, $p < .001$), and 10 (t [1610] = 2.94, $p = .003$) years, when compared to participants included in this study (n = 1383). These findings are consistent with the tendency for socially disadvantaged families to be lost to follow-up over time [47], and are considered in the Discussion.

Raine Study participants who completed only one adolescent assessment (n = 495) were also significantly more likely to be from single-parent families at age 8 (X^2 [1] = 4.60, $p = .032$), but not at ages 5 ($p = .295$) or 10 ($p = .256$) years; were significantly less likely to have employed parents at age 8 (X^2 [1] = 8.48, $p = .004$), but not at ages 5 ($p = .072$) or 10 ($p = .379$) years; had significantly lower family incomes at ages 5 (t [1696] = 3.28, $p = .001$), 8 (t [1663] = 4.10, $p < .001$), and 10 (t [1676] = 3.54, $p < .001$) years; and had significantly higher CBCL Externalising Problem scores at ages 5 (t [1705] = 2.66, $p = .008$), 8 (t [1680] = 4.31, $p < .001$), and 10 (t [1704] = 3.14, $p = .002$) years, compared to participants included in this study (n = 1383). There were no significant between-group differences in eating disorder symptom scores or the prevalence of categorical eating disorder behaviours (*ps* = .187 - .986) across participants who completed one adolescent assessment and those who completed two or more.

For participants who completed two of the three adolescent assessments, there was no evidence to suggest that missing eating disorder data were not missing at random (Little's MCAR test X^2 [1399] = 1376, $p = .664$). Nonetheless, a conservative approach was taken by imputing data prior to analysis, rather than relying on the GEE procedure, which would require data to be missing completely at random in order for reliable estimates to be obtained [48]. Data were imputed for 281 participants in total, with 141 participants at age 17 and 140 participants at age 20. Multiple imputation was conducted using eating disorder variables, BMI, depressive symptom scores and CBCL Internalising and Externalising Problem scores as predictors in the imputation model (in varying combinations ranging from few predictors to many predictors) [42]. However, this imputation approach produced marked over-estimates for rare behaviours (i.e., vomiting), irrespective of the particular combination of predictor variables. When EM imputation with maximum likelihood was conducted [43], this over-estimation did not occur. Estimated means and standard deviations for the original and EM eating disorder data were highly similar, as were symptom prevalence rates and associations between eating disorder symptoms and depressive symptoms. Thus, EM imputation was used in preference to multiple imputation. All subsequent analyses make use of the full, imputed data set.

Scores on the BDI-Y ranged from 0 to 34 for boys (M [SD] = 5.06 [5.32]) and from 0 to 50 for girls (M[SD] = 7.88 [7.80]). The proportion of participants classified as having at least mild depressive symptoms (score > 17) was 4.0% (n = 26) for boys and 12.5% (n = 83) for girls, equating to 7.9% of the sample overall (n = 109). The BDI-Y was not completed by 73 participants (36 boys and 37 girls), giving a sample size of 1310 (49% male) for analyses on the effects of depressive symptoms on eating disorder trajectories.

Changes in eating disorder symptoms over time

Mean global eating disorder symptom scores and prevalence rates for categorical eating disorder symptoms are shown in Table 1 (boys) and Table 2 (girls).

Male participants

There was a significant main effect of time on boys' global eating disorder symptom scores (F [2, 1168.36] = 11.98, $p < .001$) and on rates of binge eating (Wald X^2 [2] = 20.22, $p < .001$) and attempts to follow strict dietary rules (Wald X^2 [2] = 17.92, $p < .001$). For global eating disorder symptom scores, there was a small but statistically significant decrease in scores from age 14 to age 17, before stable symptoms from age 17 to 20 (see Table 1). The prevalence of objective binge eating also decreased significantly from age 14 to age 17 before stable symptoms from age 17 to age 20, whilst attempts to follow strict dietary rules decreased significantly from age 14 to age 17 but then increased to approximate 14-year levels at age 20. Prevalence rates are shown in Table 1 and odds ratios from generalised estimating equations are shown in Table 3, below. By age 20, binge eating was approximately one-third as likely to occur (OR = .29) as at age 14.

There were no significant main effects of time on the prevalence of purging (Wald X^2 [2] = 4.18, $p = .123$), fasting (Wald X^2 [2] = 1.38, $p = .502$) or hard exercise (Wald X^2 [2] = 6.06, $p = .500$) in boys.

Female participants

For girls, significant main effects of time were identified for all eating disorder symptoms except attempts to follow strict dietary rules (Wald X^2 [2] = 5.53, $p = .063$). There was a small but statistically significant increase in global symptom scores from age 14 to age 17, before symptoms decreased to approximate 14-year levels at age 20 (F [2, 865.18] = 14.71, $p < .001$) (see Table 2). The same pattern was observed for fasting (Wald X^2 [2] = 37.01, $p < .001$). The prevalence of binge eating was stable from age 14 to age 17 before increasing significantly to age 20 (Wald X^2

Table 1 Eating disorder symptoms and body mass index by time, for male participants (n = 680)

	14 yrs	17 yrs	20 yrs	*p*
Body mass index (M [SD])	20.91_a (3.91)	22.74_b (4.17)	24.45_c (4.59)	<.001
Global symptoms (M [SD])	0.33_a (0.35)	0.30_b (0.40)	0.31_b (0.38)	<.001
Objective binge eating (% yes)	$23.6\%_a$ (n = 160)	$15.0\%_b$ (n = 102)	$17.2\%_b$ (n = 117)	<.001
Purging (% yes)	1.2% (n = 8)	2.5% (n = 17)	2.7% (n = 18)	.123
Fasting (% yes)	9.7% (n = 66)	8.5% (n = 58)	8.1% (n = 55)	.502
Dietary rules (% yes)	$21.4\%_a$ (n = 145)	$16.2\%_b$ (n = 110)	$21.1\%_a$ (n = 143)	<.001
Hard exercise (% yes)	49.0% (n = 333)	46.5% (n = 316)	50.8% (n = 345)	.500

Note. Global symptoms refer to a global index of dietary restraint and eating, weight and shape concerns.
p values and column subscripts denote significant differences over time, as identified through generalised estimating equations or linear mixed models. Columns with different subscripts differ significantly at $p < .05$.
a,b,c indicate significant differences over time.

Table 2 Eating disorder symptoms and body mass index by time, for female participants (n = 703)

	14 yrs	17 yrs	20 yrs	*p*
Body mass index (M [SD])	21.49 (4.16)$_a$	23.11 (4.51)$_b$	24.37 (5.21)$_c$	<.001
Global symptoms (M [SD])	0.61 (0.54)$_a$	0.82 (0.64)$_b$	0.66 (0.50)$_a$	<.001
Objective binge eating (% yes)	38.5% (n = 271)$_a$	36.8% (n = 259)	43.4% (n = 305)$_b$	<.001
Purging (% yes)	3.7% (n = 26)$_a$	13.5% (n = 95)$_b$	14.0% (n = 98)$_b$	<.001
Fasting (% yes)	16.4% (n = 115)$_a$	26.5% (n = 186)$_b$	19.5% (n = 137)$_a$	<.001
Dietary rules (% yes)	33.6% (n = 236)	35.0% (n = 246)	41.0% (n = 288)	.063
Hard exercise (% yes)	56.8% (n = 399)$_a$	64.2% (n = 451)$_b$	69.4% (n = 488)$_b$	<.001

Note. Global symptoms refer to a global index of dietary restraint and eating, weight and shape concerns.
p values and column subscripts denote significant differences over time, as identified through generalised estimating equations or linear mixed models. Columns with different subscripts differ significantly at $p < .05$.
a,b,c indicate significant differences over time.

[2] = 11.99, $p < .001$), whereas prevalence rates increased significantly from age 14 to ages 17 and 20 for purging (Wald X^2 [2] = 48.64, $p < .001$) and hard exercise (Wald X^2 [2] = 33.59, $p < .001$). Prevalence rates are shown in Table 2 and odds ratios from generalised estimating equations are shown in Table 4, below. As shown, the greatest increase in prevalence was observed for purging, with this behaviour being over 4 times as likely to occur at age 20 than at age 14 (OR = 4.23).

When considering differences between male and female participants, global eating disorder symptom scores and rates of categorical eating disorder symptoms were significantly higher in females than males, for all symptoms at all time points ($p < .002$). Body mass index was greater in females than in males at age 14 only ($p = .008$).

Prospective effects of depression on eating disorder symptoms

Male participants

There was a significant main effect of 14-year depression status on boys' global eating disorder symptom scores (F [1, 1575.17] = 32.58, $p < .001$) and on rates of binge eating (Wald X^2 [1] = 6.37, $p = .012$), purging (Wald X^2 [1] = 94.72, $p < .001$), fasting (Wald X^2 [1] = 5.89, $p = .015$), attempts to follow strict dietary rules (Wald X^2 [1] = 4.14, $p = .042$), and hard exercise (Wald X^2 [1] = 6.57, $p = .010$). In all cases, symptoms were higher for boys with elevated depression at age 14, on average and across the 6-year study period, than for boys without depression at age 14. Odds ratios are shown in Table 3. Boys with elevated depressive symptoms at age 14 were nearly three times as likely to report binge

Table 3 Odds ratios (and 95% CI) for changes in eating disorder symptoms across adolescence, in relation to time (age), 14-year depression status, and the interaction between time and 14-year depression status, for male participants

	Binge eating	Purging	Fasting	Dietary rules	Exercise
Time (reference = age 14):					
Age 17	0.52**	2.15	0.82	0.65**	0.90
	(0.40 – 0.68)	(0.92 – 5.06)	(0.58 – 1.15)	(0.51 – 0.84)	(0.77 – 1.06)
Age 20	0.29**	2.29 [1]	0.87	0.91	1.08
	(0.22 – 0.37)	(1.01 – 5.16)	(0.63 – 1.19)	(0.71 – 1.17)	(0.77 – 1.06)
Depression at age 14 (reference = no depression)					
Mild or greater	2.89**	2.72**	2.80**	1.71*	2.29**
	(1.31 – 6.40)	(1.00 – 7.58)	(1.32 – 5.97)	(1.02 – 2.87)	(1.21 – 4.31)
Time x depression (reference = age 14, no depression)					
Age 17 x 14-year	0.75	0.67	1.03	0.68	1.19
depression	(0.32 – 1.79)	(0.05 – 8.58)	(0.36 – 2.89)	(0.18 – 2.50)	(0.38 – 3.68)
Age 20 x 14-year	0.67	1.53	0.41	0.92	0.74
depression	(0.24 – 1.84)	(0.11 – 10.39)	(0.10 – 1.62)	(0.24 – 3.52)	(0.26 – 2.10)

* $p < .05$ ** $p < .01$ [1] The overall effect of time on purging prevalence from 14 to 20 years was not statistically significant, but the comparison between 14 and 20 years was significant at $p = .046$.
Note. Models are adjusted for body mass index and family income. The effective sample size with these covariates was n = 678 for models with time only and n = 644 for models with depression.

Table 4 Odds ratios (and 95% CI) for changes in eating disorder symptoms across adolescence, in relation to time (age), 14-year depression status, and the interaction between time and 14-year depression status, for female participants (n = 703)

	Binge eating	Purging	Fasting	Dietary rules	Exercise
Time (reference = age 14)					
Age 17	0.93	4.07**	1.84**	1.23	1.36**
	(0.78 - 1.11)	(2.69 - 6.16)	(1.49 - 2.27)	(1.00 - 1.50)	(1.15 - 1.62)
Age 20	1.22**	4.23**	1.24	0.98	1.75**
	(1.01 - 1.47)	(2.78 - 6.43)	(0.97 - 1.58)	(0.81 - 1.19)	(1.44 - 2.11)
Depression at age 14 (reference = no depression)					
Mild or greater	3.54**	3.29**	2.89**	1.25	1.40
	(2.18 - 5.75)	(2.14 - 5.09)	(1.99 - 4.18)	(0.90 - 1.73)	(0.98 - 2.01)
Time x depression (reference = age 14, no depression)					
Age 17 x 14-year	0.51**	0.39**	0.40**	0.84	0.71
depression	(0.30 - 0.88)	(0.16 - 0.97)	(0.23 - 0.70)	(0.47 - 1.50)	(0.37 - 1.36)
Age 20 x 14-year	0.41**	0.21**	0.43**	0.43*	0.48
depression	(0.21 - 0.82)	(0.08 - 1.85)	(0.22 - 0.84)	(0.28 - 0.82)	(0.24 - 0.97)

* $p < .05$ ** $p < .01$

Note. Models are adjusted for body mass index and family income. The effective sample size with these covariates was n = 697 for models with time only and n = 619 for models with depression. Interaction effects are summarised in Figures 1 and 2.

eating (OR = 2.89), purging (OR = 2.72) and fasting (OR = 2.80) than boys without elevated depression.

There were no significant time x depression interaction effects for global eating disorder symptom scores (F [2, 918.94] = 1.71, $p = .182$), binge eating (Wald X^2 [2] = 0.64, $p = .724$), purging (Wald X^2 [1] = 0.96, $p = .756$), fasting (Wald X^2 [2] = 2.04, $p < .361$), strict dietary rules (Wald X^2 [2] = 0.35, $p = .839$), or hard exercise (Wald X^2 [2] = 0.94, $p = .623$).

Girls

There was a significant main effect of 14-year depression status on girls' global eating disorder symptom scores (F [1, 1519.48] = 68.13, $p < .001$) and on rates of binge eating (Wald X^2 [1] = 19.06, $p < .001$), purging (Wald X^2 [1] = 35.68, $p < .001$), and fasting (Wald X^2 [1] = 32.18, $p < .001$). In all cases, symptoms were higher for girls with elevated depression at age 14, on average and across the 6-year study period, than for girls without depression at age 14.

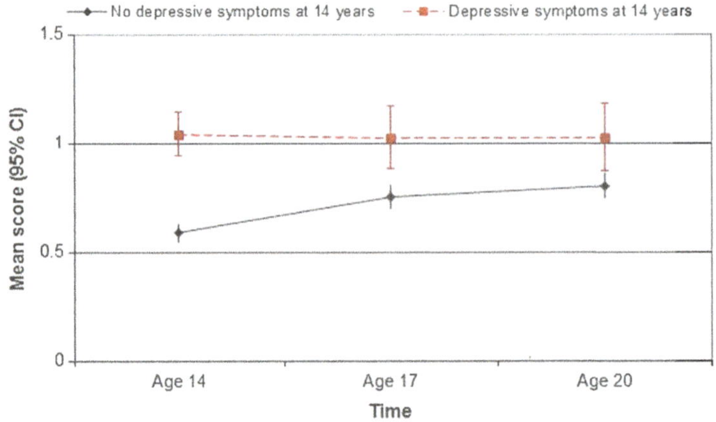

Figure 1 Changes in girls' global eating disorder symptom scores (mean scores with 95% confidence intervals), by time and 14-year depression status. There are significant main effects of time and 14-year depression status, and a significant interaction effect between time and depression.

There was no significant main effect of depression on girls' attempts to follow strict dietary rules (Wald X^2 [1] = 1.77, p = .183) or hard exercise (Wald X^2 [1] = 3.16, p = .076). Odds ratios are provided in Table 4, and show that girls with elevated depressive symptoms at age 14 were approximately three times as likely to report binge eating (OR = 3.54), purging (OR = 3.29) and fasting (OR = 2.89) than girls without elevated depression.

Significant time x depression interaction effects were also identified for global eating disorder symptom scores (F [2, 906.72] = 9.86, p < .001), binge eating (Wald X^2 [2] = 7.34, p = .025), purging (Wald X^2 [2] = 10.61, p = .005), fasting (Wald X^2 [2] = 9.59, p = .008), and attempts to follow strict dietary rules (Wald X^2 [2] = 7.04, p = .030). There was no significant time x depression interaction for hard exercise (Wald X^2 [2] = 3.60, p = .165).

The interaction effect for global eating disorder symptoms is summarised in Figure 1. Girls with elevated depressive symptoms at age 14 had higher scores at each time point than girls without depressive symptoms at age 14, but scores remained stable between age 14 and age 20 for the depressive symptom group, whereas they increased over time for the non-depressed group.

Interaction effects for the categorical variables are summarised in Figure 2. Girls with depressive symptoms at age 14 had higher prevalence rates for each eating disorder symptom at each time point, with the exception of dietary rules at age 20. However, rates for binge eating, fasting, and dietary rules decreased by approximately 10% from age 14 to age 20 for this group, and rates for purging increased from at age 14 to age 17 but then decreased to approximate 14-year levels at age 20. For girls *without* depressive symptoms at age 14, rates for binge eating, purging, fasting and dietary rules increased over time (see Figure 2).

Discussion

This study has described the prevalence and trajectory of eating disorder symptoms in male and female adolescents followed from 14 to 20 years of age. Symptom trajectories varied according to the specific eating disorder symptom studied, participant sex, and the presence of depressive symptoms in early adolescence.

For boys, eating disorder symptoms tended to be stable (for purging, fasting and hard exercise) or decreasing (for global eating disorder symptom scores and binge eating) from 14 to 17 years, and then stable to 20 years. An exception was found for strict dietary rules, where prevalence decreased from age 14 to age 17 before increasing to baseline levels by age 20. These results are consistent with findings from the small number of previous studies with adolescent males [3,5,8], which observed stable or reducing symptoms from early to middle adolescence, before an increase in symptoms in late adolescence or early adulthood. In this sample, we did not observe marked increases in eating pathology in late adolescence, suggesting that any increases in this cohort did not occur until after age 20. It is interesting to note that the one symptom that *did* increase in late adolescence was attempts to follow strict dietary rules. Cognitive-behavioural theories would suggest that an increase in strict dieting may precede a subsequent increase in binge eating, and possibly purging [22,49]. This allows for the hypothesis that male participants in this sample are at risk for these behaviours as they move in to early adulthood.

Boys who reported depressive symptoms at age 14 had higher rates of all eating disorder symptoms, on average, than boys who did not report marked depression at age 14. However, depression at age 14 did not relate significantly to symptom trajectories over the following 6 years.

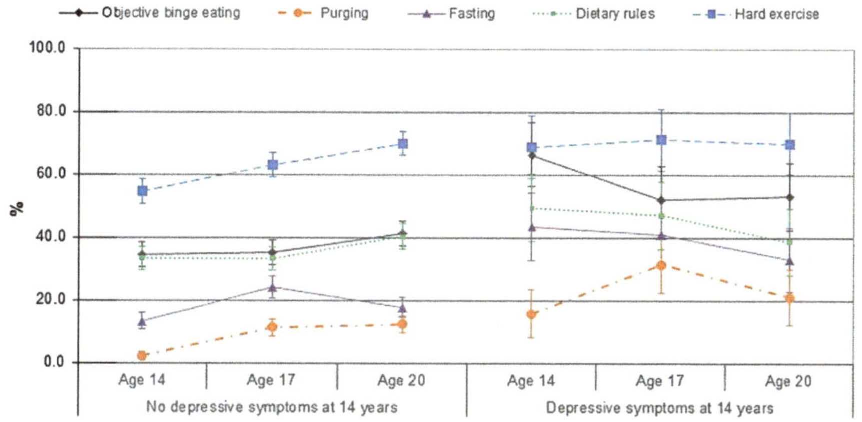

Figure 2 Prevalence rates (with 95% confidence intervals) for categorical eating disorder symptoms in girls, by time and 14-year depression status. There are significant main effects of time for binge eating, purging, fasting and driven exercise; significant main effects of 14-year depression group for binge eating, purging and fasting; and significant time x depression interaction effects for binge eating, purging, fasting and attempts to follow strict dietary rules.

If males do experience increases in eating disorder symptoms later than females, as they transition into adulthood, it is possible that depressive symptoms would be more relevant to male symptom trajectories if assessed at a later time point. Future studies may need to time male assessments accordingly, to capture changes in pathology after age 20. As relatively few studies have tested prospective associations between depression and eating pathology in males [21,23], it also seems possible that these relationships are less pronounced for males than for females. If so, it would be important to identify other factors that may influence the onset and persistence of male eating pathology.

For girls, the prevalence of strict dietary rules remained stable from 14 to 20 years but rates for all other symptoms varied significantly over time. Fasting and global eating disorder symptom scores increased from age 14 to peak in prevalence at age 17, before returning to 14-year levels at age 20. Rates of binge eating were stable from age 14 to age 17 and increased significantly thereafter, rising by approximately 6% before age 20. In contrast, rates of purging and hard exercise increased by approximately 10% from age 14 to age 17, and then remained stable through to age 20. These findings are broadly consistent with those reported elsewhere [e.g., 3,5,6], but the sequence of binge eating relative to purging was unexpected. Others have observed peaks in binge eating risk prior to peaks in purging [6,20], an order that is consistent with theories of BN development and the view that purging is a compensatory response to binge eating behaviour [49]. However, Neumark-Sztainer et al. [5] also found stable rates of binge eating in their sample of female adolescents followed from early to late adolescence, whereas rates of purging behaviour increased over that time frame. As some studies have focused on risk for symptom onset at an individual level (e.g., [6,20]), rather than changes in prevalence at a population level ([5], this study), it is possible that methodological differences may partially account for this cross-study variation. Nonetheless, additional research is indicated to clarify the relative prevalence of binge eating and purging at different time points in adolescence.

Girls' eating disorder symptom trajectories also varied significantly according to the presence or absence of depressive symptoms at age 14. On average, girls with elevated depression reported higher rates of binge eating, purging and fasting than girls without elevated depression, consistent with previous reports [19]. However, girls with elevated depression at age 14 showed decreases in binge eating, fasting and dietary rules from 14 to 20 years, whilst girls without elevated depression at age 14 showed increases in these symptoms over time. Contrasting results were observed for purging, which was the only eating disorder symptom to increase in prevalence after age 14 for the group who reported depressive symptoms at baseline. Previous studies have found depressive symptoms to predict increases in binge eating as well as purging [20], so our failure to replicate this relationship should be followed up in future research. Attention to methodology is also important here, as we considered the effects of depression at one time point on eating disorder symptom trajectories thereafter. This is different to considering reciprocal relationships between depression and eating pathology over time, which has been the focus in several past investigations (e.g., [17]). This study tested one aspect of the putative relationship between depression and eating pathology, by considering how early adolescent depression influenced later changes in eating disorder symptoms. We do not report on reverse or reciprocal relationships (i.e., the effects of eating disorder symptoms on depression) or on associations between late adolescent depression and eating disorder symptoms.

These results have four key implications for eating disorder prevention and intervention efforts in adolescence. First, boys' eating disorder symptoms appear to decrease in frequency in middle adolescence, suggesting that prevention and early intervention initiatives for males may be more beneficial in the period of transition to young adulthood, rather than earlier in adolescence. Second, the marked increase in purging behaviour in girls from age 14 to age 17 suggests that purging should be a focus of eating disorder screening and intervention programmes for early and middle adolescent females. Third, and consistent with previous findings [5,12], binge eating, strict dieting and driven exercise are reported by at least one in three female adolescents, regardless of age. There is a pressing need to identify effective and universal prevention, screening and intervention strategies for these behaviours. Fourth, the presence of depression in early adolescence does not appear to predict later increases in eating pathology, but it may be a marker of existing eating disorder symptoms. The reverse may also hold true, and joint assessment of depression and eating disorder symptoms in adolescents may be worthwhile. Similarly, coordinated intervention efforts for depression and eating pathology may be of benefit to some adolescents.

This study benefited from prospective, population-based data from male and female participants, attention to the full range of eating disorder symptoms, and attention to the effects of early adolescent depression on eating disorder symptom trajectories. Two limitations deserve note, however, including participant attrition within the Raine Study cohort and the lack of follow-up into adulthood. Regarding attrition, the loss of disadvantaged families is a well-replicated phenomenon in longitudinal cohort studies [47]. In the Raine Study, attrition has served to increase the representativeness of the cohort over time, as the study initially over-sampled socially-disadvantaged women. Previous analyses have shown that participants who remained in the study to adolescence are broadly comparable to the Western Australian population on a range of socio-demographic indicators [50]. Despite this, replication of our results in other cohorts is important and would help to strengthen the findings observed here. We also found that, even amongst participants who remained in the study to adolescence, individuals who completed one adolescent assessment (and who were consequently excluded from this study) were more socially disadvantaged in childhood than those who completed two or more assessments. Our results should be interpreted with this in mind, and with the understanding that different findings may emerge with a socially disadvantaged sample. Regarding follow-up duration, this issue is particularly relevant to male participants, who may be expected to show increases in eating pathology after age 20. The benefits of following male participants into early adulthood should be considered and planned for in future analyses.

Conclusions

This study provides new data on the prevalence and trajectory of eating disorder symptoms in males and females followed from 14 to 20 years of age. Results highlight the importance of attending to sex and depressive symptoms when considering eating disorder symptom trajectories, and confirm that different eating disorder symptoms may be expected to show different trajectories across adolescence. In this sample, females showed peaks in fasting and the global index of dietary restraint and eating, weight and shape concerns at age 17. Binge eating peaked at age 20, whilst purging and hard exercise for weight control increased between ages 14 and 17 and remained elevated at age 20. For males, global eating disorder symptom scores and binge eating decreased across adolescence, whilst the prevalence of strict dietary rules reduced from age 14 to age 17 before returning to baseline levels at age 20. Depressive symptoms at age 14 impacted on eating disorder symptom trajectories in females, but not in males.

Consent

Written informed consent was obtained from participants for their data to be used for research purposes, including publications.

Appendix A

Eating disorder questionnaire items (adapted from the Child Eating Disorder Examination [30] and Eating Disorder Examination-Questionnaire [31]).

General instructions:

- **Please read each question carefully.** Circle the most appropriate option.
- **Please take your time.** If you are uncomfortable about a question or unsure of an answer, please leave it blank and contact one of the Raine Study staff.
- **Remember all answers are STRICTLY confidential.**

Over the last four weeks (one month)...

Q1. Have you been trying hard to eat less to change your shape or weight? (even if you haven't managed to do so)

Not at all 0
Some of the time (once per week / a few times a month) 1
A lot of the time (a few times a week) 2
Most of the time (every day or nearly every day) 3

Q2. Have you gone for long periods of time (<u>8 hours or more</u>) without eating anything to try and change your shape or weight?

Not at all 0
Some of the time (once per week / a few times a month) 1
A lot of the time (a few times a week) 2
Most of the time (every day or nearly every day) 3

Q3. Have you tried not to eat certain foods (like chocolate or chips) to try to change your shape or weight? (even if you haven't been able to do so)

Not at all 0
Some of the time (once per week / a few times a month) 1
A lot of the time (a few times a week) 2
Most of the time (every day or nearly every day) 3

Q4. Have you tried to stick to any definite rules about diet or eating? For example sticking to a calorie limit, a set amount of food or rules about what or when you should eat? (even if you haven't been able to do so)

Not at all 0
Some of the time (once per week / a few times a month) 1
A lot of the time (a few times a week) 2
Most of the time (every day or nearly every day) 3

Q5. Have you been thinking about food or calories so much that you've found it hard to concentrate on things you are interested in? For example reading, watching TV or following a conversation?

Not at all 0
Some of the time (once per week / a few times a month) 1
A lot of the time (a few times a week) 2
Most of the time (every day or nearly every day) 3

Q6. Have you been afraid of losing control over your eating?
Not at all 0
Some of the time (once per week / a few times a month)1
A lot of the time (a few times a week) 2
Most of the time (every day or nearly every day) 3

Q7. Have there been times when you felt you had eaten an unusually large amount of food – much more than what most people would eat in the same situation?
Not at all 0
Some of the time (once per week / a few times a month) 1
A lot of the time (a few times a week) 2
Most of the time (every day or nearly every day) 3

Q8. Have you felt that you couldn't control what or how much you were eating?
Not at all 0
Some of the time (once per week / a few times a month) 1
A lot of the time (a few times a week) 2
Most of the time (every day or nearly every day) 3

Q9. Have you felt that you couldn't stop eating once you had started?
Not at all 0
Some of the time (once per week / a few times a month) 1
A lot of the time (a few times a week) 2
Most of the time (every day or nearly every day)3

Q10. Have you felt guilty after eating?
Not at all 0
Some of the time (once per week / a few times a month) 1
A lot of the time (a few times a week) 2
Most of the time (every day or nearly every day) 3

Q11. Have you eaten in secret because you are embarrassed by how much you eat?
Not at all 0
Some of the time (once per week / a few times a month) 1
A lot of the time (a few times a week) 2
Most of the time (every day or nearly every day) 3

Q12. Have you been afraid that you might gain weight or become fat?
Not at all 0
Some of the time (once per week / a few times a month) 1
A lot of the time (a few times a week) 2
Most of the time (every day or nearly every day) 3

Q13. Have you felt fat?
Not at all 0
Some of the time (once per week / a few times a month) 1
A lot of the time (a few times a week) 2
Most of the time (every day or nearly every day) 3

Q14. Have you had a <u>strong</u> desire to lose weight?
Not at all 0
Some of the time (once per week / a few times a month) 1
A lot of the time (a few times a week) 2
Most of the time (every day or nearly every day) 3

Q15. Have you made yourself sick (vomit) after eating to control your weight?
Not at all 0
Some of the time (once per week / a few times a month) 1
A lot of the time (a few times a week) 2
Most of the time (every day or nearly every day) 3

Q16. Have you taken any pills (like laxatives or water pills) to try to control your weight?
Not at all 0

Some of the time (once per week / a few times a month) 1
A lot of the time (a few times a week) 2
Most of the time (every day or nearly every day) 3

Q17. Have you exercised <u>hard</u> to control your weight?
Not at all 0
Some of the time (once per week / a few times a month) 1
A lot of the time (a few times a week) 2
Most of the time (every day or nearly every day) 3

People have different ideas about what sort of things are important to them in how they think about themselves. For some people doing well at school is very important to them in how they think about themselves, for others, how they are getting on with friends is very important.

We're now going to ask you to think about how important weight and shape are to you in how you think of yourself as a person.

Q18. Has your weight been important in how you think of yourself as a person?
Not at all 0
Some of the time (once per week / a few times a month) 1
A lot of the time (a few times a week) 2
Most of the time (every day or nearly every day) 3

Q19. Has your shape been important in how you think of yourself as a person?
Not at all 0
Some of the time (once per week / a few times a month) 1
A lot of the time (a few times a week) 2
Most of the time (every day or nearly every day) 3

Q20. Have you felt unhappy about your weight?
Not at all 0
Some of the time (once per week / a few times a month) 1
A lot of the time (a few times a week) 2
Most of the time (every day or nearly every day) 3

Q21. Have you felt unhappy about your shape?
Not at all 0
Some of the time (once per week / a few times a month) 1
A lot of the time (a few times a week) 2
Most of the time (every day or nearly every day) 3

Q22. Have you been concerned about other people seeing you eat?
Not at all 0
Some of the time (once per week / a few times a month) 1
A lot of the time (a few times a week) 2
Most of the time (every day or nearly every day) 3

Q23. Have you felt uncomfortable about seeing your body, for example, in the mirror, or in the bath or shower?
Not at all 0
Some of the time (once per week / a few times a month) 1
A lot of the time (a few times a week) 2
Most of the time (every day or nearly every day) 3

Q24. Have you felt uncomfortable about other people seeing your body, for example, in the change rooms, or when wearing bathers or tight clothes
Not at all 0
Some of the time (once per week / a few times a month) 1
A lot of the time (a few times a week) 2
Most of the time (every day or nearly every day) 3

Abbreviations

BDI-Y: Beck depression inventory-youth; BMI: Body mass index; ChEDE: Child eating disorder examination; EDE-Q: Eating disorder examination; KEMH: King edward memorial hospital for women; Raine study: Western australian pregnancy cohort (Raine) study.

Competing interests

The authors declare that they have no competing interests.

Authors' contributions

KA, WO and SB participated in the design of the study. RC provided guidance on the statistical analyses. KA performed the statistical analyses and drafted the manuscript. All authors read and approved the final manuscript.

Acknowledgments

We are extremely grateful to the Raine Study participants and their families who took part in this study and to the Raine Study team for cohort management and data collection.

The first author is supported by an early career research fellowship from the National Health and Medical Research Council (NHMRC) of Australia. Core funding for the Western Australian Pregnancy Cohort (Raine) Study is provided by the Raine Medical Research Foundation; The University of Western Australia (UWA); the Faculty of Medicine, Dentistry and Health Sciences at UWA; the Telethon Institute for Child Health Research; the Women's and Infant's Research Foundation; and Curtin University. Funding for the 14-year Raine Study follow-up was provided by the Raine Medical Research Foundation and NHMRC project grants. Funding for the 17-year follow-up was provided by NHMRC programme grant 35314. Funding for the 20-year follow-up was provided by the Canadian Institutes of Health Research and NHMRC project grants.

Author details

[1]Telethon Institute for Child Health Research, Centre for Child Health Research, The University of Western Australia, PO Box 855, West Perth, WA, Western Australia. [2]School of Psychology, The University of Western Australia, Crawley, Western Australia. [3]Department of Clinical Neuroscience, University of North Dakota School of Medicine and Health Sciences, Fargo, North Dakota, USA. [4]Department of Biostatistics, Neuropsychiatric Research Institute, Fargo, North Dakota, USA.

References

1. Stice E, Marti C, Shaw HE, Jaconis M: **An 8-year longitudinal study of the natural history of threshold, subthreshold, and partial eating disorders from a community sample of adolescents.** *J Abnorm Psychol* 2009, **118**:587–597.
2. Isomaa R, Isomaa A-L, Marttunen M, Kaltiala-Heino R, Bjorkqvist K: **The prevalence, incidence and development of eating disorders in Finnish adolescents–A two-step 3-year follow-up study.** *Eur Eat Disord Rev* 2009, **17**:199–207.
3. Abebe DS, Lien L, Von Soest R: **The development of bulimic symptoms from adolescence to young adulthood in females and males: a population-based longitudinal cohort study.** *Int J Eat Disord* 2012, **45**:737–745.
4. Steinhausen HC, Gavez S, Metzke CW: **Psychosocial correlates, outcome, and stability of abnormal adolescent eating behavior in community samples of young people.** *Int J Eat Disord* 2005, **37**:119–126.
5. Neumark-Sztainer D, Wall M, Larson NI, Eisenberg ME, Loth K: **Dieting and disordered eating behaviors from adolescence to young adulthood: Findings from a 10-year longitudinal study.** *J Am Diet Assoc* 2011, **111**:1004–1011.
6. Stice E, Killen JD, Hayward C, Taylor CB: **Age of onset for binge eating and purging during late adolescence: a 4-year survival analysis.** *J Abnorm Psychol* 1998, **107**:671–675.
7. Keel PK, Baxter MG, Heatherton TF, Joiner TE: **A 20-year longitudinal study of body weight, dieting, and eating disorder symptoms.** *J Abnorm Psychol* 2007, **116**:422–432.
8. Sonneville KR, Horton NJ, Micali N, Crosby RD, Swanson SA, Solmi F, Field AE: **Longitudinal associations between binge eating and overeating and adverse outcomes among adolescents and young adults.** *JAMA Pediatrics* 2013, **167**:149–155.
9. Wade TD, Wilksch S, Lee C: **A longitudinal investigation of the impact of disordered eating on young women's quality of life.** *Health Psychol* 2012, **31**:352–359.
10. Mond JM, Hay PJ: **Dissatisfaction versus over-evaluation in a general population sample of women.** *Int J Eat Disord* 2011, **44**:721–726.
11. Mond JM, Hay P, Rodgers B, Owen C, Crosby R, Mitchell JC: **Use of extreme weight control behaviors with and without binge eating in a community sample: implications for the classification of bulimic-type eating disorders.** *Int J Eat Disord* 2006, **39**:294–302.
12. Hay PJ, Mond J, Buttner P, Darby A: **Eating disorder behaviors are increasing: Findings from two sequential community surveys in South Australia.** *PLoS One* 2008, **3**(2):e1541.
13. Hudson JI, Hiripi E, Pope HGJ, Kessler RC: **The prevalence and correlates of eating disorders in the National Comorbidity Survey replication.** *Biol Psychiatry* 2007, **61**:348–358.
14. Godart NT, Perdereau F, Rein Z, Berthoz S, Wallier J, Jeammet P, Flament MF: **Comorbidity studies of eating disorders and mood disorders: critical review of the literature.** *J Affect Disord* 2007, **97**:37–49.
15. Swanson SA, Crow SJ, Le Grange D, Swendsen J, Merikangas KR: **Prevalence and correlates of eating disorders in adolescents: Results from the national comorbidity survey replication adolescent supplement.** *Arch Gen Psychiatry* 2011, **68**(7):714–723.
16. Stice E: **Risk and maintenance factors for eating pathology: a meta-analytic review.** *Psychol Bull* 2002, **128**:825–848.
17. Marmorstein NR, von Ranson KM, Iacono WG, Malone SM: **Prospective associations between depressive symptoms and eating disorder symptoms among adolescent girls.** *Int J Eat Disord* 2008, **41**(2):118–123.
18. Stice E, Bearman SK: **Body image and eating disturbances prospectively predict increases in depressive symptoms in adolescent girls: a growth curve analysis.** *Dev Psychol* 2001, **37**:597–607.
19. Silberg JL, Bulik CM: **The developmental association between eating disorders symptoms and symptoms of depression and anxiety in juvenile twin girls.** *J Child Psychol Psychiatry* 2005, **46**:1317–1326.
20. Stice E, Agras WS: **Predicting onset and cessation of bulimic behaviors during adolescence: a longitudinal grouping analysis.** *Behav Ther* 1998, **29**:257–276.
21. Gardner RM, Stark K, Friedman BN, Jackson NA: **Predictors of eating disorder scores in children ages 6 through 14: a longitudinal study.** *J Psychosom Res* 2000, **49**:199–205.
22. Stice E, Shaw HE, Nemeroff G: **Dual pathway model of bulimia nervosa: Longitudinal support for dietary restraint and affect-regulation mechanisms.** *J Soc Clin Psychol* 1998, **17**:129–149.
23. Ricciardelli LA, McCabe MP: **Dietary restraint and negative affect as mediators of body dissatisfaction and bulimic behavior in adolescent girls and boys.** *Behav Res Ther* 2001, **39**:1317–1328.
24. Stice E: **A prospective test of the dual-pathway model of bulimic pathology: mediating effects of dieting and negative affect.** *J Abnorm Psychol* 2001, **110**:124–135.
25. Allen KL, Byrne SM, McLean NJ: **The dual-pathway and cognitive-behavioural models of binge eating: prospective evaluation and comparison.** *Eur Child Adolesc Psychiatry* 2012, **21**:51–62.
26. Santos M, Richards CS, Bleckley MK: **Comorbidity between depression and disordered eating in adolescents.** *Eat Behav* 2007, **8**:440–449.
27. Kieling C, Baker-Henningham H, Belfer M, Conti G, Ertem I, Omigbodun O, Rohde LA, Srinath S, Ulkuer N, Rahman A: **Child and adolescent mental health worldwide: evidence for action.** *Lancet* 2011, **378**:1515–1525.
28. Newnham JP, Evans SF, Michael CA, Stanley FJ, Landau LI: **Effects of frequent ultrasound during pregnancy: a randomised controlled trial.** *Lancet* 1993, **342**:887–891.
29. Allen KL, Byrne SM, Forbes D, Oddy WH: **Risk factors for full- and partial-syndrome early adolescent eating disorders: a population-based pregnancy cohort study.** *J Am Acad Child Adolesc Psychiatry* 2009, **48**:800–809.
30. Bryant-Waugh RJ, Cooper PJ, Taylor CL, Lask BD: **The use of the Eating Disorder Examination with children: a pilot study.** *Int J Eat Disord* 1996, **19**:391–397.
31. Fairburn CG, Beglin SJ: **Assessment of eating disorders: interview or self-report questionnaire?** *Int J Eat Disord* 1994, **16**:363–370.
32. Mond JM, Hay PJ, Rodgers B, Owen C, Beumont PJV: **Validity of the Eating Disorder Examination Questionnaire (EDE-Q) in screening for eating disorders in community samples.** *Behav Res Ther* 2004, **42**:551–567.
33. Keel PK, Crow SJ, Davis TL, Mitchell JE: **Assessment of eating disorders: Comparison of interview and questionnaire data from a long-term follow-up study of bulimia nervosa.** *J Psychosom Res* 2002, **53**:1043–1047.
34. Berg KC, Stiles-Shields EC, Swanson SA, Peterson CB, Lebow J, Le Grange D: **Diagnostic concordance of the interview and questionnaire versions of the eating disorder examination.** *Int J Eat Disord* 2012, **45**:850–855.
35. Berg KC, Peterson CB, Frazier P, Crow SJ: **Psychometric evaluation of the eating disorder examination and eating disorder examination-questionnaire: a systematic review of the literature.** *Int J Eat Disord* 2012, **45**:428–438.
36. Berg KC, Peterson CB, Frazier P, Crow SJ: **Convergence of scores on the interview and questionnaire versions of the eating disorder examination: a meta-analytic review.** *Psychol Assess* 2011, **23**:714–724.
37. Goldschmidt AB, Doyle AC, Wilfley DE: **Assessment of binge eating on overweight youth using a questionnaire version of the child eating disorder examination with instructions.** *Int J Eat Disord* 2007, **40**:460–467.

38. Walsh BT: *Report of the DSM-5 Eating Disorders Work Group.* Virginia: American Psychiatric Association DSM-5 Development; 2009.
39. Beck S, Beck AT, Jolly J: *Beck Youth Inventory.* New York: Psychological Corporation; 2001.
40. Beck AT, Steer RA, Brown GK: *Beck Depression Inventory.* 2nd edition. San Antonio: The Psychological Corporation; 1996.
41. Eack SM, Singer JB, Greeno CG: **Screening for anxiety and depression in community mental health: the Beck anxiety and depression inventories.** *Community Ment Health J* 2008, **44:**465–474.
42. Kenwood MG, Carpenter J: **Multiple imputation: current perspectives.** *Stat Methods Med Res* 2007, **16:**199–218.
43. Schafer JL, Graham JW: **Missing data: our view of the state of the art.** *Psychol Methods* 2002, **7:**141–177.
44. Zhou XH, Eckert GJ, Tierney WM: **Multiple imputation in public health research.** *Stat Med* 2001, **20:**1541–1549.
45. Liang KY, Zeger S: **Longitudinal data analysis using generalized linear models.** *Biometrika* 1986, **73:**13–22.
46. Wang YG, Carey V: **Working correlation structure misspectification, estimation and covariate design: Implications for generalised estimating equations performance.** *Biometrika* 2003, **90:**29–41.
47. Wolke D, Waylen A, Samara M, Steer C, Goodman R, Ford T: **Selective drop-out in longitudinal studies and non-biased prediction of behaviour disorders.** *Br J Psychiatry* 2009, **195:**249–256.
48. Chen HY, Little R: **A test of missing completely at random for generalised estimating equations with missing data.** *Biometrika* 1999, **86:**1–13.
49. Fairburn CG, Marcus MD, Wilson GT: **Cognitive-behavioural therapy for binge eating and bulimia nervosa: a comprehensive treatment manual.** In *Binge eating: Nature, assessment and treatment.* Edited by Fairburn CG, Wilson GT. New York: Guilford Press; 1993:361–404. edn.
50. Li J, Kendall GE, Henderson S, Downie J, Landsborough L, Oddy WH: **Maternal psychosocial wellbeing in pregnancy and breastfeeding duration.** *Acta Paediatr* 2008, **97:**221–225.

11

Enhancing quality of life in people with disordered eating using an online self-help programme

Sau F Leung[1*], Joyce LC Ma[2] and Janice Russell[3]

Abstract

Background: Eating disorders are serious mental illnesses that have a significant effect on afflicted individuals' quality of life. Evidence has shown that they can be improved with treatment. Internet-based interventions are useful in engaging individuals with eating disorders in self-management and treatment. This study aimed primarily to identify the change in quality of life of individuals with disordered eating after participating in an open trial of an Internet-based self-help programme, and compared their quality of life at assessment with that of healthy controls. Factors affecting their quality of life were examined. Secondary outcomes related to symptom improvement were also reported.

Methods: This study included 194 individuals with disordered eating and 50 healthy controls. The former group was recruited from eating disorder outpatient clinics and treatment units, as well as via information disseminated through various Internet websites, while the healthy controls were recruited from university student newspapers and university campuses. The Medical Outcomes Study Short Form Survey (SF-36v2) was used to assess participants' quality of life. Other measures were used to assess their symptoms and motivational stages of change to recover from an eating disorder. The Wilcoxon signed ranks test and one-way repeated measures ANOVA were used to identify the change in quality of life of individuals with disordered eating from baseline to 1-, 3- and 6-month follow-ups. The Mann–Whitney *U* test was employed to compare the difference in quality of life between participants with disordered eating and the healthy controls. Spearman rank order correlations were performed to examine the factors associated with quality of life.

Results: The participants with disordered eating had significantly poorer quality of life than the healthy controls in both physical and psychological domains. The factors associated with their poor quality of life included dieting behaviour, use of laxatives, severe eating disorder psychopathology, depression and anxiety. Over a six-month follow-up period, a significant number of participants engaged in self-help behaviours using the Internet-based programme. They experienced improvements in their quality of life, eating disorder psychopathology, depression severity, anxiety level and motivational stages of change.

Conclusions: Internet-based self-help programmes have the potential to enhance quality of life in individuals with disordered eating and could be useful adjuncts to professional treatment.

Keywords: Quality of life, Eating disorders, Internet-based self-help programme

* Correspondence: sau.fong.leung@polyu.edu.hk
[1]School of Nursing, The Hong Kong Polytechnic University, Hung Hom, Kowloon, Hong Kong, China
Full list of author information is available at the end of the article

Background

Eating disorders are serious mental illnesses that impair cognitive function, judgment and emotional stability, and limit the life activities of the sufferers [1]. Such disorders have a significant impact on individuals' quality of life, and can seriously affect their physical, social and psychological well-being [2,3]. The severity and chronicity of the illnesses are likely to exert negative effects on various life domains, such as physical functioning, performance at work or school, finances, interpersonal relationships, and social and role functioning [4-6]. Some factors in eating disorders have been reported to be associated with poorer quality of life, such as binge eating, vomiting, laxative use, use of diet pills, excessive exercise, severe psychopathology, extremes of BMI, and presence of psychiatric comorbidity [7-10].

Individuals with eating disorders have substantial impairment in quality of life, worse than those with other psychiatric disorders (e.g., alcohol abuse and somatoform disorder) [11], physical illnesses (e.g., angina and cystic fibrosis) [12], and healthy controls [2,13]. In a study comparing current and former eating disorder patients, current patients were shown to have poor quality of life in most domains, including sense of belonging, work/education, coping with disease-specific psychopathology, leisure activities, life skills, sense of purpose or meaning, financial situation, living condition, and particularly self-image and well-being [14]. Former eating disorder patients had better quality of life than current patients, but their ratings in different domains were only slightly above average. Another study found that former eating disorder patients had poorer quality of life than a normal reference group, even though they had recovered from their illnesses [2]. The findings of these studies underscore the impact of eating disorders on individuals' quality of life, even following recovery.

There is some evidence showing that quality of life can be improved with face-to-face treatment [7,15], but this is limited to individuals who have access to professional services or who are willing to receive treatment. Internet-based interventions could be a viable alternative to reach out to individuals with eating disorders and engage them in self-management and treatment. Numerous European studies using a self-help approach have shown that Internet-based interventions can improve eating disorder symptoms, general psychopathology, self-esteem, depression and general life satisfaction [16-20]. However, little is known about their use in the Asia-Pacific region. It is important to replicate similar studies from the West and expand this innovative approach to therapy in the Asia-Pacific region, as it may have the potential to enhance the quality of life of individuals with eating disorders.

This study aimed primarily to i) identify the change in quality of life of individuals with disordered eating after using an Internet-based self-help programme developed in the Asia-Pacific region, ii) compare their quality of life with healthy controls at baseline assessment, and iii) identify the factors affecting their quality of life. Other secondary outcomes related to the improvement in eating disorder psychopathology, depression severity, anxiety level and motivational stages of change were also examined.

Methods

Design

This study was an open trial of an Internet-based self-help programme, the "Smart Eating" programme, developed in the Asia-Pacific region by the first author. A randomised controlled design was not used due to the difficulty of recruiting a large number of participants with eating disorders. This difficulty can be related to the ego-syntonic nature of the disorders, ambivalence toward treatment and poor acceptability of treatments [21,22]. The study was conducted in Hong Kong and Sydney, and was approved by the University of Sydney Human Research Ethics Committee and the relevant health service ethics committees. Participation in the study was voluntary. All participants were provided with a detailed information sheet when they logged into the self-help programme on the Internet. They were informed that further explanation of the study could be obtained from the investigators, either through direct personal contact or by e-mail. Written consent was obtained from each participant online through the self-help programme, and they were informed that they could withdraw from the study at any time.

Participants were required to complete an online registration in the self-help programme, and to choose their own usernames and passwords to log in to the programme. The online registration form elicited demographic information including gender, date of birth, body weight, body height, nationality, country of current residence, e-mail address, marital status, educational attainment, occupation, health history and treatments related to eating disorders, and assessment scores of the SCOFF questionnaire and EDE-Q, 5th edition (EDE-Q5). For security purposes, the demographic information and data provided by the users were protected by password and a special Web maintenance service.

The SCOFF questionnaire is a 5-item quick screening tool that addresses the core features of anorexia nervosa and bulimia nervosa [23]. A score of 2 or above in the SCOFF questionnaire indicates a high risk of having an eating disorder. The EDE-Q is a 28-item self-report questionnaire that focuses on symptoms that occurred within the previous 28 days [24]. Some items in the

EDE-Q identify the behavioural features of eating disorders in terms of frequency or days the behaviour has occurred, and others assess the severity of eating disorder symptoms on four subscales: dietary restraint, eating concern, weight concern, and shape concern. The items on each subscale are rated on a 7-point rating scale (0–6). A mean score of 4–6 on any subscale is interpreted as meaning a greater likelihood of clinical severity.

Assessment questionnaires

The Medical Outcomes Study Short Form Survey (SF-36 version 2) was administered through the Smart Eating programme to assess the participants' quality of life. It is the most widely used generic quality of life measure for individuals with eating disorders [12]. It contains 36 questions on eight scales to measure physical functioning, physical role functioning, bodily pain, general health, vitality, social functioning, emotional role functioning, and mental health [25]. The score of each scale ranges from 0–100, with higher scores indicating a better state of health. The eight scales can be summarised into the Physical Component Summary scale (PCS) and the Mental Component Summary scale (MCS).

In a large U.S. population study, SF-36 version 2 was identified to have high internal consistency reliability coefficients for all scales (well above 0.8) [25]. The SF-36 can be used to assess functional capacity and well-being across a wide variety of medical and psychiatric conditions, to monitor changes in functioning over time, and to evaluate treatment options [26]. The measure has been adapted for use in numerous large-scale studies and across different healthcare settings in Australia since 1992. In a random sample of 855 subjects from the general population, the SF-36 was reported to have good internal consistency reliability for all scales (Cronbach's alpha = 0.81-0.92) and good construct validity in factor analysis, supporting the accuracy of both the physical and mental health dimensions [27]. In the first Australian national household panel survey involving 13,055 respondents, SF-36 was shown to be psychometrically sound, with good internal consistency, discriminant validity and high reliability across its eight scales [28]. The psychometric properties of SF-36 were further established in Australia from the data drawn from five studies with 41,338 participants aged 45 to 97 years in the Dynamic Analyses to Optimise Ageing (DYNOPTA) project [29]. These results confirmed the structural validity and good internal consistency reliability of SF-36, and were comparable with those found in younger Australian and international samples.

Other health assessment questionnaires offered by the Smart Eating programme include the Eating Disorder Examination Questionnaire (EDE-Q5) [24], the Eating Disorder Inventory-3 (EDI-3) [30], the Beck Depression Inventory (BDI-II) [31], the Beck Anxiety Inventory (BAI) [32], and the Motivational Stages of Change for Adolescents Recovering from an Eating Disorder (MSCARED) [33], which could be administered to both adolescents and adults in this study. EDE-Q5 is different from EDI-3, since EDE-Q5 measures the behavioural features of eating disorders, dietary restraint and concerns over eating, weight and shape [24], whereas the EDI-3 assesses the attitudes, behaviours and psychological traits of individuals with eating disorders [30]. Permission was obtained from the developers or authorities for online use of the questionnaires. All questionnaires demonstrated good psychometric properties in terms of internal consistency reliability [34-37], test-retest reliability [30,34-36,38], convergent validity [37], and concurrent validity [38].

Higher scores on the EDE-Q5, EDI-3, BDI-II, and BAI indicate more severe eating disorder psychopathology and associated psychological symptoms. Higher scores on the SF-36 and MSCARED indicate better perceived quality of life and higher motivation to change disordered eating behaviour.

Participants

The participants were recruited by the first author. Those with disordered eating were recruited through personal approach or promotional leaflets distributed in two outpatient eating disorder clinics and two eating disorder treatment units, and information disseminated through various Internet websites. The healthy controls were recruited from two universities through university student newspapers and the on-campus distribution of promotional leaflets. Individuals were able to participate in the study if they were aged 16 to 50 years old (male or female) and identified themselves as healthy controls or suffering from an eating disorder as shown by the assessment scores of the SCOFF questionnaire or the EDE-Q5.

Participants who successfully registered in the programme were invited via e-mail to complete six self-assessment questionnaires available in the self-help programme. After completing this baseline assessment, they received an e-mail with instructions on using the programme. The participants were reminded via e-mail to complete the six self-assessment questionnaires at the 1- and 3-month follow-up periods, as well as at the 6-month follow-up if possible. Participants with disordered eating were also followed up monthly through e-mail correspondence. The e-mails were standardised, enquiring about individual progress in using the programme and encouraging them to continue.

Materials

The smart eating self-help programme

The Smart Eating self-help programme comprises several components relating to healthy eating, family education, health assessment, motivation enhancement, self-help strategies, and psychological health promotion. The motivation enhancement component encourages individuals' motivation to change and recover from an eating disorder. The self-help strategies introduced in the programme help individuals restore healthy weight; normalise eating patterns; manage dieting, bingeing, and purging; challenge negative automatic thoughts and thinking errors; develop problem-solving abilities; and prevent relapse. The psychological health promotion component covers strategies for coping with stress, body image alteration, low self-esteem, depression, and anxiety. The content of the programme incorporates expert input from eating disorder specialists and is consistent with treatment recommendations for eating disorders from different eating disorder practice guidelines, including those of the American Psychiatric Association (APA) [39], the National Institute for Clinical Excellence (NICE) [40] and the Royal Australian and New Zealand College of Psychiatrists [41,42]. Before its launch, the programme was examined in a usability test on 15 female inpatients to demonstrate its usefulness, satisfactory information quality and good interface quality.

To acquire the maximum benefit from the Smart Eating programme, participants with disordered eating were recommended to go through its individual components in the following pattern as prescribed in the programme:

1. Browse through the information on healthy eating
2. Solicit support from family members to overcome an eating disorder, and ask them to view the information about family education
3. Complete all health assessment questionnaires at baseline
4. Work through the worksheets on motivational enhancement
5. Follow the steps in the self-help strategies to overcome eating disorders
6. Use different strategies to promote psychological health
7. Complete all health assessment questionnaires again at 1-, 3- and 6-month follow-up intervals to monitor personal progress

The healthy controls in this study had access limited to the programme components of healthy eating, family education and health assessment. They could use the programme to find out whether they had an eating disorder or an associated psychological problem (e.g. anxiety or depression). Participants with disordered eating had access to all components of the programme, and used it to learn and apply various self-help strategies and perform online self-assessments to monitor their progress in eating disorder psychopathology, motivational stage of change, and psychological health. They also used the programme privately at a time and pace convenient to themselves. A tracking system was implemented to determine compliance with the programme regarding health assessment, motivation enhancement, self-help strategies and psychological health promotion.

Data analysis

The data were analysed using the Predictive Analytics Software (PASW 17.0) statistical package. Descriptive analysis was performed to identify participants' demographic characteristics. The Wilcoxon signed ranks test and one-way repeated measures ANOVA were used to identify changes in the quality of life of individuals with disordered eating from baseline to the 1-, 3- and 6-month follow-ups. The Mann–Whitney *U* test was employed to compare the differences in quality of life between participants with disordered eating and the healthy controls. Spearman rank order correlations were performed to examine the factors affecting individuals' quality of life.

Results

Participant characteristics

A total of 362 individuals who identified themselves as having an eating disorder and 88 healthy controls registered in the programme from August 2006 to May 2012. The former group is referred to as the participants with disordered eating in this study. Among them, 194 (53.6%) participants with disordered eating and 50 (56.8%) healthy controls initiated their baseline health assessment with the Smart Eating programme, and their findings are reported in this paper (Figure 1). Reminders were sent to those individuals who did not initiate the programme, but they did not respond.

The 194 participants with disordered eating comprised 191 females and 3 males. Their ages ranged from 16 to 50 years (mean age 26.9). Their mean body mass index (BMI) was 21.25 (SD 5.99; range 13.05-57.81). Among them, 82 (42.3%) were not receiving any specialist treatment for eating disorders, and 112 (57.7%) were receiving treatment. The treatment was provided by psychiatrists/medical practitioners (86/194, 44.3%), psychologists/counsellors (44/194, 22.7%), dieticians (28/194, 14.4%) or a mental health nurse specialist (1/194, 0.5%). Some of the participants reported taking medication (50/194, 25.8%), and a few were using Chinese herbal medicine (1/194, 0.5%), acupuncture (1/194, 0.5%), naturopathy (1/194, 0.5%), or nutritional supplements (2/194, 1%) in their treatment. Among the healthy controls, there were 45 females and 5 males. Their ages ranged from 17 to 48

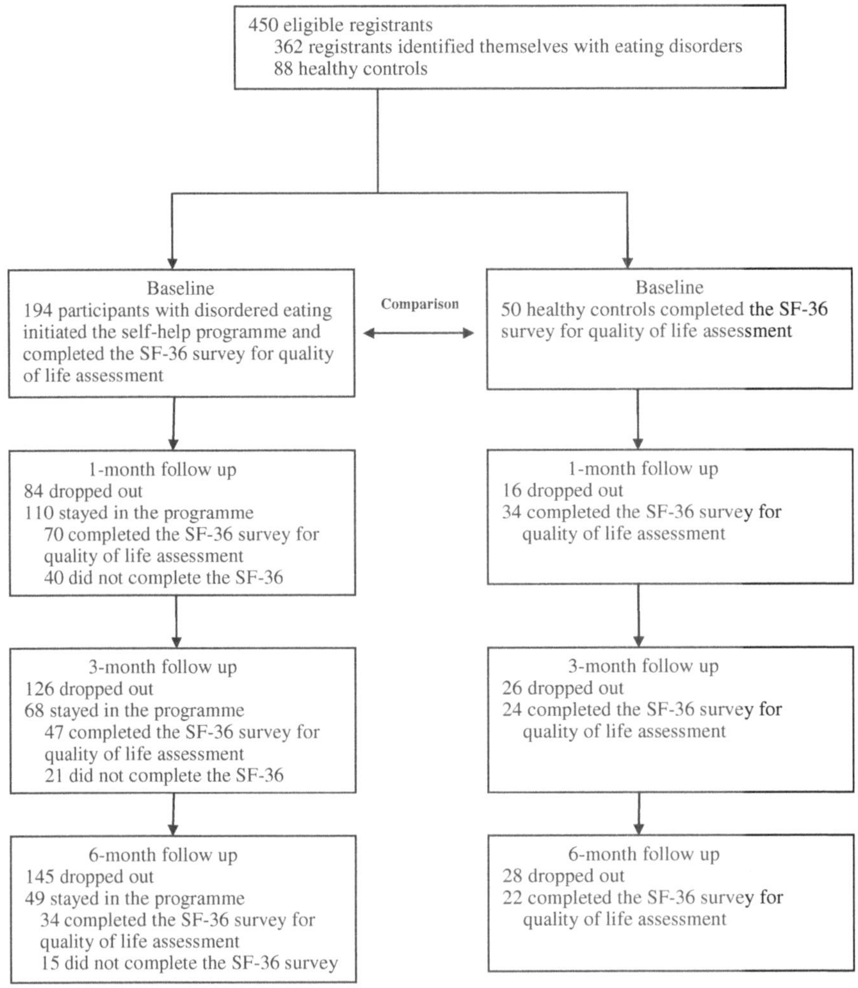

Figure 1 Flow of participants in the Smart Eating self-help programme.

years (mean age 24.7). Their mean BMI was 20.7 (SD 3.14; range 16.2-31.3). Most of the participants were Australian or Hong Kong Chinese. A majority of them had a secondary education or higher. Table 1 shows detailed demographic information.

Online health assessment scores of the participants

The eating disorder psychopathology of the participants was examined by the online self-administered SCOFF questionnaire and the Eating Disorder Examination Questionnaire (EDE-Q 5th edition) when they registered in the Smart Eating programme. According to the assessment scores, 191 participants with disordered eating scored at least 2 on the SCOFF questionnaire or had at least one subscale score on the EDE-Q5 falling in the clinically significant range (≥ 4). The three remaining participants had non-significant assessment scores but reported participating in treatment for their eating disorders, and two had low BMI (15.59 and 16.53). Thus, all 194 participants with disordered eating had a clinically significant eating disorder based on their SCOFF questionnaire/EDE-Q5 scores or their treatment for an eating disorder. The participants with disordered eating had significantly higher mean scores in the SCOFF questionnaires (3.36) and the Eating Disorder Examination Questionnaire (≥4 for each subscale) than the healthy controls (Table 2). At baseline assessment, the former group also had significantly higher scores on EDI-3, BDI-II, and BAI, indicating more severe eating disorder psychopathology, depressive symptoms and anxiety level than the latter group.

SF-36 measured the quality of life of the participants. Those with disordered eating were identified as having significantly poorer quality of life than the healthy controls in both physical (physical functioning, physical role

Table 1 Demographic characteristics of participants (n=244)

Variables	Participants with disordered eating (n=194)		Healthy controls (n=50)	
	Number	Percentage	Number	Percentage
Gender				
Female	191	98.5	45	90
Male	3	1.5	5	10
Educational level				
No schooling	3	1.5	0	0
Secondary	62	32	4	8
Tertiary	128	66	45	90
Unknown	1	0.5	1	2
Marital status				
Single	134	69.1	45	90
Married	32	16.5	5	10
Cohabiting	22	11.3	0	0
Divorced	5	2.6	0	0
Widowed	1	0.5	0	0
Employment status				
Full-time employment	92	47.4	11	22
Unemployed	13	6.7	0	0
Homemaker	8	4.1	0	0
Student	81	41.8	39	78
Nationality/National group				
Australian	142	73.2	3	6
Chinese	12	6.2	41	82
Other Asian	9	4.6	0	0
European	12	6.2	2	4
New Zealander	10	5.1	1	2
Canadian	4	2.1	0	0
American	4	2.1	2	4
Others	1	0.5	1	2

functioning, bodily pain and general health) and mental health domains (vitality, social functioning, emotional role functioning and mental health). Their quality of life in the mental health domains was also worse than in the physical health domains. This was also shown from the lower score in the Mental Component Summary scale (MCS) than the Physical Component Summary scale (PCS) of SF-36. Table 2 compares the differences in all the health assessment scores at baseline between the participants with disordered eating and the healthy controls.

Factors affecting the quality of life of participants with disordered eating

To identify the factors associated with poor quality of life in participants with disordered eating, Spearman rank order correlations were performed among various variables concerning eating disorder psychopathology, depression severity, anxiety level, motivational stages of change and quality of life. The findings revealed that quality of life (SF-36 score; mean scores of both physical and mental health domains) had a significant negative correlation with dieting behaviour ($r_{s=}$-0.165, $p<0.05$) and use of laxatives ($r_{s=}$ -0.167, p=<0.05) (Table 3). Also, quality of life was significantly affected by the increase in eating disorder psychopathology, depression severity and anxiety level, as shown from the negative correlation between SF-36 scores and those on the SCOFF questionnaire (r_s= −0.204, $p<0.01$), Global EDE-Q5 (r_s= −0.428, $p<0.01$), EDI-3 (r_s= −0.573, $p<0.01$), BDI-II (r_s= −0.715, $p<0.01$) and BAI (r_s= −.592, $p<0.01$) (Table 3). However, there was a significant positive correlation between individuals' motivational stages of change and the quality of life domains of physical function (r_s= 0.168, $p<0.05$), general health (r_s= 0.208, $p<0.01$), vitality (r_s= 0.209, $p<0.01$) and mental health (r=0.146, $p<0.05$).

Change in the quality of life of participants with disordered eating in this open trial study

The tracking system of the Smart Eating programme found that 194 participants with disordered eating engaged in various self-help behaviours, such as completing at least one baseline health assessment (177/194, 91.2%), working through motivation enhancement exercises (108/194, 55.7%), learning how to improve body image (91/194, 46.9%), and using self-help strategies to overcome eating disorders (63/194, 32.5%). Other self-help behaviours included identifying strategies for overcoming depression (55/194, 28.4%), managing anxiety (53/194, 27.3%), coping with stress (50/194, 25.8%), and boosting self-esteem (47/194, 24.2%).

Seventy participants (36.1%) used the programme for at least 1 month. The Wilcoxon signed ranks test identified significant improvement in their quality of life (Z= −2.581, $p<0.05$), particularly in the domains of bodily pain (Z= −2.167, $p<0.05$), general health (Z= −2.623, $p<0.01$), social functioning (Z= −2.475, $p<0.05$) and emotional role functioning (Z= −2.382, $p<0.05$) from baseline to 1-month follow up. The improvement in quality of life continued at the 3-month follow up for 47 participants (F=6.532, $p<0.01$), who also experienced significant improvements in their general health (F=5.655, $p<0.01$), social functioning (F=10.69, $p<0.001$), emotional role functioning (F=11.877, $P<0.001$) and mental health (F=7.746, $p<0.01$), as shown by the result of the one-way repeated measures ANOVA. At the 6-month follow up, 34 participants were still using the programme. Table 4 shows that these participants had significant improvement in their quality of life, eating disorder psychopathology, depression level and motivational stages of change from baseline assessment to the 1-month, 3-month and

Table 2 Comparison of health assessment scores of participants with disordered eating and healthy controls at baseline using the Mann–Whitney *U* test

Variables	Participants with disordered eating (n=194)		Healthy controls (n=50)		Z	P value
	(M)	(SD)	(M)	(SD)		
SCOFF score	3.36	0.95	0.63	0.83	−10.45	<0.001
EDE-Q5 (global score)	4.47	0.97	0.92	0.78	−10.58	<0.001
Dietary restraint	4.08	1.24	0.55	0.75	−10.44	<0.001
Eating concern	4.15	1.25	0.42	0.59	−10.61	<0.001
Shape concern	4.91	1.15	1.70	1.27	−9.89	<0.001
Weight concern	4.66	1.24	1.25	1.20	−9.94	<0.001
SF-36v2*	52.40	16.14	75.82	11.89	−8.14	<0.001
PCS	65.35	18.20	79.26	11.74	−4.97	<0.001
Physical functioning	84.66	18.10	89.80	16.57	−2.32	0.021
Physical role functioning	67.05	28.75	85.64	17.46	−4.22	<0.001
Bodily pain	64.71	23.81	82.12	20.95	−4.66	<0.001
General health	44.98	23.42	59.48	19.26	−4.02	<0.001
MCS	39.45	18.27	72.38	16.05	−8.74	<0.001
Vitality	31.18	19.25	57.72	18.04	−7.38	<0.001
Social functioning	40.74	26.17	83.58	19.32	−8.59	<0.001
Emotional rolefunctioning	45.45	26.43	80.52	19.69	−7.55	<0.001
Mental health	40.44	18.60	67.70	20.18	−7.39	<0.001
EDI-3	16.29	4.11	6.70	2.78	−9.99	<0.001
Drive for thinness	22.42	5.40	5.80	5.48	−9.89	<0.001
Bulimia	16.50	9.43	3.74	3.52	−7.86	<0.001
Body dissatisfaction	29.75	8.46	14.15	8.90	−8.15	<0.001
Low self-esteem	15.19	5.49	5.35	3.59	−8.99	<0.001
Personal alienation	15.06	5.88	6.00	4.95	−8.02	<0.001
Interpersonal insecurity	13.96	5.86	6.28	4.33	−7.32	<0.001
Interpersonal alienation	12.53	5.46	5.74	3.86	−7.18	<0.001
Interoceptive deficits	19.17	7.67	6.30	5.65	−8.56	<0.001
Emotional dysregulation	10.22	6.64	4.61	3.99	−5.51	<0.001
Perfectionism	14.51	6.20	7.09	4.58	−6.86	<0.001
Asceticism	13.78	5.74	4.17	2.74	−9.09	<0.001
Maturity fears	12.37	7.33	11.20	5.10	−0.71	0.478
BDI-II	32.51	13.28	7.19	7.94	−9.41	<0.001
BAI	19.66	12.10	4.71	4.05	−8.82	<0.001
MSCARED #	2.89	0.98	0	0	−11.00	<0.001

SCOFF, The SCOFF Questionnaire; EDE-Q5, Eating Disorder Examination Questionnaire version 5.
SF-36v2*, Mean score of physical and mental health domains of the 36-item Short Form Health Survey version 2.
PCS, SF-36 Physical Component Summary scale; MCS, SF-36 Mental Component Summary scale.
EDI-3, Eating Disorder Inventory version 3; BDI-II, Beck Depression Inventory version 2.
BAI, Beck Anxiety Inventory.
MSCARED, The Motivational Stages of Change for Adolescents Recovering from an Eating Disorder.
# Motivational stages of change.
0=Not applicable, 1=Pre-contemplation, 2=Contemplation, 3=Preparation, 4=Action, 5=Maintenance, 6=Recovery.

6-month follow-ups. They had significant increases in their SF-36 and MSCARED scores, and significant decreases in their EDE-Q5, EDI-3 and BDI-II scores.

Intention-to-treat analysis

In view of the number of participants with disordered eating who did not complete the follow-up health assessment and self-help programme, an intention-to-treat analysis was also performed. This type of analysis is used for clinical trial data in which the outcomes of all participants, including those who drop out prematurely, are included in the analysis. The last observation carried forward (LOCF) method was used, in which the missing values of the outcome variables are

Table 3 Spearman's rank-order correlations between quality of life and eating disorder psychopathology, eating disorder behaviours, depression severity, anxiety level and motivational stages of change

	SF-36 v2	*Physical functioning*	*Physical role functioning*	*Bodily pain*	*General health*	*Vitality*	*Social functioning*	*Emotional role functioning*	*Mental health*
SCOFF	−0.204**	−0.002	−0.141*	−0.129	−0.154*	−0.120	−0.204**	−0.189**	−0.204**
Global EDE-Q5	−0.428**	−0.254**	−0.276**	−0.239**	−0.327**	−0.341**	−0.350**	−0.323**	−0.418**
Dieting	−0.165*	−0.069	−0.066	−0.118	−0.149*	−0.170*	−0.118	−0.104	−0.208**
Vomiting	−0.036	0.019	−0.002	−0.051	−0.025	−0.012	−0.032	−0.088	−0.040
Bingeing	0.084	0.120	0.109	0.190*	0.185*	0.107	0.051	−0.153*	−0.038
Laxative misuse	−0.167*	−0.172*	−0.109	−0.249**	−0.094	−0.060	−0.061	−0.122	−0.113
Compulsive exercise	−0.053	0.256**	0.017	−0.163*	0.036	0.048	−0.262**	−0.059	−0.098
EDI-3	−0.573**	−0.266**	−0.354**	−0.295**	−0.421**	−0.476**	−0.424**	−0.472**	−0.602**
BDI-II	−0.715**	−0.375**	−0.437**	−0.314**	−0.537**	−0.611**	−0.553**	−0.561**	−0.742**
BAI	−0.592**	−0.292**	−0.393**	−0.409**	−0.372**	−0.379**	−0.482**	−0.493**	−0.567**
MSCARED	0.113	0.168*	0.018	0.071	0.208**	0.209**	0.017	−0.037	0.146*

*Significance P<0.05, ** Significance P<0.01.
SF-36v2, The 36-item Short Form Health Survey version 2; SCOFF, The SCOFF Questionnaire.
EDE-Q5, Eating Disorder Examination Questionnaire version 5; EDI-3, Eating Disorder Inventory version 3.
BDI-II, Beck Depression Inventory version 2; BAI, Beck Anxiety Inventory.
MSCARED, The Motivational Stages of Change for Adolescents Recovering from an Eating Disorder.

replaced by the most recent known values before the participants were lost to follow up [43]. This is based on the rationale that participants with eating disorders are unlikely to improve further in the absence of treatment.

The intention-to-treat analyses revealed significant increases in their SF-36 and MSCARED scores from baseline to 1-, 3- and 6-month follow-ups and significant decreases in their EDE-Q5, EDI-3 and BDI-II scores (Table 5). These findings indicate a significant improvement in their quality

Table 4 Comparison of health assessment scores of participants with disordered eating from baseline to 1-, 3- and 6-month follow-ups using one-way repeated measures ANOVA

N=34	Time 1 (baseline)	Time 2 (1-month FU)	Time 3 (3-month FU)	Time 4 (6-month FU)	F	Partial eta squared	P value
	Mean ± s.d.	Mean ± s.d.	Mean ± s.d.	Mean ± s.d.			
SF-36v2*	45.60±15.84	50.23±19.58	55.72±22.41	59.23±24.27	4.93	0.323	**0.007**
PCS	59.67±21.05	61.34±24.38	64.15±24.17	68.95±25.34	2.30	0.182	0.097
Physical functioning	79.71±21.46	79.56±25.74	82.06±23.59	82.35±20.12	0.26	0.025	0.852
Physical role functioning	57.32±33.57	57.18±33.87	62.94±29.68	69.29±32.93	1.80	0.148	0.168
Bodily pain	59.71±25.72	63.35±25.93	61.38±29.90	70.38±29.31	2.01	0.162	0.134
General health	41.94±29.26	45.26±28.59	50.24±30.17	53.76±31.06	2.51	0.196	0.077
MCS	31.54±13.81	39.12±18.78	47.28±24.18	49.51±26.70	8.40	0.448	**<0.001**
Vitality	27.18±20.58	32.29±22.36	36.00±27.29	38.53±27.65	2.61	0.202	0.069
Social functioning	29.38±21.17	38.94±26.60	49.71±31.25	50.03±32.03	5.78	0.359	**0.003**
Emotional role functioning	34.29±22.51	46.56±23.79	56.65±24.95	59.76±32.34	9.40	0.476	**<0.001**
Mental health	35.29±14.92	38.68±17.42	46.76±23.25	49.71±23.90	6.40	0.382	**0.002**
Global EDE-Q5	4.63±0.83	3.99±1.25	3.34±1.53	3.26±1.72	12.52	0.540	**<0.001**
EDI-3	17.44±3.44	16.08±4.67	14.45±5.68	13.43±5.92	11.05	0.517	**<0.001**
BDI-II	37.29±12.48	31.71±15.33	26.26±16.60	23.82±17.43	8.53	0.452	**<0.001**
BAI	20.63±10.47	19.34±11.99	18.17±13.53	16.94±14.09	1.07	0.091	0.377
MSCARED	3.18±0.90	3.53±1.05	3.91±1.22	4.03±1.38	4.57	0.307	**0.009**

FU, follow up; s.d., standard deviation.
SF-36v2*, Mean score of physical and mental health domains of the 36-item Short Form Health Survey version 2.
PCS, SF-36 Physical Component Summary scale; MCS, SF-36 Mental Component Summary scale.
EDE-Q5, Eating Disorder Examination Questionnaire version 5; EDI-3, Eating Disorder Inventory version 3.
BDI-II, Beck Depression Inventory version 2; BAI, Beck Anxiety Inventory.
MSCARED, The Motivational Stages of Change for Adolescents Recovering from an Eating Disorder.

Table 5 Comparison of health assessment scores of participants with disordered eating from baseline assessment to 1-, 3- and 6-month follow-ups in the intention-to-treat analyses using one-way repeated measures ANOVA

N=194	Time 1 (baseline)	Time 2 (1-month FU)	Time 3 (3-month FU)	Time 4 (6-month FU)	F	Partial eta squared	P value
	Mean ± s.d.	Mean ± s.d.	Mean ± s.d.	Mean ± s.d.			
SF-36v2*	52.40±16.14	53.87±17.19	55.00±18.06	55.62±18.53	5.29	0.077	**0.002**
PCS	65.35±18.20	66.48±19.16	67.07±19.55	67.92±19.77	3.33	0.050	**0.021**
Physical functioning	84.66±18.10	84.38±20.17	84.87±19.60	84.92±18.93	0.31	0.005	0.816
Physical role functioning	67.05±28.75	68.18±29.08	69.48±28.07	70.60±28.53	2.57	0.039	0.056
Bodily pain	64.71±23.81	66.68±23.50	66.13±25.17	67.79±25.06	2.89	0.043	**0.037**
General health	44.98±23.42	46.68±23.45	47.80±23.92	48.37±24.15	4.04	0.060	**0.008**
MCS	39.45±18.27	41.30±19.63	42.98±20.77	43.35±21.37	5.97	0.086	**0.001**
Vitality	31.18±19.25	32.03±20.33	33.18±21.22	33.65±21.43	2.63	0.040	0.051
Social functioning	40.74±26.17	43.57±27.43	45.33±28.22	45.32±28.29	4.87	0.071	**0.003**
Emotional role functioning	45.45±26.43	48.03±26.38	50.18±26.67	50.76±28.21	5.30	0.077	**0.002**
Mental health	40.44±18.60	41.57±19.31	43.22±20.63	43.69±20.84	5.09	0.074	**0.002**
Global EDE-Q5	4.47±0.97	4.16±1.19	4.00±1.33	3.97±1.39	14.27	0.194	**<0.001**
EDI-3	16.29±4.10	15.81±4.39	15.48±4.68	15.29±4.80	9.40	0.131	**<0.001**
BDI-II	32.51±13.28	30.57±13.76	29.44±14.31	28.99±14.62	9.07	0.127	**<0.001**
BAI	19.66±12.10	19.10±11.94	18.87±12.36	18.64±12.49	1.25	0.020	0.292
MSCARED	3.22±0.89	3.36±0.92	3.43±0.98	3.44±1.05	6.41	0.093	**<0.001**

FU, follow up; s.d., standard deviation.
SF-36v2*, Mean score of physical and mental health domains of the 36-item Short Form Health Survey version 2.
PCS, SF-36 Physical Component Summary scale; MCS, SF-36 Mental Component Summary scale.
EDE-Q5, Eating Disorder Examination Questionnaire version 5; EDI-3, Eating Disorder Inventory version 3.
BDI-II, Beck Depression Inventory version 2; BAI, Beck Anxiety Inventory.
MSCARED, The Motivational Stages of Change for Adolescents Recovering from an Eating Disorder.

of life revealed by the SF-36, particularly in their bodily pain, general health, social functioning, emotional role functioning and mental health. Also there was a significant reduction in their eating disorder psychopathology as measured by the EDE-Q5 and the EDI-3. In addition, there were significant decreases in their depression levels, assessed by the BDI-II, along with an increase in their motivational stages of change, measured by the MSCARED. Although the BAI scores from baseline to 6-month follow-up showed a decrease in participants' anxiety levels, the change was non-significant.

Discussion

The Smart Eating programme engaged a significant number of individuals with disordered eating in self-help behaviour and also reached out to a number of those not receiving eating disorder treatment. Over a period of time using the programme, the participants saw an improvement in their quality of life, particularly in general health, social functioning, emotional role functioning and mental health as demonstrated by the increase in domain scores from baseline to the 1-, 3- and 6-month follow-ups. Improvement was also identified in participants' eating disorder psychopathology, depression severity, anxiety level and motivational stages of change. There were significant decreases in the EDE-Q5, EDI-3 and BDI-II scores and increases in their MSCARED scores. The intention-to-treat analyses produced similar results to the completer analyses at the 3- and 6-month follow-ups. The self-help programme appears to have the potential to enhance quality of life in individuals with disordered eating by reducing their eating disorder symptoms, depression and anxiety, and improving their motivational stages of change. A significant number of participants in this study (112/194, 57.7%) were already in treatment, but they also used the programme. This implies that the programme could be a useful adjunct to their professional treatment.

As expected, there was a significant difference in the clinical features between participants with disordered eating and the healthy controls. The difference was recognised in their assessment scores on the SCOFF questionnaire, EDE-Q5, EDI-3, BDI-II, BAI and SF-36, which showed that participants with eating disorders had severe eating disorder symptoms, depression and anxiety, resulting in poorer quality of life. Their quality of life was much worse than that of healthy controls in all the domains studied in the SF-36. Consistent with earlier findings, this study confirmed several associated factors affecting individuals' quality of life, including dieting, use of laxatives, severe eating disorder psychopathology and the existence of psychiatric comorbidity such as anxiety and depression [7-9]. A significant negative correlation was observed between quality of life and these factors in the study sample. Similar to the findings of other studies, eating disorders caused more impairment in the mental health domains of the participants' quality of life than in the physical health domains, and the impairment was more noticeable in vitality, mental health and social functioning in the SF-36 [2,44-46].

This study had several limitations. One was the convenience (non-random pragmatic) sampling method. Another was the open trial design of the self-help programme. The third limitation was the difficulty of recruiting a large sample of healthy controls due to the lack of incentives for them to initiate the programme for health assessment. In addition, there was a high attrition rate, although the majority of participants used the programme for at least a month. High attrition rates are common in studies using self-help treatments for eating disorders (0–69.7%) [47] and natural in Internet-based trials, particularly those with self-help applications [48]. The last limitation was the demographic differences between the disordered eating participants and the healthy controls. The former group was mostly Australian, whereas the latter group was mostly Chinese. This difference may not have had much impact on the findings of this study. Recent studies identified that the eating disorder psychopathology was similar between westernised Chinese and Australians [49,50], and the clinical presentation of eating disorders in Hong Kong Chinese has increasingly been found to conform to that in Western countries [51].

Future studies using the Smart Eating programme are recommended. The effectiveness of the programme in enhancing quality of life in individuals with eating disorders could be further evaluated in a randomised controlled study. Also, the effect of the programme could be compared with specialist treatment only and the condition of combining both specialist treatment and the programme.

Conclusions

Eating disorders have a significant impact on individuals' quality of life. Sufferers of eating disorders report significantly poorer quality of life than healthy controls in all physical and mental health domains. This poor quality of life can be associated with eating disordered behaviours, symptom severity, depression and anxiety. The Smart Eating online self-help programme developed in the Asia-Pacific region for people with eating disorders has the potential benefit of engaging individuals in self-help behaviour and treatment, and improving their quality of life. It could be a useful adjunct to professional treatment.

Competing interests

The authors declare that they have no competing interests.

Authors' contributions

SL, JM and JR contributed to the design of the study and data collection. SL analysed the findings and drafted this paper. All authors read and approved the final manuscript.

Acknowledgements

The authors would like to thank Dr. John Morgan, Professor Christopher Fairburn and Dr. Joanne Gusella for permission to use the SCOFF questionnaire, the Eating Disorder Examination-Questionnaire and the Motivational Stages of Change for Adolescents Recovering from an Eating Disorder (MSCARED) in this study. The authors would also like to acknowledge the valuable contribution of the subjects in this study.

Author details

[1]School of Nursing, The Hong Kong Polytechnic University, Hung Hom, Kowloon, Hong Kong, China. [2]Department of Social Work, The Chinese University of Hong Kong, Shatin, New Territories, Hong Kong, China. [3]Discipline of Psychiatry, Faculty of Medicine, Sydney Medical School, University of Sydney, Sydney, NSW 2006, Australia.

References

1. Klump KL, Bulik CM, Kaye WH, Treasure J, Tyson E: **Academy for eating disorders position paper: eating disorders are serious mental illnesses.** *Int J Eat Disord* 2009, **42**:97–103.
2. de la Rie S, Noordenbos G, van Furth EF: **Quality of life and eating disorders.** *Qual Life Res* 2005, **14**:1511–1522.
3. Doll HA, Petersen SE, Stewart-Brown SL: **Eating disorders and emotional and physical well-being: Associations between student self-reports of eating disorders and quality of life as measured by the SF-36.** *Qual Life Res* 2005, **14**:705–717.
4. Mitchell JE, Hatsukami D, Eckert ED, Pyle RL: **Characteristics of 275 patients with bulimia.** *Am J Psychiat* 1985, **142**:482–485.
5. Engel SG, Adair CE, Hayas CL, Abraham S: **Health-related quality of life and eating disorders.** *Int J Eat Disord* 2009, **42**:179–181.
6. Bamford B, Sly R: **Exploring quality of life in the eating disorders.** *Eur Eat Disord Rev* 2010, **18**:147–153.
7. Padierna A, Quintana JM, Arostegui I, Gonzalez N, Horcajo MJ: **Changes in health related quality of life among patients treated for eating disorders.** *Qual Life Res* 2002, **11**:545–552.
8. Mond JJ, Hay PJ, Rodgers B, Owen C, Mitchell J: **Correlates of the use of purging and non-purging methods of weight control in a community sample of women.** *Aust NZ J Psychiat* 2006, **40**:136–142.
9. Mond JJ, Hay PJ, Rodgers B, Owen C, Mitchell J: **Correlates of self-induced vomiting and laxative misuse in a community sample of women.** *J Nerv Ment Dis* 2006, **194**:40–46.
10. Jenkins PE, Hoste RR, Meyer C, Blissett JM: **Eating disorders and quality of life: A review of literature.** *Clin Psychol Rev* 2011, **31**:113–121.
11. Spitzer RL, Kroenke K, Linzer M, Hahn SR, Williams JB, DeGruy FV, Brody D, Davies M: **Health-related quality of life in primary care patients with mental disorders: results from the PRIME-MD 1000 study.** *J Am Med Assn* 1995, **274**:1511–1517.
12. Keilen M, Treasure T, Schmidt U, Treasure J: **Quality of life measurements in eating disorders, angina, and transplant candidates: Are they comparable?** *J Roy Soc Med* 1994, **87**:441–444.
13. Mond JM, Hay PJ, Rodgers B, Owen C, Beumont PJV: **Assessing quality of life in eating disorder patients.** *Qual Life Res* 2005, **14**:171–178.
14. de la Rie S, Noordenbos G, Donker M, van Furth EF: **The patient's view on quality of life and eating disorders.** *Int J Eat Disord* 2007, **40**:13–20.
15. Halvorsen I, Heyerdahl S: **Girls with anorexia nervosa as young adults: Personality, self-esteem, and life satisfaction.** *Int J Eat Disord* 2006, **39**:285–293.
16. Carrard I, Rouget P, Fern'andez-Arandab F, Volkart A-C, Damoiseau M, Lam T: **Evaluation and deployment of evidence-based patient self-management support program for bulimia nervosa.** *Int J Med Inform* 2006, **75**:101–109.

17. Liwowsky I, Cebulla M, Fichter M: **New ways to combat eating disorders – evaluation of an internet-based self-help program in bulimia nervosa.** *MMW Fortschr Med* 2006, **148:**31–33.
18. Nevonen L, Mark M, Levin B, Lindström M, Paulson-Karlsson G: **Evaluation of a new Internet-based self-help guide for patients with bulimic symptoms in Sweden.** *Nord J Psychiat* 2006, **60:**463–468.
19. Ljotsson B, Lundin C, Mitsell K, Carlbring P, Ramklint M, Ghaderi A: **Remote treatment of bulimia nervosa and binge eating disorder: A randomized trial of Internet-assisted cognitive behavioural therapy.** *Behav Res Ther* 2007, **45:**649–661.
20. Carrard I, Fernandez-Aranda F, Lam T, Nevonen L, Liwowsky I, Volkart AC, Rouget P, Golay A, Van der Linden M, Norring C: **Evaluation of a guided internet self-treatment programme for bulimia nervosa in several European countries.** *Eur Eat Disor Rev* 2011, **19:**138–149.
21. Halmi KA, Agras WS, Crow S, Mitchell J, Wilson GT, Bryson SW, Kraemer HC: **Predictors of treatment acceptance and completion in anorexia nervosa.** *Arch Gen Psychiatry* 2005, **62:**776–781.
22. Treasure J, Claudino AM, Zucker N: **Eating disorders.** *Lancet* 2010, **375:**583–593.
23. Morgan JF, Reid F, Lacey JH: **The SCOFF questionnaire: assessment of a new screening tool for eating disorders.** *Brit Med J* 1999, **319:**1467–1468.
24. Fairburn CG, Beglin SJ: **Assessment of eating disorders: Interview or self-report questionnaire?** *Int J Eat Disord* 1994, **16:**363–370.
25. Ware JE, Kosinski M, Dewey JE: *How to score version 2 of the SF-36 Health Survey.* Lincoln, RI: QualityMetric Incorporated; 2002.
26. Rush AJ, Pincus HA, First MB, Blacker D: *Handbook of psychiatric measures.* Washington, DC: American Psychiatric Association; 2000.
27. Sanson-Fisher RW, Perkins JJ: **Adaptation and validation of the SF-36 health survey for use in Australia.** *J Clin Epidemiol* 1998, **51:**961–967.
28. Butterworth P, Crosier T: **The validity of the SF-36 in an Australian national household survey: demonstrating the applicability of the household income and labour dynamics in Australia (HILDA) survey to examination of health inequalities.** *BMC Public Health* 2004, **4:**44.
29. Bartsch LJ, Butterworth P, Byles JE, Mitchell P, Shaw J, Anstey KJ: **Examining the SF-36 in an older population: analysis of data and presentation of Australian adult reference scores from the Dynamic Analyses to Optimise Ageing (DYNOPTA) project.** *Qual Life Res* 2011, **20:**1227–1236.
30. Garner DM: *Eating disorder inventory –3: professional manual.* U.S.A: Psychological Assessment Resources, Inc; 2004.
31. Beck AT, Steer RA, Brown GK: *Beck depression inventory - second edition: manual.* New York: The Psychological Corporation; 1996.
32. Beck AT, Steer RA: *Beck anxiety inventory – manual.* New York: The Psychological Corporation; 1993.
33. Gusella JL: *Manual for the MSCARED – motivational stages of change for adolescents recovering from an eating disorder.* Canada: Eating Disorders Clinic, IWK Health Centre; 2002.
34. Beck AT, Steer RA, Garbin MG: **Psychometric properties of the beck depression inventory: twenty-five years of evaluation.** *Clin Psychol Rev* 1988, **8:**77–100.
35. Luce KH, Crowther JH: **The reliability of the eating disorder examination – self-report questionnaire version (EDE-Q).** *Int J Eat Disord* 1999, **25:**349–351.
36. Osman A, Hoffman J, Barrios FX, Kopper BA, Breitenstein JL, Hahn SK: **Factor structure, reliability, and validity of the beck anxiety inventory in adolescent psychiatric inpatients.** *J Clin Psychol* 2002, **58:**443–456.
37. Dum M, Pickren J, Sobell LC, Sobell MB: **Comparing the BDI-II and the PHQ-9 with outpatient substance abusers.** *Addict Behav* 2008, **33:**381–387.
38. Gusella J, Butler G, Nichols L, Bird D: **A brief questionnaire to assess readiness to change in adolescents with eating disorders: Its applications to group therapy.** *Eur Eat Disor Rev* 2003, **11:**58–71.
39. Anonymous: **Treatment recommendations for patients with eating disorders.** *Am J Psychiat* 2006, **163**(July Supplement).
40. National Collaborating Centre for Mental Health: *Eating disorders: Core interventions in the treatment and management of anorexia nervosa, bulimia nervosa and related eating disorders.* London: National Institute for Clinical Excellence; 2004:1–28.
41. Beumont P, Hay P, Beumont R: **Summary Australian and New Zealand clinical practice guideline for the management of anorexia nervosa.** *Australas Psychiat* 2003, **11:**129–133.
42. Royal Australian and New Zealand College of Psychiatrists Clinical Practice Guidelines Team for Anorexia Nervosa: **Australian and New Zealand clinical practice guidelines for the treatment of anorexia nervosa.** *Aust NZ J Psychiat* 2004, **38:**659–670.
43. Mazumdar S, Liu KS, Houck PR, Reynolds CF: **Intent-to-treat analysis for longitudinal clinical trials: coping with the challenge of missing values.** *J Psychiatr Res* 1999, **33:**87–95.
44. Latner JD, Vallance JK, Buckett G: **Health-related quality of life in women with eating disorders: Association with subjective and objective binge eating.** *J Clin Psychol Med S* 2008, **15:**148–153.
45. Hay P: **Quality of life and bulimic eating disorder behaviors: Findings from a community-based sample.** *Int J Eat Disord* 2003, **33:**434–442.
46. González-Pinto A, Inmaculada F, Cristina R, de Corres Blanca F, Sonsoles E, Fernando R, Purificacion L: **Purging behaviors and comorbidity as predictive factors of quality of life in anorexia nervosa.** *Int J Eat Disord* 2004, **36:**445–450.
47. Sysko R, Walsh BT: **A critical evaluation of the efficacy of self-help interventions for the treatment of bulimia nervosa and binge-eating disorder.** *Int J Eat Disord* 2008, **41:**97–112.
48. Eysenbach G: **The law of attrition.** *J Med Internet Res* 2005, **7:**e11.
49. Soh NL, Touyz S, Dobbins TA, Surgenor LJ, Clarke S, Kohn MR, Lee EL, Leow V, Rieger E, Ung KE, Walter G: **Restraint and eating concern in North European and East Asian women with and without eating disorders in Australia and Singapore.** *Aust NZ J Psychiat* 2007, **41:**536–545.
50. Mond JM, Chen A, Kumar R: **Eating-disordered behavior in Australian and Singaporean women: A comparative study.** *Int J Eat Disord* 2010, **43:**717–723.
51. Lee S, Ng KL, Kwok K, Fung C: **The changing profile of eating disorders at a tertiary psychiatric clinic in Hong Kong (1987–2007).** *Int J Eat Disord* 2010, **43:**307–314.

Perceived psychosocial impairment associated with eating disorder features: responses to a mental health literacy intervention

Caroline Bentley[1*], Kassandra Gratwick-Sarll[1] and Jonathan Mond[1,2]

Abstract

Background: Whether and to what extent young adults are aware of the adverse impact of eating disorder features (EDF) on psychosocial functioning is unclear, although such awareness may affect the experience and behavior of sufferers. The aim of the current study was to examine young adults' perceptions of psychosocial impairment associated with EDF, and the potential effect on these perceptions of an eating disorders "mental health literacy" (ED-MHL) intervention.

Methods: Undergraduate students (male: $n = 35$; female: $n = 141$) completed self-report questionnaires prior to, immediately following, and 3 months after completion of a 3-h ED-MHL intervention. Perceived psychosocial impairment associated with EDF–binge eating, purging, extreme dietary restriction, overvaluation of weight/shape, and excessive exercise–was assessed at each time point.

Results: At all 3 time points, EDF were considered to have a 'slightly negative' to 'very negative' impact on psychosocial functioning. Prior to the intervention, binge eating, purging and extreme dietary restriction were generally considered to have a greater negative impact than excessive exercise and overvaluation of weight/shape. Three months after the ED-MHL intervention, participants reported greater perceived impairment associated with excessive exercise and overvaluation; while perceptions of psychosocial impairment associated with binge eating, purging and dietary restriction remained largely unchanged. Females perceived greater impairment associated with EDF than males did immediately after the intervention, but not at the 3-month follow-up.

Conclusions: The adverse effects on psychosocial functioning of binge eating, purging and extreme dietary restriction appear to be readily recognized by young people. Awareness of the adverse effects of excessive exercise and overvaluation may be poorer, but amenable to improvement by means of a relatively simple intervention. These features may warrant particular attention in health promotion programs.

Keywords: Eating disorder features, Psychosocial functioning, Mental health literacy

* Correspondence: Caroline.Bentley@anu.edu.au
[1]Research School of Psychology, Australian National University, Canberra, ACT 0200, Australia
Full list of author information is available at the end of the article

Background

In recent years, evidence has accumulated concerning the negative impact of eating disorder features, namely, binge eating, extreme weight-control behaviors, and key cognitive features, such as the overvaluation of body weight/shape, on individuals' quality of life [1–3]. Increasing focus on eating disorder features (EDF) is appropriate, given broad acceptance of the transdiagnostic model of eating disorder psychopathology [4] and increasing awareness of the need for a dimensional, symptom-based approach to diagnostic criteria for mental disorders [5, 6]. Assessing EDF rather than eating disorders can provide more stable construct definitions over time and accommodate individuals who might otherwise be excluded by virtue of overly restrictive diagnostic criteria [5, 6]. For these reasons, it is increasingly recognized that reducing the adverse impact of EDF on individuals' quality of life should be a key target of preventive interventions [6–8].

One way to reduce the adverse impact of EDF on individuals' quality of life is to improve public awareness and understanding of the nature of these features and of the distress and disability that they engender [9]. Improving these and other aspects of eating disorders "mental health literacy" (ED-MHL) would have, potentially, at least two benefits. First, improved community awareness and understanding of the nature and adverse impact of EDF may be conducive to improved uptake of mental health care, where this is needed, among sufferers [10–12]. Improved uptake of mental health care would be expected to follow from improvements in the ED-MHL not only of individuals who have or may develop symptoms, but also of these individuals' family and friends and members of their social networks more generally [9, 13, 14]. Evidence suggests that appropriate interventions may be effective in improving awareness and understanding of the nature and treatment of mental health problems as well as confidence in assisting–and willingness to assist–sufferers to seek appropriate help, including interventions designed to improve ED-MHL [13, 15]. Second, improved awareness of the nature and adverse impact of EDF may be conducive to lower levels of stigma towards, and, in turn, among sufferers. Lower levels of internalized stigma would be expected to have a direct benefit in terms of improved quality of life, while also being conducive to improved uptake of mental health care where this is needed [16].

Available evidence suggests that the public is generally sympathetic toward individuals with eating disorders–anorexia nervosa and bulimia nervosa at least–in that people generally recognize the seriousness and distressing nature of these conditions [17]. However, it is also apparent that a substantial minority (around one third) of people, young adults in particular, hold attitudes that may trivialize and otherwise stigmatize eating disorders, such as the beliefs that having an eating disorder 'might not be too bad' [17] and that individuals with an eating disorder 'only have themselves to blame' and should 'pull themselves together' [18]. Further, attitudes of this kind may be more common in young men than in young women [19, 20].

There is some evidence that individuals' beliefs about the adverse impact of eating disorders vary as a function of the features comprising the disorder [19–21]. Thus, the perception that eating disorders are mild or even trivial may be more commonly ascribed to individuals with binge eating disorder than individuals with anorexia nervosa or bulimia nervosa [19, 21]. That is, in the absence of extreme weight-control behaviors and/or low body weight, the adverse impact of binge eating may be underestimated. Perceived impairment associated with "non-purging" extreme weight-control behaviors, namely, extreme dietary restriction and excessive exercise, may also tend to be underestimated, given that these behaviors are more "normative" and socially sanctioned, whereas the distress caused by purging behaviors may be more likely to be recognized [22, 23]. The negative impact of weight/shape overvaluation may also be underestimated, given the overlap of this construct with body dissatisfaction [24], despite its status as a core feature of eating disorder psychopathology [4] and despite evidence suggesting it may be a better predictor of mental health impairment than other EDF [7, 8].

To our knowledge, no study has examined individuals' perceptions of impairment associated with different EDF. Research of this kind may be helpful in indicating which EDF may be more or less susceptible to trivialization. Ideally, research of this kind would be conducted in young adults, given that eating disorders–and EDF–typically have their onset in adolescence or early adulthood [5]. Further, it would be helpful not only to document young adults' perceptions of the impairment associated with EDF, but also to determine whether a brief intervention might be effective in improving this aspect of ED–MHL, should it be found to be problematic. The goal of the current study was, therefore, to examine young adults' perceptions of psychosocial impairment associated with EDF prior to and following an ED-MHL intervention. A secondary aim of the study was to examine sex differences in perceptions of impairment over time. In view of the paucity of existing evidence, our only a priori hypotheses were that purging behaviors would be seen to be associated with greater impairment in psychosocial functioning than non-purging behaviors and that young men would perceive at least some EDF to be associated with lower levels of impairment than young women at one or more time points.

Method

Study design and recruitment of participants

Participants were 141 female and 35 male ($N = 176$) third-year undergraduate psychology students from the

Australian National University who opted in to the voluntary research component of the 'Should I Say Something?' workshop, which was offered through a laboratory class. Of the students enrolled in the laboratory classes, 94.6 % volunteered to participate in the study at baseline. The dropout rate across time was 8.0 %. 'Should I Say Something?' is a 3-h interactive workshop developed by Hart et al. [13], with promising preliminary findings regarding its effectiveness in promoting ED-MHL [15]. The workshop is designed to improve participants' understanding of the nature and treatment of eating disorders and to provide them with the skills to assist someone close to them (or themselves) to seek early and appropriate treatment for an eating disorder or other mental health issue. The workshop was conducted by the first and second author and included a slide presentation, a vignette on the lived experience of a young woman with anorexia nervosa, and individual and group activities throughout (cf. [13, 15]). No remuneration or other incentives to participation were provided. Participants completed questionnaires immediately before and after participating in the workshop (Time 1 and Time 2, respectively) and at a 3-month follow-up (Time 3). Questionnaires assessed participants' perceptions of psychosocial impairment associated with different EDF; as well as ascertaining participants' sociodemographic information and experience with eating disorders (Table 1). The questionnaires also included other measures not relevant to the present study which are detailed elsewhere [15]. The vast majority of participants (98 %) were aged 18 to 26 years at baseline. Participants reported that 31.8 % had studied eating disorders at university and 42.0 % believed they had known someone personally with an eating disorder. The study design and methods were approved by the Australian National University Human Research Ethics Committee (protocol no. 2012/523).

Table 1 Demographic characteristics of study participants (Time 1)

	Women (n = 141) %	Men (n = 35) %	Total Sample (N = 176) %
Sex	80.1	19.9	100
Born in Australia	61.7	65.7	62.5
English as first language	75.2	82.9	76.7
Studied eating disorders at university	31.9	31.4	31.8
Knew/knows someone with an eating disorder	44.0	34.3	42.0
	Mean (SD)	Mean (SD)	Mean (SD)
Age (years)	20.00 (2.90)	21.09 (4.79)	20.22 (3.38)

Study measures

Perceived psychosocial impairment associated with different EDF was assessed by asking participants: "How do you think [a specific EDF] would impact on someone's [psychosocial functioning]?" Psychosocial functioning was defined by two items which were subsequently combined: "emotional wellbeing" and "social relationships (with friends, family & partners)". Participants responded to each item on a five-point, Likert-type scale (1 = 'very positive impact'; 2 = 'slightly positive impact'; 3 = 'impact neither positive nor negative'; 4 = 'slightly negative impact'; 5 = 'very negative impact'). Cronbach's alphas in the present study for psychosocial functioning (Time 1) were 0.76 for female participants and 0.75 for male participants.

Specific EDF were defined as follows. Purging was defined as "Inducing vomiting, weekly or more, in order to influence one's body weight and/or shape" and/or " Taking laxatives, weekly or more, in order to influence one's body weight and/or shape". Extreme dietary restriction was defined as "Going for long periods of time (8 h + during the day) without eating anything, on most days, in order to influence one's body weight and/or shape" [25, 26]. Binge eating was defined as "Eating what other people would think was a very large amount of food given the situation and feeling a loss of control over eating at the time, weekly or more" [5]. Excessive exercise was defined as "Exercising really hard in a driven or compulsive way, on most days, in order to influence one's body weight and/or shape" [25, 26]. Overvaluation of weight/shape was defined as "Thinking one's body weight and/or shape is very important to their self-esteem".

Statistical analysis

Data were stratified by sex for the purpose of descriptive statistics (mean ratings of perceived impairment associated with each EDF at each time point) and in all analyses. Tests of significant differences between ratings of different EDF at each time point, and across different time points were conducted using Friedman tests and post-hoc Bonferroni-corrected Wilcoxon Signed Rank tests. Mann Whitney U tests were employed to test for sex differences in ratings for each EDF at each time point. A significance level of .05 was adopted for all tests where a Bonferroni correction is not specified. All analysis was conducted using SPSS version 22.0.

Results

Mean ratings of perceived psychosocial impairment associated with different EDF across the three time points are presented in Fig. 1 (females) and Fig. 2 (males). It can be seen that all mean ratings-across time points and for both sexes-reflect perceptions of EDF as having a 'slightly negative' to 'very negative' impact on psychosocial functioning (i.e., mean range is 3.5 to 4.7).

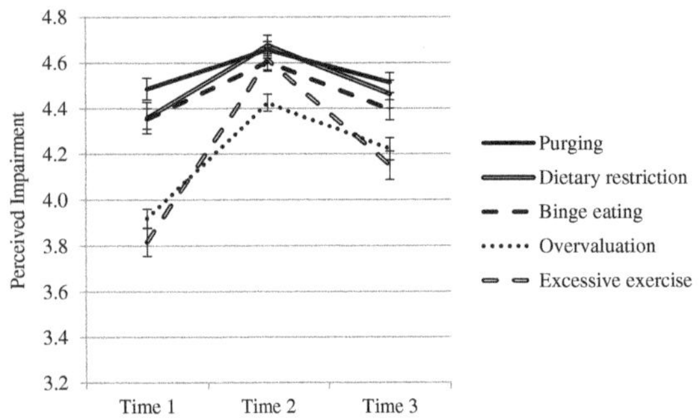

Fig. 1 Mean ratings of perceived impairment associated with eating disorder features across time points (females)

Perceived impairment associated with EDF

Friedman tests of differences in mean ratings of perceived impairment associated with different EDF (for both sexes, at three time points) were all significant (all $p < .01$). Post-hoc Bonferroni-corrected Wilcoxon Signed Rank tests identified the source of these significant differences, which are reported in text for the sake of brevity. At Time 1, females' mean ratings of impairment associated with purging, dietary restriction and binge eating were significantly higher than their mean ratings associated with overvaluation and excessive exercise (all $p < .001$). For males at Time 1, mean ratings of impairment associated with purging and dietary restriction were significantly higher than mean ratings associated with overvaluation and excessive exercise; mean ratings associated with binge eating were significantly higher than mean ratings associated with excessive exercise (all $p < .001$).

At Time 2, females' mean ratings of impairment associated with purging, dietary restriction, binge eating and excessive exercise were significantly higher than mean ratings associated with overvaluation (all $p < .005$). For males at Time 2, mean ratings of impairment associated with purging, dietary restriction and binge eating were significantly higher than mean ratings associated with overvaluation (all $p < .005$).

At Time 3, females' mean ratings of impairment associated with purging, dietary restriction and binge eating were significantly higher than mean ratings associated with excessive exercise; mean ratings associated with purging and dietary restriction were significantly higher than mean ratings associated with overvaluation (all $p < .005$). For males at Time 3, mean ratings of impairment associated with purging and dietary restriction were significantly higher than mean ratings associated with excessive exercise (all $p < .005$).

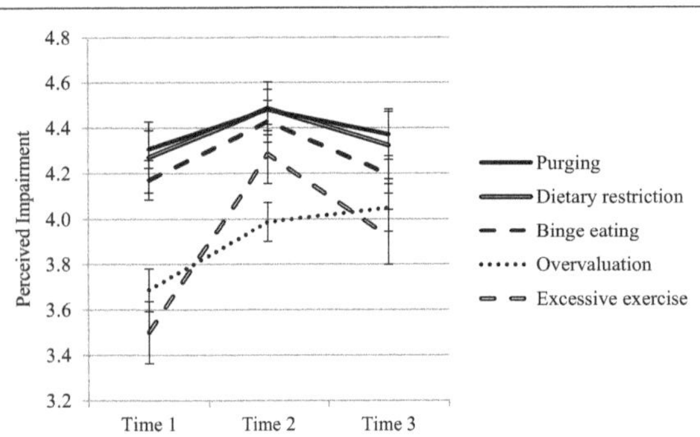

Fig. 2 Mean ratings of perceived impairment associated with eating disorder features across time points (males)

Change over time in perceived impairment associated with EDF

Results of Friedman tests of differences across time for mean ratings of perceived impairment associated with specific EDF, by sex, are presented in Table 2. Results of post-hoc Bonferroni-corrected Wilcoxon Signed Rank tests are also presented in Table 2, to identify the source of significant differences (where applicable). It can be seen that females' mean ratings of impairment associated with all five EDF significantly increase immediately post intervention, then significantly decrease by 3-month follow-up. This resulted in no significant difference between baseline and follow-up for female ratings of impairment associated with purging, dietary restriction and binge eating; while female ratings of impairment associated with overvaluation and excessive exercise remained significantly higher at follow-up than baseline.

For males, there were no significant changes across time points for ratings of impairment associated with purging, dietary restriction and binge eating. For perceived impairment associated with excessive exercise, males significantly increased their ratings between baseline and post intervention ($p < .001$) and sustained this change (relative to baseline) at 3-month follow-up ($p = .012$). For perceived impairment associated with overvaluation, males appeared to increase their ratings between baseline and post intervention and sustain this change at follow-up, however these results were not significant (both $p = .033$; Bonferroni-corrected $\alpha = .017$).

Sex differences in perceived impairment associated with EDF

Sex differences in ratings of perceived psychosocial impairment associated with different EDF at each of the three time points are presented in Table 3. As can be seen, at Times 1 and 3 there were no significant sex differences regarding participants' ratings of the perceived psychosocial impairment associated with EDF. At Time 2, female participants rated psychosocial impairment associated with EDF as significantly greater than male participants did for purging ($p < .05$), dietary restriction

Table 2 Results of Friedman tests and post-hoc Wilcoxon signed rank tests (where applicable) for perceived impairment associated with eating disorder features (across time points, split by sex)

		Friedman	Time 1 *vs.* Time 2	Time 2 *vs.* Time 3	Time 1 *vs.* Time 3
		χ^2	z	z	z
Females	Purging	15.29**	−3.92**	−3.19**	−0.71
	Dietary restriction	44.57**	−6.17**	−4.70**	−1.35
	Binge eating	28.66**	−5.04**	−4.15**	−0.68
	Overvaluation	54.45**	−7.10**	−3.51**	−4.06**
	Excessive exercise	111.55**	−8.86**	−6.31**	−4.51**
Males	Purging	3.66	-	-	-
	Dietary restriction	4.88	-	-	-
	Binge eating	5.49	-	-	-
	Overvaluation	7.34*	−2.13*	−0.22	−2.13*
	Excessive exercise	19.60**	−4.55**	−2.01*	−2.51*

* < .05; ** < .001

($p < .05$), overvaluation ($p < .01$) and excessive exercise ($p < .01$).

Discussion

Summary of main findings

This study examined individuals' perceptions of psychosocial impairment associated with EDF and the potential effects of an ED-MHL intervention on these perceptions. EDF included binge eating, purging, extreme dietary restriction, excessive exercise and overvaluation of weight/shape. Prior to the intervention, participants reported, on average, perceptions of each EDF as having a 'slightly negative' to 'very negative' impact on psychosocial functioning. Generally, binge eating, purging and dietary restriction were considered to have a greater adverse impact on psychosocial functioning than excessive exercise and overvaluation. None of these findings differed by sex. Immediately following the intervention, females' ratings of perceived impairment associated with EDF were higher than males' ratings for all EDF except binge eating. Females' ratings of perceived impairment associated with EDF increased for all five EDF, whereas males' ratings increased only for excessive exercise. At the 3-month follow-up, perceptions of impairment associated with binge eating, purging and dietary restriction did not differ from those observed at baseline, whereas perceptions of impairment associated with excessive exercise were greater than at baseline. In females, but not males, perceptions of impairment associated with overvaluation were greater at the 3-month follow-up than at baseline. No sex differences were observed at the 3-month follow-up.

Study implications

Several of these findings are encouraging. First, it is encouraging that participants generally perceived the EDF considered to have a negative impact on psychosocial functioning. Second, it is encouraging that the degree of impairment attributed to EDF was similar among male and female participants. This finding contrasts with those of previous studies suggesting that young men are more prone to trivialize eating disorders than young women [19, 20]. Third, it is encouraging that participants appeared to be aware that dietary restriction may be associated with impairment in psychosocial functioning comparable to that of binge eating and purging. Concerns have been expressed that impairment associated with extreme dietary

Table 3 Results of Mann Whitney U tests of sex differences in mean scores for perceived impairment associated with eating disorder features across time points

	Time 1 $N = 141$ (f) + 35 (m)		Time 2 $N = 140$ (f) + 35 (m)		Time 3 $N = 131$ (f) + 31 (m)	
	z	r[i]	z	r	z	r
Purging	−1.87	0.14	−1.99*	0.15	−1.50	0.11
Dietary restriction	−1.25	0.09	−2.01*	0.15	−1.24	0.09
Binge eating	−1.87	0.14	−1.79	0.13	−1.95	0.15
Overvaluation	−1.58	0.12	−3.42**	0.26	−1.58	0.12
Excessive exercise	−1.81	0.14	−2.79**	0.21	−1.59	0.12

* < .05; ** < .01

[i]Small effect size = .1; medium effect size = .3; large effect size = .5

restriction (e.g., [7, 27]) may be minimized due to the fact that it may be seen to be "normative" or even desirable, particularly in the context of concerns surrounding the "obesity epidemic" [28]. Fourth, it is encouraging that participants' perceptions of impairment associated with excessive exercise and overvaluation increased following the ED-MHL intervention, and that pre-post differences in this regard were still apparent at the 3-month follow-up. This finding adds to a small but growing literature on the utility of ED-MHL interventions [13, 15].

Certain other findings were, however, less encouraging. First, the benefits of the intervention in terms of increasing awareness of the negative impact were largely confined to female participants. The content of the intervention (e.g., vignette depicting only a female sufferer), the sex of the presenters (both female) and female participants being more prone to social desirability effects [29], may all have been factors in this regard. Second, these differential benefits appeared to be short-lived, since sex differences were no longer apparent at the 3-month follow-up, although as noted above some changes were maintained at follow-up by both males and female participants. The tendency for post-intervention changes in knowledge and beliefs concerning eating-disordered behavior to diminish over time, which was observed in early studies of eating disorder prevention trials [30], highlights the importance of including follow-up assessments and, perhaps, the need for booster sessions, in future trials of this kind. Third, perceptions of impairment associated with overvaluation and excessive exercise were lower than for other EDF at baseline and, to a lesser degree, at follow-up. Although this finding may not be surprising, it is concerning given that overvaluation is a core component of eating disorder psychopathology [4] and known to be strongly associated with impairment in mental health and quality of life in both males and females [3, 7, 8]. Findings relating to perceived impairment associated with excessive exercise are more difficult to interpret, given the lack of any agreed-upon operational definition of this term [28], but there is good evidence that certain exercise behaviors, such as exercising primarily as means of controlling weight or shape, are strongly associated with eating disorder psychopathology and, in turn, impairment in quality of life, in young women [31]. Further, there is growing concern about the adverse physical and mental health consequences of excessive exercise–that aimed at developing muscle mass in particular–in young men [6]. Hence, efforts may be needed to improve community ED-MHL relating to the adverse effects of overvaluation and excessive exercise in particular.

Study strengths and limitations

A limitation of the current study is the relatively small number of male participants ($n = 35$) and, in turn, relatively lower statistical power to detect effects involving males and differences between males and females. The use of psychology students as participants might also be considered a limitation of the current study, given the greater potential for ceiling effects regarding ED-MHL in this population and other characteristics of student samples that may limit the generalizability of the findings to the broader population. On the other hand, interventions of this kind may be particularly important among psychology students and in student populations more generally, given that EDF and other mental health problems may be over-represented in these populations [32–34]. Strengths of the current study include the recruitment of male and female participants, assessment of perceptions of impairment associated with a broad range of EDF, assessment immediately following and 3 months following the intervention, and the low rates of dropout. This is, to our knowledge, the first study to examine individuals' perceptions of psychosocial impairment associated with different EDF and potential changes in these perceptions in response to an ED-MHL intervention.

Conclusion

Findings from the current study suggest that ED-MHL concerning awareness of the adverse effects of EDF on quality of life among male and female psychology students may generally be acceptable. Adverse effects of extreme dietary restriction, binge eating and purging at least appear to be readily recognized in this population. Awareness of the adverse effects of excessive exercise and overvaluation was initially poorer, but improved somewhat following an ED-MHL intervention. These features may warrant particular attention in health promotion programs. Future trials of ED-MHL interventions may benefit from the inclusion of vignettes depicting male sufferers and/or male facilitators.

Competing interests

The authors declare that they have no competing interests.

Authors' contributions

CB and JM designed the study, CB and KGS conducted the intervention and data collection, CB conducted data analysis and interpretation (with input from JM) and CB prepared the manuscript (with input from JM and KGS). All authors read and approved the final manuscript.

Author details

[1]Research School of Psychology, Australian National University, Canberra, ACT 0200, Australia. [2]Department of Psychology, Macquarie University, Sydney, Australia.

References

1. Bentley C, Gratwick-Sarll K, Harrison C, Mond J. Sex differences in psychosocial impairment associated with eating disorder features: A schools-based study. Int J Eat Disord. 2015;48:633–40.
2. Bentley C, Mond J, Rodgers B. Sex differences in psychosocial impairment associated with eating-disordered behavior: What if there aren't any? Eat Behav. 2014;15:609–14.

3. Mitchison D, Mond J, Slewa-Younan S, Hay P. Sex differences in health-related quality of life impairment associated with eating disorder features: A general population study. Int J Eat Disord. 2013;46:375–80.
4. Fairburn CG. Cognitive Behavior Therapy and Eating Disorders. New York: Guildford Press; 2008.
5. American Psychiatric Association (APA). Diagnostic and Statistical Manual of Mental Disorders. 5th ed. Washington, DC: American Psychiatric Association; 2013.
6. Mitchison D, Mond J. Epidemiology of eating disorders, eating disordered behaviour, and body image disturbance in males: A narrative review. J Eat Disord. 2015;3:20.
7. Mond JM, Hay PJ, Rodgers B, Owen C. Mental health impairment associated with eating-disorder features in a community sample of women. J Ment Health. 2011;20:456–66.
8. Latner JD, Mond JM, Vallance JK, Gleaves DH, Buckett G. Quality of life impairment and the attitudinal and behavioral features of eating disorders. J Nerv Ment Dis. 2013;201:592–7.
9. Mond JM. Eating disorders "mental health literacy": An introduction. J Ment Health. 2014;23:51–4.
10. Mond JM, Hay PJ. Functional impairment associated with bulimic behaviors in a community sample of women and men. Int J Eat Disord. 2007;40:391–8.
11. Mond JM, Hay PJ, Darby A, Paxton SJ, Quirk F, Buttner P, et al. Women with bulimic eating disorders: When do they receive treatment for an eating problem? J Consult Clin Psychol. 2009;77:835–44.
12. Clement S, Schauman O, Graham T, Maggioni F, Evans-Lacko S, Bezborodovs N, et al. What is the impact of mental health-related stigma on help-seeking? A systematic review of quantitative and qualitative studies. Psychol Med. 2015;45:11–27.
13. Hart L, Jorm A, Paxton S. Mental health first aid for eating disorders: Pilot evaluation of a training program for the public. BMC Psychiatry. 2012;12:98–116.
14. Mond JM, Hay PJ, Paxton SJ, Rodgers B, Darby A, Nillson J, et al. Eating disorders "mental health literacy" in low risk, high risk and symptomatic women: Implications for health promotion programs. Eat Disord. 2010;18:267–85.
15. Gratwick-Sarll K, Bentley C. Improving eating disorders mental health literacy: A preliminary evaluation of the "Should I Say Something?" workshop. Eat Disord. 2014;22:405–19.
16. Griffiths S, Mond JM, Murray SB, Touyz S. The prevalence and adverse associations of stigmatization in people with eating disorders. Int J Eat Disord. 2015;48:767–74.
17. Mond J, Hay PJ, Rodgers B, Owen C, Beumont PJV. Beliefs of women concerning the severity and prevalence of bulimia nervosa. Soc Psychiatry Psychiatr Epidemiol. 2004;39:299–304.
18. Crisp AH, Gelder MG, Rix S, Meltzer HI, Rowlands OJ. Stigmatisation of people with mental illnesses. Br J Psychiatry. 2000;177:4–7.
19. Anderson R, Gratwick-Sarll K, Bentley C, Harrison C, Mond J. Adolescents' perception of the severity of binge eating disorder: A population-based study. J Ment Health. (In press).
20. Mond JM, Arrighi A. Gender differences in perceptions of the severity and prevalence of eating disorders. Early Interv Psychiatry. 2011;5:41–9.
21. Ebneter DS, Latner JD. Stigmatizing attitudes differ across mental health disorders: A comparison of stigma across eating disorders, obesity, and major depressive disorder. J Nerv Ment Dis. 2013;201:281–5.
22. Gratwick-Sarll K, Mond J, Hay P. Self-recognition of eating-disordered behavior in college women: Further evidence of poor eating disorders "mental health literacy"? Eat Disord. 2013;21:310–27.
23. Mond J, Hay P, Rodgers B, Owen C. Self-recognition of disordered eating among women with bulimic-type eating disorders: A community-based study. Int J Eat Disord. 2006;39:747–53.
24. Mond JM, Hay PJ. Dissatisfaction versus over-evaluation in a general population sample of women. Int J Eat Disord. 2011;44:721–6.
25. Fairburn CG, Beglin SJ. Assessment of eating disorders: interview or self-report questionnaire? Int J Eat Disord. 1994;16:363–70.
26. Mond J, Hall A, Bentley C, Harrison C, Gratwick-Sarll K, Lewis V. Eating disorder features in adolescent boys: Eating Disorder Examination Questionnaire norms. Int J Eat Disord. 2014;47:335–41.
27. Brown CS, Kola-Palmer S, Dhingra K. Gender differences and correlates of extreme dieting behaviours in US adolescents. J Health Psychol. 2015;20:569–79.
28. Mond J, Mitchison D, Hay P. Eating disordered behavior in men: Prevalence, impairment in quality of life, and implications for prevention and health promotion. In: Cohn L, Lemberg R, editors. Current findings on males with eating disorders. New York: Routledge; 2014. p. 195–215.
29. Hebert JR, Ma Y, Clemow L, Ockene IS, Saperia G, Stanek 3rd EJ, et al. Gender differences in social desirability and social approval bias in dietary self-report. Am J Epidemiol. 1997;146:1046–55.
30. Franko DL, Orosan-Weine P. The prevention of eating disorders: Empirical, methodological, and conceptual considerations. Clin Psychol Sci Prac. 1998;5:549–477.
31. Mond JM, Hay PJ, Rodgers B, Owen C. An update on the definition of "excessive exercise" in eating disorders research. Int J Eat Disord. 2006;39:147–53.
32. Lavender JM, De Young KP, Anderson DA. Eating Disorder Examination Questionnaire (EDE-Q): Norms for undergraduate men. Eat Behav. 2010;11:119–21.
33. Luce KH, Crowther JH, Pole M. Eating Disorder Examination Questionnaire (EDE-Q): Norms for undergraduate women. Int J Eat Disord. 2008;41:273–6.
34. Stallman HM. Psychological distress in university students: A comparison with general population data. Aust Psychol. 2010;45:249–57.

In the parents' view: weight perception accuracy, disturbed eating patterns and mental health problems among young adolescents

Liv Sand[1*], Bryan Lask[2], Mari Hysing[1] and Kjell Morten Stormark[1]

Abstract

Background: An accurate weight perception has been associated with motivation to change eating habits in the case of under- or overweight. However, recent studies have reported frequent misperceptions among parents and their offspring, both in the form of under- and overestimation of weight status. The aim of the present study was to investigate weight perception accuracy among parents of young adolescents in relation to reports on disturbed eating patterns and mental health problems.

Methods: Weight perception accuracy was assessed among parents of young adolescents (N = 5,781, aged 11 - 13 years) who participated in the ongoing Bergen Child Study (BCS). Parental weight perception was classified in overestimation, underestimation and accurate. Other measures included demographic variables, the parents' evaluations of disturbed eating patterns and mental health problems among their offspring as well as the adolescents' own weight perception accuracy.

Results: The parents accurately perceived more than 80% of normal weight adolescents, but nearly 60% of the underweight adolescents were overestimated, and a substantial proportion of overweight girls (34. 8%) and boys (12.8%) were underestimated. In general, parents who were aware of deviations from average weight in their child also reported higher levels of disturbed eating patterns, emotional problems, and behavioral problems. After controlling for demographic factors, the risk of parental over- and underestimation was significantly predicted by weight status, the adolescents' weight perception accuracy as well as disturbed eating patterns reported by the parents ($p < .05$).

Conclusions: Adolescents with under- or overweight proved most likely to be misperceived by their parents in this study. The pattern of perceptually correcting deviations from normal weight was interpreted as a positivity bias among the parents. These results suggest that weight perception accuracy should be targeted in family-focused interventions in order to strengthen adequate weight control among young adolescents.

Keywords: Weight perception, Parent reports, Adolescence, Eating patterns, Mental health

Background

Weight control in children and adolescents has become an important challenge to public health. Despite efforts to fight the obesity epidemic, a substantial proportion of overweight adolescents are not engaging in appropriate weight reducing behaviors [1], thereby increasing the risk for prolonged obesity and poor emotional well-being into adulthood [2]. In contrast, a growing number of non-overweight adolescents make efforts to reduce their weight by unsupervised diets [3] that may develop into more serious eating pathology. Weight perception has been proposed as an important factor for explaining the relationship between weight status and weight control behavior [4]. An inaccurate weight perception can take the form of both over- and underestimation of personal weight status. Both misperceptions can challenge healthy weight maintenance, as overestimation has been associated with unwarranted and unsafe dieting among adolescents [5],

* Correspondence: liv.sand@uni.no
[1]Regional Centre for Child and Youth Mental Health and Welfare, Uni Health, PO Box 7810, N-5020 Bergen, Norway
Full list of author information is available at the end of the article

while underestimation among overweight or obese individuals may result in low motivation to reduce excessive weight [6].

Parental attitude and behavior can influence the formation of body image and eating behavior among children and adolescents [7], possibly by modelling effects [8], particularly around meals and initiatives to physical exercise or sedentary activities [9]. Parents' ability to take action with regard to weight problems is again dependent upon being aware of the weight status of their children [10]. An important basis for this awareness is that parents recognize weight deviations in their offspring [11], and addressing parental weight perception seems important in preventing under- and overweight among children and adolescents.

Earlier research on the accuracy of parent's weight perceptions has focused mainly on their recognition of *overweight* in children. A review concludes that more than 60% of children with overweight were perceived by their parents of being of normal weight [12]. Comparable results have been reported for samples including both children and adolescents with overweight or obesity [13], although it has been suggested that the accuracy of parental weight perception increases with the age of the offspring [14]. There are mixed findings with regard to the offspring's gender, as some studies show that overweight boys are more likely to be underestimated than girls [15], while others show either the opposite [16] or no gender effect [17]. The likelihood of parents' underestimation seem to increase with higher Body Mass Index (BMI) of the offspring [16], and this may increase the risk of maintaining unhealthy eating patterns for children and youth who are already at the upper levels of the weight distribution.

Some studies have also investigated how accurate parents are in estimating the BMI of children who are *under-* or of *normal* weight. While parental estimates of children with normal weight were accurate in the vast majority of the cases, nearly half of the underweight children were overestimated [18]. The high frequency of overestimation for underweight children has been replicated by other studies with Swedish [19] and Norwegian [20] samples. Although there are fewer studies on this specific misperception, the high prevalence found so far and possible risks of not recognizing underweight with regard to development and growth [21] make this an important research topic in addition to the underestimation of excessive weight.

Thus, previous research has shown substantial discrepancies between actual and perceived weight reported by parents that parallel the misperceptions among children and adolescents themselves [22]. Parents generally seem to be least accurate for children who differ most from average weight, as they tend to overestimate if the child is underweight and underestimate if the child is overweight [20]. This implies that parents tend to correct from deviations from average weight, and Akerman and colleagues [19] have proposed that this skewedness can be understood as a *positivity bias*. The general function of this bias is to protect and maintain a positive image of oneself and close ones [23]. From this perspective, under- and overestimation among parents serve to experience their children as less skewed than in reality for their gender and age, thereby challenging a realistic view of the weight status of the offspring.

Parents' weight misperception seems to affect how worried they are about the weight status of their children [24]. More specifically, parents who underestimate the weight status of overweight children are less concerned with their weight than those who recognize their children as overweight [25]. It has also been reported that parents of obese children, who do not recognize weight problems in their offspring, are less likely to let their child be a part of an intervention program for obesity [26]. In line with this, it has been suggested that parents with an inaccurate weight perception also report less concerns about their children's lifestyle in terms of eating habits, physical activity and fitness level [18]. However, to our knowledge, no previous studies have investigated how parental weight perception relates to evaluation of more general emotional and behavioral problems, in addition to disturbed eating patterns. There is also a need to investigate the relation between parent- and self-reported weight perceptions in order to get a better understanding of the informant effects involved. It has been reported that weight perception accuracy among children and parents is significantly related [27]. Another study found that although the parents were slightly more accurate than their teens, both informants were poor at recognizing obesity [28]. Yet, this study focused solely on the perception of excessive weight, and it would be interesting to investigate the relation between self- and parent-report with a broader range of weight categories in a sample of young adolescents.

Aims and hypotheses

This study aimed to explore the weight perception accuracy among parents of young adolescents. The purpose was three-fold:

1) To assess the distribution of parental over- and underestimation in contrast to a more accurate perception, the latter defined as a 'control condition', across gender and weight status.
2) To investigate whether the parent's weight perception accuracy was related to their reports on their offspring's disturbed eating patterns and mental health problems.

3) To identify risk factors for parental over- and underestimation across gender, including weight status, the adolescents' own weight perception accuracy and parent reports on disturbed eating patterns as possible predictors.

All data were based on parent reports besides weight perception accuracy, which was also assessed for the adolescents. Following the notion of a positivity bias among parents, we expected highest perceptual inaccuracies for adolescents with under- or overweight. We also hypothesized that weight misperception would be related to the parents' reports on disturbed eating patterns and mental health problems of the adolescents, with lower symptom scores for those with under- or overweight who were misperceived as being of normal weight. Finally, we assumed that over- and underestimation among parents would be predicted by BMI, their concerns about eating patterns and mental health problems as well the adolescents' own weight perception accuracy.

Methods

Participants

The study is part of the longitudinal Bergen Child Study (BCS) in Norway, where a cohort of children born between 1993 and 1995 from all public and private schools in the municipality of Bergen were followed up over a ten-year period. Among the aims of the BCS is to estimate prevalence data for a broad specter of mental health problems, and use of health and school services. The ethics of the study as a whole and the different waves of the project were approved by the Regional Committee for Medical Research in Western Norway. The procedure of the BCS is described in more detail elsewhere [29].

The present analyses are drawn from the first phase of the second wave of the study administered during spring 2006. A four-page screening questionnaire was handed out from the schools to the children as well as their parents and teachers, and written informed consent was attained from all parents whose children were included in the study. The sample consisted of 5,781 subjects aged 11–13 years equally divided between 5th, 6th and 7th grade in elementary school. There were slightly more girls (52.5%) than boys. The questionnaires were usually completed by the mother (63.9%) or by both parents (17.8%).

The number of participants reflected a participation rate from the total population of 61%. Previous reports on the representativeness of the study have concluded that there was a significant non-response bias with respect to the measures on emotional and behavioral problems in the first wave of the BCS [30], although this difference was small in magnitude.

Measures

Demographic variables

The participants were asked to mark their gender (girl or boy), school grade (5–7), and pubertal timing. The latter was assessed by the statement "How would you describe your pubertal development" which could be rated on a Likert scale from 1 (*a lot earlier than my peers*) to 5 (*a lot later than my peers*). SES was based individual indicators rather than an aggregated measure [31] and included parent-reported ratings of family economy from 1 (*very poor*) to 5 (*very good*) and parental education from elementary school (1) to university level (5).

Weight status

Body Mass Index (BMI) was calculated as weight/height^2 based on parents' report of their children's weight and height. The continuous BMI measure was recoded to three weight categories (underweight, normal weight and overweight) based on international guidelines for age- and gender specific BMI percentiles [32]. Accordingly, BMI of less than 5th percentile was classified as underweight, from 5th to less than 85th as normal weight, from 85th to less than 95th percentile as overweight, and more than 95th percentile as obesity. Obese subjects were included in the overweight group.

Parents' weight perception

The parents' score on "How would you evaluate the child's weight?" on a scale from 1 (*too thin*) to 5 (*too fat*) was contrasted with the children's BMI status to define three weight perception groups: overestimation, accurate and underestimation. Adolescents with underweight could be either overestimated or correctly perceived, while adolescents with normal weight could also be underestimated. Overweight adolescents could be either underestimated or correctly perceived. An accurate weight perception defined a control condition.

Adolescents' weight perception

The adolescent's score on the statement "I feel too fat" on a scale from 1 (*not true*) to 4 (*certainly true*) was contrasted with parent reported BMI and classified in three weight perception groups. Subjects with actual under- or normal weight and feeling too fat were placed in the overestimation group, while subjects with actual overweight and not feeling overweight defined the underestimation group. Only the extreme scores were used in the categorization to avoid misinterpretations of the results. This implied that subjects with under- and normal weight who rated the question of feeling too fat as "certainly true" were included in the overestimation group, while those rating this question more moderately as "true" were included in the control condition. Likewise, only overweight subjects who rated this question as "not true" were included in the underestimation group. Participants with an accurate weight perception were included as controls for each weight category.

Disturbed eating patters

Eating patterns were assessed by four adjusted items from the Eating Disorders Scale (EDS-5) and six supplementary items regarding eating attitudes and behaviours (see Tables 1 and 2). EDS-5 was developed by Rosenvinge and colleagues for screening use [33] and has in its complete form been shown to be sensitive (0.90) and specific (0.89) in detecting symptoms of eating disorders when compared to DSM-IV criteria. The scale usually collects self-report data, but was adjusted to parent reports in this study. The items included from EDS-5 addressed comfort eating, feeling too fat, feeling guilty after eating, and needing strict diets to feel in control of eating among the adolescents. Supplementary items covered whether the adolescents have deliberately lost weight, have disturbed thoughts about weight or shape, are a vegetarian and/or have chosen a diet different from the rest of the family. All items were rated on a 3-point Likert scale from *not true* to *certainly true.*

Mental health problems

General mental health, defined by emotional and behavioral problems, was assessed by the parent reports on the symptom scales in the Strength and Difficulties Questionnaire (SDQ). This widely applied questionnaire was developed by Goodman for use in non-clinical samples [34,35]. Each scale consists of five items formulated as statements that the subjects rate on a 3-point Likert scale from *not true* to *certainly true*. The scales have been validated in several epidemiological studies and found to have good psychometric qualities, also in the Bergen Child Study [29] as well as other comparable Norwegian samples [36].

The four symptom scales included in the present study are denoted a) Emotional problems (SDQ-Emo), b) Conduct problems (SDQ-Con), c) Hyperactivity-Inattention problems (DQ-Hyp), and d) Peer problems (SDQ-Peer). The total problem score range from 0 to 10 for all four scales.

Design and statistical analyses

Statistical analyses were performed with SPSS package, version 17.0. Distribution of categorical variables was presented as percentages and continuous variables as mean with standard deviations. All analyses were done separately for girls and boys, and missing data was replaced by the item's mean score for subjects of same gender. Preliminary correlation analyses were run to test concordance between parental weight evaluation and related variables for girls and boys, using Pearson's two-tailed tests. The correspondence between the weight perception among parents and adolescents was also investigated by correlation analyses. We assessed both the concordance for weight perception per se split by gender, and the weight perception accuracy among the informants split by gender and weight status.

The weight perception groups were compared on demographic and clinical variables split by gender and weight status by independent samples *t* tests. Logistic regression analyses were performed to identify variables related to the risk of over- and underestimation split by gender. These analyses were organized in three blocks; block 1 included the demographic variables age, pubertal development and SES, block 2 included weight status and the adolescents' own weight perception accuracy, and block 3 included parent-reported eating patterns. In block 2, 'normal weight' and 'control' defined the reference categories for weight status and weight perception, respectively. Goodness-of-fit was tested for each block of the analyses using the Hosmer-Lemeshow test. The estimates in the regressions analyses were reported as Odds Ratio (OR) with 95% Confidence Interval (CI), and the total explained variance of each model (R^2) was calculated with Nagelkerke R Square.

Results

Descriptive statistics

Sample characteristics

With regard to BMI status, 7.8% of the girls were classified as underweight, 82.7% as normal weight and 9.5% as overweight. For boys, the distribution was 6.0% underweight, 90.3% normal weight, and 3.7% overweight.

The participants formed an ethnically homogenous and socioeconomically advantaged sample. The majority of the parents were born in Norway (> 85%), and more than 40% of the parents reported education on university level. Furthermore, 68% of the parents rated their family income as good, 29% as moderate, and 3% as poor. The adolescents' health was generally described as good by the parents (> 95%).

Weight perception accuracy

Regardless of gender and BMI, 81.75% of the parents showed an accurate weight perception while 9.8% overestimated and 8.45% underestimated the weight status of their offspring. The weight perception accuracy among the parents varied by gender and weight status (see Table 3). The parents overestimated more than half of the underweight girls and boys. Among normal weight subjects, less than 10% of the girls and boys were estimated as either over- or underweight by their parents. More than one third of the parents of overweight girls

Table 1 Clinical characteristics of girls with underweight, normal weight, and overweight by weight perception accuracy[n] presented as means (SD)

	Underweight		Normal weight			Overweight	
Weight perception accuracy	**Accurate**	**Overestimation**	**Underestimation**	**Accurate**	**Overestimation**	**Accurate**	**Underestimation**
Background variables							
Grade	1.91 (0.83)	1.97 (0.83)	1.87 (0.81)	1.98 (0.82)	1.86 (0.81)	1.70 (0.77)	1.80 (0.68)
Pubertal timing	3.51 (0.71)	3.31 (0.82)	3.15 (0.73)**	2.93 (0.72)	2.85 (0.63)	2.67 (0.83)	2.64 (0.84)
Family economy	2.14 (0.67)	2.15 (0.73)	2.22 (0.79)	2.15 (0.74)	2.19 (0.75)	2.26 (0.73)	2.45 (0.84)
Parental education	3.38 (1.16)	3.46 (1.15)	3.45 (1.04)	3.48 (1.11)	3.21 (1.13)*	3.20 (1.09)	2.93 (1.11)
Disturbed eating patterns							
Consciously lost weight	0.03 (1.62)	0.00 (0.00)	0.07 (0.29)*	0.03 (0.19)	0.10 (0.30)**	0.16 (0.44)	0.11 (0.31)
Disturbed thoughts about weight/shape	0.09 (0.34)	0.02 (0.14)*	0.13 (0.36)***	0.04 (0.22)	0.14 (0.41)***	0.17 (0.45)	0.11 (0.35)
Shows comfort eating	0.01 (0.12)	0.03 (0.17)	0.03 (0.23)	0.02 (0.14)	0.18 (0.47)***	0.38 (0.64)	0.07 (0.25)***
Feels guilty after eating	0.01 (0.1)	0.01 (0.10)	0.06 (0.27)*	0.02 (0.16)	0.17 (0.44)***	0.26 (0.53)	0.07 (0.25)**
Follows strict diets/rituals	0.01 (0.12)	0.01 (0.10)	0.04 (0.20)***	0.00 (0.07)	0.04 (0.21)***	0.06 (0.26)	0.00 (0.00)
Is a vegetarian	0.04 (0.20)	0.04 (0.24)	0.05 (0.29)	0.02 (0.17)	0.00 (0.00)	0.02 (0.19)	0.00 (0.00)
Provokes vomiting	0.00 (0.00)	0.02 (0.14)	0.00 (0.00)	0.00 (0.04)	0.00 (0.00)	0.01 (0.17)	0.00 (0.00)
*Is happy about physical appearance^*	0.47 (0.58)	0.39 (0.53)	0.54 (0.62)	0.45 (0.62)	0.80 (0.66)***	0.88 (0.60)	0.57 (0.58)***
Says he/she feels too fat	0.11 (0.39)	0.07 (0.26)	0.08 (0.30)**	0.20 (0.45)	0.73 (0.73)***	0.99 (0.77)	0.63 (0.63)***
Has chosen own diet	0.05 (0.23)	0.00 (0.00)*	0.06 (0.24)**	0.02 (0.16)	0.05 (0.27)*	0.05 (0.25)	0.01 (0.12)
Mental health problems							
Emotional problems	1.60 (2.11)	1.22 (1.56)	2.03 (2.09)***	1.09 (1.58)	1.65 (1.75)**	2.03 (2.14)	1.67 (1.83)
Conduct problems	0.79 (1.03)	0.76 (1.00)	0.88 (1.56)*	0.66 (0.97)	0.99 (1.26)**	1.15 (1.33)	0.83 (1.31)
Hyperactivity/inattention	2.03 (1.85)	1.97 (1.69)	2.18 (1.90)*	1.82 (1.73)	2.00 (1.83)	2.28 (1.96)	2.45 (1.04)
Peer problems	1.11 (1.76)	1.09 (1.66)	1.42 (1.85)***	0.74 (1.31)	1.39 (1.89)	1.71 (2.00)	1.09 (1.51)*

[n]*Note.* Group differences relative to correspondence significant at $^*p < .05$, $^{**}p < .01$ and $^{***}p < .001$.
^Scores reversed.

Table 2 Clinical characteristics of boys with underweight, normal weight, and overweight by weight perception accuracy[n] presented as means (SD)

	Underweight		Normal weight			Overweight	
Weight perception accuracy	**Accurate**	**Overestimation**	**Underestimation**	**Accurate**	**Overestimation**	**Accurate**	**Underestimation**
Background variables							
Grade	1.93 (0.81)	1.85 (0.86)	2.04 (0.83)	1.98 (0.81)	1.99 (0.79)	1.82 (0.79)	1.88 (0.64)
Pubertal timing	3.15 (0.68)	3.02 (0.67)	2.97 (0.68)	2.91 (0.59)	2.95 (0.79)	2.80 (0.89)	2.50 (0.71)
Family economy	2.19 (0.74)	2.08 (0.80)	2.26 (0.80)	2.16 (0.72)	2.35 (0.80)**	2.45 (0.86)	2.30 (0.82)
Parental education	3.33 (1.20)	3.47 (1.10)	3.27 (1.11)	3.45 (1.10)	3.07 (1.16)***	2.98 (1.06)	3.21 (1.29)
Disturbed eating patterns							
Consciously lost weight	0.02 (0.13)	0.00 (0.00)	0.06 (.28)	0.03 (0.19)	0.11 (0.33)***	0.19 (0.50)	0.19 (0.50)
Disturbed thoughts about weight/shape	0.08 (0.28)	0.00 (0.00)*	0.06 (0.23)*	0.02 (0.17)	0.09 (0.30)***	0.21 (0.48)	0.40 (0.52)
Shows comfort eating	0.00 (0.00)	0.00 (0.00)	0.03 (0.19)	0.02 (0.15)	0.19 (0.43)***	0.38 (0.60)	0.20 (0.42)
Feels guilty after eating	0.07 (0.31)	0.00 (0.00)	0.04 (0.19)*	0.01 (0.12)	0.13 (0.35)***	0.22 (0.46)	0.20 (0.42)
Follows strict diets/rituals	0.03 (0.26)	0.00 (0.00)	0.00 (0.00)	0.01 (0.11)	0.04 (0.23)**	0.10 (0.31)	0.10 (0.32)
Is a vegetarian	0.00 (0.00)	0.02 (0.13)	0.04 (0.25)***	0.00 (0.06)	0.00 (0.00)	0.00 (0.00)	0.10 (0.32)**
Provokes vomiting	0.00 (0.00)	0.00 (0.00)	0.01 (0.16)	0.00 (0.06)	0.02 (0.18)*	0.04 (0.21)	0.10 (0.32)
*Is happy about physical appearance^*	0.47 (0.60)	0.27 (0.60)	0.32 (0.54)	0.30 (0.56)	0.71 (0.67)***	0.90 (0.56)	0.60 (0.52)
Says he/she feels too fat	0.05 (0.22)	0.05 (0.28)	0.04 (0.23)	0.08 (0.31)	0.65 (0.70)***	1.12 (0.77)	0.60 (0.84)
Has chosen own diet	0.07 (0.25)	0.02 (0.13)	0.08 (0.34)***	0.02 (0.15)	0.06 (0.26)**	0.04 (0.21)	0.10 (0.32)
Mental health problems							
Emotional problems	2.08 (2.09)	0.78 (1.35)***	1.43 (1.81)***	0.93 (1.40)	1.86 (2.22)***	1.62 (2.03)	3.20 (2.94)*
Conduct problems	1.41 (1.78)	0.62 (0.89)**	1.02 (1.34)**	0.77 (1.12)	1.45 (1.75)***	1.09 (1.47)	1.10 (1.66)
Hyperactivity/inattention	4.15 (2.89)	2.32 (1.93)***	2.82 /2.51)*	2.46 (2.09)	3.33 (2.52)***	3.10 (2.19)	4.00 (2.94)
Peer problems	1.76 (2.28)	0.65 (1.08)**	1.29 (1.71)*	0.97 (1.55)	1.93 (2.35)***	2.41 (2.05)	2.50 (2.17)

[n]*Note.* Group differences relative to correspondence significant at $^*p < .05$, $^{**}p < .01$ and $^{***}p < .001$.
^Scores reversed.

Table 3 Parental weight perception accuracy (%) by weight status among girls and boys

	Weight status	n	Weight perception accuracy		
			Underestimation	Accurate	Overestimation
Girls	Underweight	237	0.0	42.4	57.6
	Normal weight	2509	6.2	88.9	4.9
	Overweight/obese	289	34.2	65.8	0.0
Boys	Underweight	165	0.0	48.4	59.6
	Normal weight	2480	8.8	82.3	8.9
	Overweight/obese	101	12.8	87.2	0.0

underestimated the weight of their child, while this was the case for only around 12% of the boys.

The adolescents' own weight perception accuracy also varied by gender and weight status. A total of 5.9% of the girls and 3.7% of the boys with under- or normal weight overestimated their own body size, while 19.3% of the girls and 20.5% of the boys with overweight showed a pattern of underestimation.

The correspondence between weight perception per se among parents and adolescents was significantly associated for both genders, with a correlation between the parental weight perception and the adolescents' perception of being overweight of $r = .368$ for girls and $r = .394$ for boys, with $p < .01$ for both measures. The parents' and adolescents' weight perception accuracy regardless of weight status was only significantly associated for girls ($r = .088$, $p < .01$). However, performing the analyses split by weight status revealed that the weight perception accuracy among the informants was significantly associated for both overweight girls ($r = .257$, $p < .01$) and boys ($r = .242$, $p < .05$).

Parental weight perception, demographic factors and clinical variables

The weight perception groups were compared on demographic and clinical variables split by actual weight status, and the results of these comparative analyses are presented separately for girls and boys in Tables 1 and 2.

Underweight adolescents

Comparisons between underweight adolescents who were overestimated and accurately perceived by their parents are presented in Table 1 for girls and Table 2 for boys. All reported comparisons were significant at $p < .05$. Girls with underweight who were overestimated girls were reported to choose their own diet less frequently than those who were accurately perceived, while overestimated boys were reported to have less mental health problems than the accurate group. For both genders, parents who overestimated also reported less disturbed thoughts about food/weight on behalf of their offspring.

Normal weight adolescents

Comparisons between normal weighted adolescents who were underestimated, accurately perceived, and overestimated by their parents are presented in Table 1 for girls and Table 2 for boys. Girls of normal weight who were underestimated were also reported to have later pubertal development, higher levels of feeling guilty after eating, following strict diets/rituals, and choosing their own diet, but lower scores on feeling too fat, relative to the accurate group. Boys with normal weight who were underestimated were viewed as having more disturbed eating patterns on 4 of 10 items when compared to the accurate group. For both genders, underestimation was associated with significantly higher mental health problems than the accurate group.

For girls with normal weight, overestimation was associated with lower parental education level and higher scores on disturbed eating patterns on 8 out of 10 items. For boys with normal weight, overestimation was associated with better family income, lower parental education as well as higher scores on disturbed eating patterns on 9 out of 10 items relative to the accurate group. For both genders, overestimation was associated with significantly higher scores on all mental health problems based on the parent-reports.

Overweight adolescents

Comparisons between overweight adolescents who were overestimated and accurately perceived by their parents are presented in Table 1 for girls and Table 2 for boys. These comparisons revealed few significant differences. However, overweight girls who were underestimated were also scored lower on comfort eating, feeling guilty after eating, not being happy with physical appearance, feeling too fat, and having peer problems than the controls. Overweight boys who were underestimated more often tended to be vegetarian and showed higher emotional problems than the control group according to the parents' reports.

Predictors of parental weight misperception

Variables related to overestimation

Variables related to the risk of overestimation among the parents varied partly by gender. After controlling for demographic variables, parents of both genders were more likely to overestimate if their offspring was underweight (girls: OR 16.64, CI 11.18 - 24.77, $p < .001$, boys: OR 5.85, CI 2.92 – 11.71, $p < .001$), and if the adolescents themselves overestimated their weight status (girls: OR 3.47, CI 1.60 – 7.51, $p < .01$, boys: OR 3.39, CI 1.11 – 10.37, $p < .05$). In addition, some aspects of disturbed eating patterns were related to the risk of overestimation; parent reports on comfort eating in both genders (girls: OR 4.42, CI 1.96 - 10.01, $p < .001$), boys: OR 3.04, CI 1.10 – 8.43, $p < .05$) as well as feeling too fat among boys (OR 1.65, CI 1.01 – 2.69, $p < .05$). The regression models explained considerably more variance for boys ($R^2 = .702$) than for girls ($R^2 = .275$).

Variables related to underestimation

For parents of underweight girls, the risk of underestimation increased with overweight (OR 6.63, CI 3.84 – 11.43, $p < .001$), underestimation among the adolescents themselves (OR 2.54, CI 1.07 – 6.03, $p < .05$), and parental reports on disturbed thoughts about food/weight (OR 3.31, CI 1.80 – 6.08, $p < .001$). Underestimation on behalf of girls was also negatively associated with underweight (OR 0.13, CI 0.02 – 0.99, $p < .05$) as well as parental reports on comfort eating (OR 0.29, CI 0.13 – 0.65, $p < .001$) and feeling too fat (OR 0.46, CI 0.31 – 0.70, $p < .001$).

Among the boys, neither the weight status nor the adolescents' own weight perception accuracy were significant predictors. Only a low level of feeling too fat (OR 0.32, CI 0.14 – 0.72, $p < .01$) as reported by the parents was related to the risk of underestimation after controlling for demographic factors. However, other disturbed eating patterns approached significance, for instance if the offspring has consciously lost weight (OR 2.17, CI 0.97 – 4.88, $p = .060$) or showed disturbed thoughts about food/weight (OR 2.70, CI 0.98 – 7.41, $p = .054$) according to the parents. The total models for underestimation explained more variance for girls ($R^2 = .142$) than for boys ($R^2 = .080$).

Discussion

This study aimed to add to the knowledge on weight perception by addressing the accuracy of parent reports in relation to a broad range of demographic and clinical variables. There were three main findings. Firstly, a substantial proportion of the parents misperceived the weight status of adolescents classified as under- or overweight, correcting for deviations from the average as a possible positivity bias. Secondly, parents who accurately perceived their offspring as under- or overweight were most concerned as regarded disturbed eating patterns and mental health problems on behalf of the adolescents. Third, after controlling for demographic factors, significant predictors of over- and under-estimation by the parents were the weight status of the offspring, the adolescents' own weight perception accuracy, as well as some disturbed eating patterns. Together, the multiple findings of this study support a positivity bias among parents, especially with regard to offspring classified with under- or overweight, and emphasize the reciprocal influence between the weight perception among the adolescents and their parents.

The finding that over half of the *underweight* adolescents were overestimated by the parents is compatible with findings from previous studies [18]. However, it has also been reported that up to 70% of parents of underweight children tend to overestimate their weight status [19]. Age differences in the offspring can be an explanation for these varied findings, as parental weight misperception generally seems to be higher for younger children [12]. A positivity bias among the parents might explain this pattern of overestimating on behalf of offspring with underweight, and thereby minimizing the deviation from normal weight. In addition, the masking effect of clothes could make it especially difficult for parents to estimate the size of underweight children [19] and thereby explain the relatively high frequency of this misperception.

Parents of *normal* weight adolescents either over- or underestimated their weight status in about one fifth of the cases. This proportion is moderate when compared to the over- and underestimation that appeared in the other weight categories. It may demonstrate that parents generally struggle with estimating the weight status of their adolescents, but that inaccuracies increase when the actual weight status is below or above average. This is also in accordance with a possible positivity bias, as there is less likelihood of distorting the weight of normal weight children.

With regard to gender differences, parents more frequently overestimated boys (8.9%) than girls (4.9%) of normal weight. As the body ideal for males is currently muscular rather than slim, this could be another expression of a skewed perception among parents adjusting the view of their offspring towards positive and attractive features for their gender.

Among *overweight* adolescents, parents underestimated 34.8% of the girls and 12.8% of the boys, respectively. Although this shows a substantial misperception, underestimation of overweight has been reported to be even more common for younger overweight children [37]. Parental underestimation was more common for girls than boys in the present sample, and other authors have reported the same gender difference [16,38]. If a positivity bias is driving the perceptual inaccuracy, it is reasonable that the underestimation of overweight is especially salient for girls due to the dominant ideal of being slim for females and the stigma related to being overweight.

The reports on eating patterns and mental health problems varied considerably across the actual weight categories as well as the accuracy of the parents' weight perception. For the underweight adolescents, the most consistent differences emerged on mental health problems among boys, as parents who overestimated the weight status of their sons also described significantly lower symptom scores. Normal weight adolescents who were overestimated presented more disturbed eating patterns than those who were underestimated when compared to the controls, but both misperceptions were related to elevated scores on mental health problems based on the parent reports.

For overweight adolescents, there were few significant differences between those who were underestimated and the controls, apart from lower scores on some aspects of disturbed eating patterns and peer problems among the girls. Overweight boys who were underestimated also presented more emotional problems than the controls, according to the parents. Seen together, the results suggest a pattern in which those parents who perceived their offspring to be closer to normal weight than their BMI suggests, also believed they had less disturbed eating patterns and mental health problems than the controls. Mathieu and colleagues [18] reported a comparable trend where the description of the lifestyle profile of children depended systematically on the parents' weight perception accuracy. One possible interpretation of this might be that positivity biases influencing the parents' weight estimates also skew the beliefs about the psychosocial well-being of the adolescents in an optimistic way. However, the results for the normal weight adolescents were less consistent in the present sample, and this supports the idea that the biases in parental perception are most visible with actual deviation from normal weight. In addition, the emotional problems reported on behalf of overweight boys who were underestimated suggest that parents are able to recognize some problems among their offspring even if they are not aware of their specific weight problems.

Overall, the regression analyses supported the hypotheses that the parents' weight misperceptions varied systematically with the weight status of the offspring. Accordingly, the risk of overestimation was significantly predicted by being underweight, which replicates the parents' tendency to minimize deviations from average weight [20]. In addition, the adolescents' own perception accuracy proved a significant predictor, as underestimation among the offspring increased the odds by threefold for the same misperception among parents. This concordance is interesting for the understanding of the sociocultural mechanisms involved in weight misperception and highlights the reciprocal influence between parents and children regarding distortions in body perception. Comfort eating also affected overestimation significantly for both genders, increasing the odds of this misperception by more than threefold. To our knowledge, the relation between parental overestimation and reports on comfort eating among adolescents has not previously been reported. Moreover, boys whose parents believed that they felt too fat showed a higher likelihood of being overestimated. These findings may add to knowledge of distinct eating patterns and concerns among adolescents that are related to overestimation among parents besides body weight.

In sum, the regression models for overestimation were best able to predict misperception on behalf of the boys, with over 70% of the variance explained for boys relative to less than 30% for girls. This may support the notion that body image among boys is influenced by more distinct variables than girls [39], and that the same mechanisms might come into play with regard to parents' estimates of the weight status of adolescents. The diverse results in the present study suggest that there is need for more knowledge on factors relevant to parental overestimation, both with regard to prevalence, gender differences as well as consequences for the parents' concerns about the mental health of their children and engagement in healthy weight control.

The regression models for underestimation revealed more gender differences than for overestimation with regard to significant predictors. Weight status defined as overweight and self-reported underestimation only predicted parental underestimation for girls in the sample. In addition, underestimation among girls was significantly related to high scores on disturbed thoughts about food/weight as well as low scores on comfort eating and feeling too fat. In contrast, neither the weight status nor the adolescents' own weight perception accuracy significantly affected underestimation among boys.

After controlling for demographic factors, only low scores on feeling too fat were related to the risk of underestimation among parents of adolescent boys. This factor proved to be significant for both genders, implying that parents who reported little concern about being too fat among their offspring also tended to underestimate their weight. As noted earlier, the opposite association was reported for overestimation among boys, as high scores on feeling too fat increased the likelihood of this misperception. These findings add support to the idea of a reciprocal influence between parents and their children with regard to body image and weight misperceptions. This highlights that eating patterns and attitudes conveyed by adolescents may affect the way the parents' view of their weight status, in addition to the biases that tend to minimize deviation from average.

The regression models were best able to predict underestimation among girls, with an explained variance of about 14% relative to 8% for boys. This might be due to the generally higher frequency of parental underestimation for girls reported in other samples [16]. Yet, the relatively low explained variance for both genders suggest that there are variables besides the ones included in the present study that contribute to parents' tendency to minimize the weight status of their children.

Strengths and limitations

The study has limitations that should be noted. First, as a cross-sectional design, the results are not open for causal interpretations. Second, BMI was based on parent-reported weight and height instead of direct measures due to the large sample size and practical challenges with individual assessments. One could argue that the parents were biased in both their report on specific weight and height in addition to the perception of the adolescents' weight status, but the results showed substantial discrepancies between the weight and height that was reported and the perception of the BMI status of the adolescents. If the reports on actual BMI were consistently biased, we would most likely not have found the patterns of over- and underestimation that is comparable with previous studies on parental weight perception. One could therefore argue that the results are even more striking for the parents who misperceived the weight status of their offspring despite having reported a height and weight that suggested deviations from the average.

A third limitation is the lack of a complete measure for the parents' concerns about body image and eating concerns on behalf of the adolescents. We used ten items, of which four were adjusted from the EDS-5. Ideally, this scale should have been used in its complete form and included in the regression analyses as a sum score, as well as being compared with the reports from the adolescents. On the other hand, single questionnaire items have been used in comparable studies in order to get a more detailed understanding of factors related to parental weight misperception [37,38]. The items that were chosen in the present study also seemed to be specifically related to over- and underestimation across the different weight categories, and this gives valuable insights for preventive and clinical work. Yet, although the EDS-5 is one of the few screening instruments for eating disturbances developed in Norway [40], it has so far only been validated in samples with 18 year olds and above [33]. Further studies needs to be done in order to establish norms for younger samples as well.

A further possible problem is that the study employed different measures for weight perception accuracy, as weight perception was assessed by a rating of weight status among the parents and by feeling overweight among the adolescents, respectively. Furthermore, which of the parents who completed the interview was not included in the analyses, and it is possible that the results were influenced by the dominance of mothers' reports in the study.

Possible strengths include that, to our knowledge, this is the first study of parental over- and underestimation across different weight categories for girls and boys in relation to disturbed eating patterns, emotional problems, and behavioral problems. With data from an ongoing epidemiological study with a large and representative sample, we could draw well-grounded conclusions regarding weight misperception among the parents and its' association with concerns about psychosocial problems among their offspring. The adolescent's own weight perception accuracy was also included in order to evaluate the concordance between the two informants.

Implications for future research and preventive interventions

Research on weight perception accuracy among adolescents and their parents is relatively new, and knowledge in this field is important in the face of the common eating and weight concerns in modern culture. Future research on parental weight misperceptions should ideally be longitudinal to allow for causal explanations for the different misperceptions and to formulate a more thorough theoretical understanding of the psychological mechanisms involved. It is also essential to include all weight categories as both the distribution and factors that influence the inaccuracy seem to vary according to the BMI of the children. Although most studies have focused on underestimation of excessive weight, overestimation of under- and normal weight should be further investigated in order to get a more comprehensive picture of the body perception among youth and their parents.

The notion of a positivity bias was to a large part supported by the present study, but more research is needed to establish how these biases operate and to which extent they modify the experience of the psychosocial health of the offspring in addition to physical features as weight status. In this sample, there was a pattern of lower symptom scores for adolescents who were erroneously perceived as normal weight, and this suggest that parents who minimize weight problems are also inclined to report less eating concerns and mental health problems in their offspring. Positivity biases can have an adaptive function by preserving a stable and optimistic impression of self and others, but if they also lower parents' awareness of real problems in their offspring, the skewedness in perception could challenge parent's ability to meet the needs of their children and thereby impair healthy development. Future studies on parental weight estimates might also take account of the degree of perceptual inaccuracy in order to define nuanced subgroups in the samples and to provide reference points for the clinical significance of the various misperceptions.

Based on these multiple findings, preventive and clinical interventions should target weight perception among not only children and adolescents, but also their parents. This perspective is essential for supporting parents' ability to estimate the weight status of their offspring in a realistic way, and subsequently, seek help early and initiate appropriate interventions if needed. The high frequency of weight misperception of under- and overweight adolescents suggests that interventions should be directed towards the whole family, including education on weight perception accuracy [15] as well as supporting health literacy in general [41]. Strategies for improving parental weight perception has been shown to be successful [42], and parents tend to be more worried about the weight status of their child if their doctor express similar concerns [13]. This gives hope for interventions directed at improving the parents' awareness of weight deviations in their children and offering a counterbalance to the positivity bias that might skew the parents' perceptions of the physical and emotional well-being of their offspring.

Conclusion

The findings suggest that parents misperceive the weight status of young adolescents in line with the adolescents themselves. Parents were inclined to overestimate the weight status of underweight adolescents and underestimate the weight status of overweight adolescents. The low awareness of deviations from normal weight among parents may challenge healthy weight maintenance efforts as well as responsiveness to psychosocial problems on behalf of adolescents. Family-oriented interventions should target potential positivity biases and work towards a realistic perception of self and others in order to encourage healthy weight control and adequate emotional support.

Competing interests

The authors declare that they have no competing interests.

Authors' contributions

LS participated in the design of the study, performed the statistical analyses and was responsible for drafting the manuscript. BL participated in the formulation of the aims of the study, interpretation of the main findings and drafting the manuscript. MH participated in the planning of statistical analyses and commented on written drafts. KMS participated in the design and coordination of the study and helped to formulate the research questions and draft the manuscript. All authors read and approved of the final manuscript.

Acknowledgements

This study was supported by "The National Program for Integrated Clinical Specialist and PhD-training for Psychologists" in Norway. The program is a joint cooperation between the Universities of Bergen, Oslo, Tromsø, The Norwegian University of Science and Technology (Trondheim), the Regional Health Authorities, and the Norwegian Psychological Association. The program is funded jointly by The Ministry of Education and Research and The Ministry of Health and Care Services. This study is also a part of the Bergen Child Study, hosted by the Centre for Child and Youth Mental Health Welfare at Uni Health in Bergen, Norway, and we would like to thank the research group and department for support and cooperation.

Author details

[1]Regional Centre for Child and Youth Mental Health and Welfare, Uni Health, PO Box 7810, N-5020 Bergen, Norway. [2]Gt Ormond St Hospital for Children NHS Foundation Trust, Great Ormond Street, London WC1N 3JH, UK.

References

1. Yost J, Krainovich-Miller B, Budin W, Norman R: **Assessing weight perception accuracy to promote weight loss among U.S. female adolescents: a secondary analysis.** *BMC Public Health* 2010, **10**(465):11.
2. Loth KA, Mond J, Wall M, Neumark-Sztainer D: **Weight status and emotional well-being: longitudinal findings from Project EAT.** *J Pediatr Psychol* 2011, **36**(2):216–225.
3. Olesti-Baiges M, Martin-Vergara N, Riera-Sole A, de la Fuente-Garcia M, Bofarull-Bosch JM, Ricoma-de Castellarnau G, Pinol Moreso JL: **Assessment of self-perceived body image in female adolescents aged 12–21 years in the city of Reus (Spain).** *Enferm Clin* 2007, **17**(2):78–84.
4. Kim KH: **Religion, weight perception, and weight control behavior.** *Eat Behav* 2007, **8**(1):121–131.
5. Liechty JM: **Body image distortion and three types of weight loss behaviors among nonoverweight girls in the United States.** *J Adolesc Health* 2010, **47**(2):176–182.
6. Brug J, Wammes B, Kremers S, Giskes K, Oenema A: **Underestimation and overestimation of personal weight status: associations with socio-demographic characteristics and weight maintenance intentions.** *J Hum Nutr Diet* 2006, **19**(4):253–262.
7. Powell MR, Hendricks B: **Body schema, geder, and other correlates in nonclinical populations.** *Genet Soc Gen Psychol Monogr* 1999, **125**(4):333–412.
8. Brown R, Ogden J: **Children's Eating attitudes and behaviour: a study of the modeling and control theories of parental influence.** *Health Educ Res* 2004, **19**(3):261–271.
9. Lau R, Quadrel MJ, Hartman KA: **Development and change of young adult's preventive health beliefs and behaviours: influence from parents and peers.** *J Health Soc Psychol* 1990, **31**(3):240–259.
10. Moore LC, Harris CV, Bradlyn AS: **Exploring the relationship between parental concern and the management of childhood obesity.** *Matern Child Health J* 2012, **16**(4):902–908.
11. Tremblay L, Rinaldi CM, Lovsin T, Zecevic C: **Parent's Perceptions of children's weight: the accuracy of ratings and associations for strategies for feeding.** *Early Child Dev Care* 2011, **182**(8):1027–1040.
12. Rietmeijer-Mentink M, Paulis WD, van Middelkoop M, Bindels PJ, van der Wouden JC: **Difference between parental perception and actual weight status of children: a systematic review.** *Matern Child Nutr* 2013, **9**(1):3–22.
13. Eckstein KC, Mikhail LM, Ariza AJ, Thomson S, Millard SC, Binns HJ: **Parent's perceptions of their child's weight and health.** *Pediatrics* 2006, **117**(3):681–690.
14. Valdes XL, Nota MF, Franco SM: **Parental perception of children's weight as a function of ethnicity/race, gender, and age.** *J Ky Med Assoc* 2009, **107**(12):485–489.
15. Wald ER, Ewing LJ, Cluss P, Goldstrohm S, Cipriani L, Colborn DK, Weissfeld L: **Parental perception of children's weight in a paediatric primary care setting.** *Child Care Health Dev* 2007, **33**(6):738–743.
16. Souto-Gallardo MC, Jimenez-Cruz A, Bacardi-Gascon M: **Parents perception of weight status of Mexican preschool children using different tools.** *Arch Latinoam Nutr* 2011, **61**(4):382–388.
17. Nazario Rodriguez IJ, Figueroa WI, Rosado J, Parrilla Idel C: **Perception of parents regarding their children's weight.** *Bol Asoc Med P R* 2008, **100**(2):33–38.

18. Mathieu EM, Drapeau V, Tremblay A: Parental misperception of their child's body weight status impedes the assessment of child lifestyle behaviours. *Int J Pediatr* 2010, **2010**(2010):9.
19. Akerman A, Williams ME, Meunier J: Perception versus reality: an exploration of children's measures body mass in relation to Caregiver's estimates. *J Health Psychol* 2007, **12**(6):871–882.
20. Juliusson PB, Roelants M, Markestad T, Bjerknes R: Parental perception of overweight and underweight in children and adolescents. *Acta Paediatr* 2011, **100**(2):260–265.
21. de Onis M, Blössner E, Borghi EAF, Morris R: Estimates of global prevalence of childhood underweight in 1990 and 2015. *J Am Med Assoc* 2004, **291**(21):2600–2606.
22. Chaimovitz R, Issenman R, Moffat T, Persad R: Body perception: do parents, their children, and their children's physicians perceive body image differently? *J Pediatr Gastroenterol Nutr* 2008, **47**(1):76–80.
23. Mezulis AH, Abramson LY, Hyde JS, Hankin BL: Is there a universal positivity bias in attributions? A meta-analytic review of individual, developmental, and cultural differences in the self-serving attributional bias. *Psychol Bull* 2004, **130**(5):711–747.
24. Bossink-Tuna HN, L'Hoir MP, Beltman M, Boere-Boonekamp MM: Parental perception of weight and weight-related behaviour in 2- to 4-year-old children in the eastern part of the Netherlands. *Eur J Pediatr* 2009, **168** (3):333–339.
25. Tschamler JM, Conn KM, Cook SR, Halterman JS: Underestimation of children's weight status: views of parents in an urban community. *Clin Pediatr (Phila)* 2010, **49**(5):470–476.
26. Taveras EM, Hohman KH, Price SN, Rifas-Shiman SL, Mitchell K, Gortmaker SL, Gillman MW: Correlates of participation in a pediatric primary care-based obesity prevention intervention. *Obesity (Silver Spring)* 2011, **19**(2):449–452.
27. Huang JS, Donohue M, Becerra K, Ronghui X: Relationship between parents' and children's weight perception: Results of a survey. *Infant Child Adolesc Nutrit* 2009, **1**(1):15–20.
28. Goodman E, Hinden BR, Khandelwal BS: Accuracy of teen and parental reports of obesity and body mass index. *Pediatrics* 2000, **106**(1):52–58.
29. Heiervang E, Stormark KM, Lundervold AJ, Heimann M, Goodman R, Posserud MB, Ullebo AK, Plessen KJ, Bjelland I, Lie SA, Gillberg C: Psychiatric disorders in Norwegian 8- to 10-year-olds: an epidemiological survey of prevalence, risk factors, and service use. *J Am Acad Child Adolesc Psychiatry* 2007, **46**(4):438–447.
30. Stormark KM, Heiervang E, Heimann M, Lundervold A, Gillberg C: Predicting nonresponse bias from teacher ratings of mental health problems in primary school children. *J Abnorm Child Psychol* 2008, **36**(3):411–419.
31. Boe T, Overland S, Lundervold AJ, Hysing M: Socioeconomic status and children's mental health: results from the Bergen Child Study. *Soc Psychiatry Psychiatr Epidemiol* 2012, **47**(10):1557–1566.
32. Cole TJ, Bellizzi MC, Flegal KM, Dietz WH: Establishing a standard definition for child overweight and obesity worldwide: international survey. *BMJ* 2000, **320**(7244):1240–1243.
33. Rosenvinge JH, Perry JA, Bjørgum L, Bergesen TD, Silvera D, Holte A: A new instrument measuring disturbed eating patterns in community populations: development and initial validation of a five-item scale (EDS-5). *Eur Eat Disord Rev* 2001, **9**(2):123–132.
34. Goodman R: The extended version of the strengths and difficulties questionnaire as a guide to child psychiatric caseness and consequent burden. *J Child Psychol Psychiatry* 1999, **40**(5):791–799.
35. Goodman R: Psychometric properties of the strengths and difficulties questionnaire. *J Am Acad Child Adolesc Psychiatry* 2001, **40**(11):1337–1345.
36. Van Roy B, Groholt B, Heyerdahl S, Clench-Aas J: Self-reported strengths and difficulties in a large Norwegian population 10–19 years : age and gender specific results of the extended SDQ-questionnaire. *Eur Child Adolesc Psychiatry* 2006, **15**(4):189–198.
37. Etelson D, Brand DA, Patrick PA, Shirali A: Childhood obesity: do parents recognize this health risk? *Obes Res* 2003, **11**(11):1362–1368.
38. Vanhala ML, Keinänen-Kiukaanniemi S, Kaikkonen KM, Laitinen JH, Korpelainen RI: Factors asociated with parental recognition of a child's overweight status - a cross sectional study. *BMC Public Health* 2011, **11**(665):7.
39. Carlson Jones D: Body image among adolescent girls and boys: a longitudinal study. *Dev Psychol* 2004, **40**(5):823–835.
40. Reas DL, Bang L, Øverås M, Lask B, Rø Ø: Oversettelse og kulturell tilpasning av psykometriske instrumenter: erfaringer fra tester som brukes ved spiseforstyrrelser. *Tidsskr Nor Laegeforen* 2012, **49**(3):260–264.
41. Garrett-Wright D: Parental perception of preschool child body weight. *J Pediatr Nurs* 2011, **26**(5):435–445.
42. Perrin EM, Jacobson Vann JC, Benjamin JT, Skinner AC, Wegner S, Ammerman AS: Use of a pediatrician toolkit to address parental perception of children's weight status, nutrition, and activity behaviors. *Acad Pediatr* 2010, **10**(4):274–281.

The relationship between obsessive-compulsive personality disorder traits, obsessive-compulsive disorder and excessive exercise in patients with anorexia nervosa: a systematic review

Sarah Young[1*], Paul Rhodes[1], Stephen Touyz[1] and Phillipa Hay[2,3]

Abstract

Objective: Obsessive-compulsive personality disorder (OCPD) traits and obsessive-compulsive disorder (OCD) are commonly associated with patients with Anorexia Nervosa (AN). The aim of this review was to systematically search the literature to examine whether OCPD and OCD are positively associated with excessive exercise in patients with AN.

Method: A systematic electronic search of the literature (using PsycInfo, Medline and Web of Knowledge) was undertaken to identify relevant publications until May 2012.

Results: A total of ten studies met criteria for inclusion in the review. The design of the studies varied from cross-sectional to retrospective and quasi-experimental. Seven out of the ten studies reviewed demonstrated a positive relationship between OCPD and/or OCD in AN patients who exercise excessively, whilst three studies found a lack of relationship, or a negative relationship, between these constructs.

Conclusion: There is evidence from the literature to suggest that there is a positive relationship between OCPD and excessive exercise in patients with AN. However, the relationship between OCD and excessive exercise is less clear and further research is required to qualify the strength of such relationships. Future research should utilise the most comprehensive and reliable clinical assessment tools, and address prognostic factors, treatment factors and specific interventions for patients with OCPD and/or OCD and excessive exercise.

Keywords: Anorexia nervosa, Exercise, Obsessive-compulsive disorder, Obsessive-compulsive personality, Excessive

Review

Anorexia Nervosa (AN) is recognised as one of the most serious chronic mental illnesses, with significant physical and psychosocial consequences [1]. In order to reduce burden of illness, increased understanding of developmental and maintaining factors of AN is required. The relationship between obsessionality and AN has been observed for a number of decades. However, research is yet to determine the distinct nature of this relationship and the putative moderating effect of excessive exercise [2].

Rothenberg [3] proposed that eating disorders are a "variant" of Obsessive-Compulsive Disorder (OCD), evidenced by high comorbidity between OCD and AN [4-6] and reporting of obsessional symptoms in AN patients [7]. AN patients follow strict food and exercise routines, and commonly present with obsessions of contamination and symmetry as well as compulsions of checking and counting [8-10]. There is also some neurochemical evidence for the relationship, with altered serotonergic function (5-HT) apparent in OCD and AN [11]. Although Obsessive-Compulsive Personality Disorder (OCPD) and OCD are recognised as distinct clinical syndromes, research has shown they significantly overlap in the risk profile for AN [12,13]. Yet, in their genetic studies, Lilenfeld, Kaye and colleagues demonstrated that while there was no shared causative factor for OCD and eating disorders within families, OCPD traits were demonstrated to be a specific familial risk factor for anorexia nervosa [14]. AN patients demonstrate personality traits which are

* Correspondence: syou5950@uni.sydney.edu.au
[1]Clinical Psychology Unit, Mackie Building K01, School of Psychology, University of Sydney, Sydney, NSW 2006, Australia
Full list of author information is available at the end of the article

highly concordant with OCPD- perfectionism, rigidity, higher impulse control and emotional restraint [15,16]. However, causal inferences are difficult to determine with obsessionality compounded by starvation effects [17]. AN patients show minimal changes in obsessional personality characteristics following weight restoration [18], suggesting that such pre-morbid personality traits play a role in the pathogenesis of AN [2].

Excessive exercise plays a detrimental role in the pathogenesis and maintenance of AN [19-21], and features in up to 80% of patients with AN [22]. The inverse relationship between reduced dietary intake and increased physical activity or hyperactivity- referred to as "activity anorexia" [23] was proposed as a bio-behavioural model of AN [21]. The presence of feeling "guilty" if an exercise session is missed is central to an eating disorder, signifying the obligatory nature of the behaviour [24] (also see [25,26] for models of the relationship between exercise dependence and eating pathology). Excessive exercise in AN has been associated with detrimental factors including: higher energy requirements for re-feeding/weight-gain [27]; elevated psychopathology [28]; and higher rates of relapse after recovery [29]. Based on the prognostic characteristics of excessive exercise, research has aimed to identify personality and psychological variables associated with this construct. AN patients who exercise excessively report higher levels of depression, anxiety and perfectionism [30,31], but potential relationships between excessive exercise and other psychological variables are thus far unclear.

Rationale for the current review

The reviewed research suggests that AN is associated with increased OCD symptomatology and a higher prevalence of OCPD traits. Research is warranted to determine personality and psychological variables for excessive exercise, in particular those that may be remedial to interventions [32]. The aims are to critically examine evidence as to whether OCPD traits and/or OCD are associated with excessive exercise in AN, and to determine the nature of such relationships between these constructs in patients with AN.

Method

Search strategy

The search strategy was designed to identify all studies of patients with AN, in which OCPD or its traits, or OCD and its features were formally assessed, and in which excessive exercise was formally measured through clinical interview or clinical judgement.

The following databases were systematically searched from April-beginning of May 2012: PsycINFO (1806-present), Medline (1950-present) and Web of Knowledge (1864-present). Reference lists from relevant articles were also manually searched for additional studies. The following search terms were used: (anorexia* OR anore* OR eating disorder*) AND (exercise* OR excessive exercise* OR exercise abuse* OR over-exercise* OR compulsive exercise* OR exercise dependen* OR physical activit*) AND (personalit* OR obsessiv* OR obsessive compulsiv* OR compulsiv* OR OCD). Peer-reviewed research articles that focused on the relationship between exercise and obsessive compulsive disorder and/or obsessive compulsive personality traits in patients with anorexia nervosa were included. A total of 443 papers were retrieved from the electronic search. The titles and abstracts were screened to assess the suitability of papers. A second reviewer also screened a proportion of the titles and abstract to reduce selection bias. 79 papers were excluded from their title, and 302 papers were excluded from their abstract. The full text of 62 papers was read, and 54 were excluded. The reference lists of the final full text papers were searched manually, and a further two articles were retrieved. The second reviewer also read full texts of papers meeting the inclusion criteria, and there were no discrepancies in the inclusion of articles, thus a total of 10 studies were included in the review.

Selection of studies

A detailed map of the search strategy can be seen in Figure 1. Papers were selected if: a) study was written (or available) in English; b) participants fulfilled standard DSM-IV-TR, DSM-IV, DSM-III or ICD-10 current or lifetime diagnosis criteria for AN; c) participants were assessed as having excessive exercise as a feature of their eating disorder; d) participants were assessed for OCPD traits or OCD symptoms/features using established scales/interview methods. Papers had to be published in peer reviewed journals, thus abstracts and dissertations were not included. There were no restrictions made on publication year, age or gender of participants, although the literature's focus on females was aligned with current and historical low prevalence rates of AN in males. No restrictions were placed on participant's Body Mass Index (BMI), the chronicity of illness in the sample, or the type of treatment received. Studies were excluded if the sample did not contain a group of patients with AN (if sample only included patients with Bulimia Nervosa or Eating Disorder Not Otherwise Specified). Studies were also excluded if they did not include a clinical sample: for example, only community samples, samples from university population or athlete samples without a sample of patients with diagnosed eating disorders.

Quality assessment

The final retrieved articles underwent quality assessment utilising an amended version of the original Quality

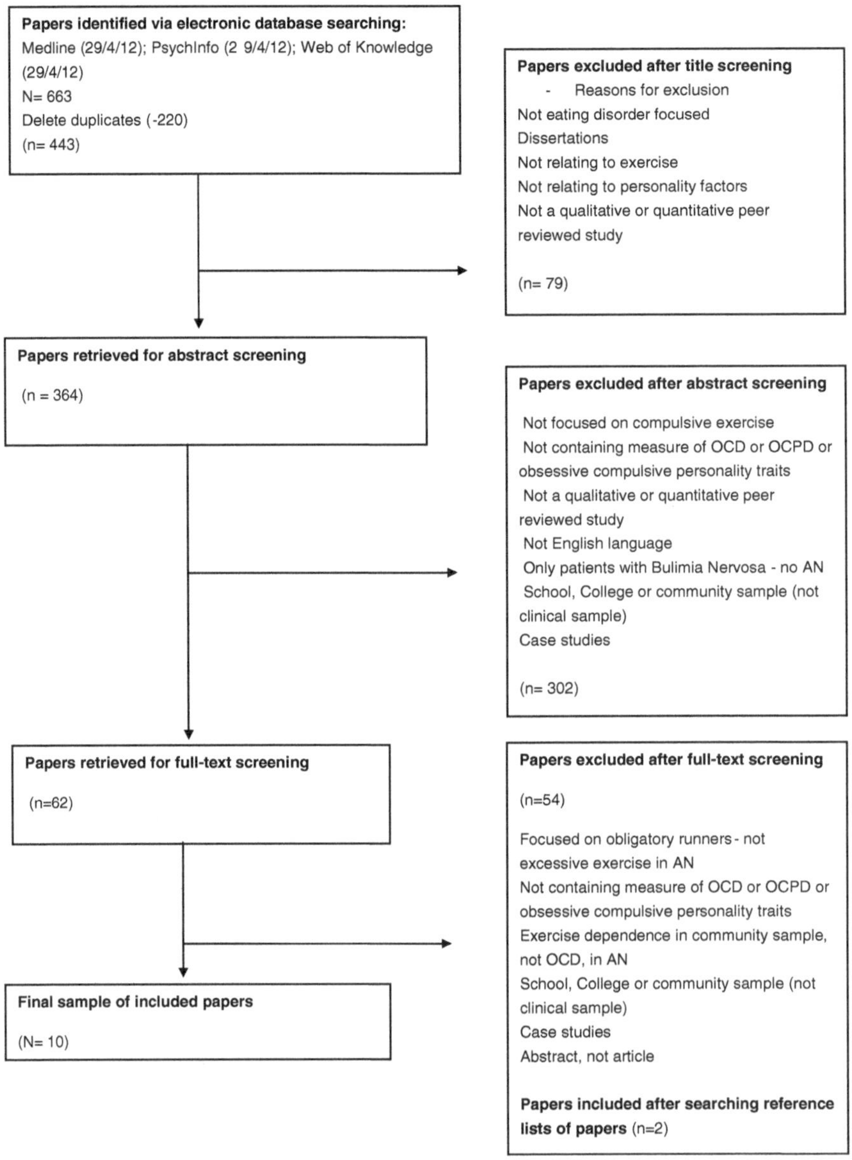

Figure 1 Flow chart of article retrieval process.

Index by Downs and Black [33]. The Quality Index is a reliable tool for measuring the methodological quality of epidemiological and health research [33]. This index had been amended by Ferro and Speechley [34] for their systematic review in the health science field. For their review, they excluded the assessment of quality items addressing characteristics of intervention studies, such as blinding, randomisation, withdrawals and drop-outs and integrity of intervention. The amended version resulted in 15 items (see Table 1). Each checklist item was scored 0 (No or Unable to Determine), or 1 (Yes). The maximum score was 15. A higher score indicated greater methodological rigour.

Results

Description of studies

A total of ten studies were reviewed: four studies utilised AN participants who were receiving inpatient treatment; three studies used inpatients and outpatients; one study used outpatients only, whilst another study stated that they recruited from four eating disorder services, but did not specify the settings. The final study included patients

Table 1 Quality index of included studies (Ferro &Speechley, 2009, amended from Downs & Black, 1998)

	Hypothesis clearly described	*Main outcomes clearly described*	*Characteristics of patients described*	*Main findings clearly described*	*Estimates of random variability*	*Actual probability values used*	*Response rate clearly described*	*Patients - represent population*	*Patients prepared- represent population*	*Staff, place and facilities*	*Data dredging*	*Statistical tests appropriate*	*Outcome measures valid/ reliable*	*Adjustment for confounding*	*Sample size or power calculation*	*Total*
Anderluh et al. (2009) [35]	1	1	1	1	0	1	0	0	0	0	1	1	1	1	0	9
Bewell-Weiss & Carter (2010) [36]	1	1	1	1	1	1	0	0	0	1	1	1	1	1	0	11
Davis & Claridge (1998) [37]	1	1	1	1	1	1	0	0	0	1	1	1	1	1	0	11
Davis & Kaptein (2006) [38]	1	1	1	1	1	1	0	0	0	1	1	1	1	1	0	11
Davis et al. (1998) [2]	1	1	1	1	1	1	0	0	0	1	1	1	1	1	0	11
Davis et al. (1995) [39]	1	1	1	1	1	1	0	1	0	1	1	1	1	1	0	12
Holtkamp et al. (2004) [40]	1	1	1	1	1	1	0	0	0	1	1	1	1	1	0	11
Naylor et al. (2011) [41]	1	1	1	1	1	1	1	0	0	1	1	1	1	1	0	12
Penas-Lledo et al. (2002) [31]	1	1	1	1	1	0	0	1	0	1	1	1	1	1	0	11
Shroff et al. (2006) [42]	1	1	1	1	1	1	0	1	0	1	1	1	1	1	1	13

with AN who were from the multisite international Price Foundation Study of AN, BN and AN Trios studies, and their affected relatives who met lifetime diagnosis of AN (see Tables 2 and 3 for a summary of the studies). Studies were conducted in a number of countries, including USA, Canada, Germany and Spain. Two other studies were conducted across more than one treatment site, such as in Slovenia and the UK. The majority of studies employed cross-sectional designs. One paper utilised a prospective design [38] and two used a retrospective design [31,35]. The final study was quasi-experimental [2].

Quality assessment

The total mean score on the Quality Index was 11.2/15 and scores ranged from 9–13. Refer to Table 1 for the quality assessment of each study. The mean subscale scores were 5.9/7.0 (range 5–7) for reporting, 1.2/3.0 (range 0–2) for external validity and 4.0/4.0 for internal validity. One study reported a power calculation.

Measures used

Objective measures of height and weight were collected in all studies. Structured interview schedules for exercise behaviours included different versions of the Eating Disorder Examination (EDE) interview [44]. These structured interviews assessed the exercise behavior of the participant over the past three months, asking about exercise that was "obligatory" or "obsessive" or "driven", and engaged in for the purpose of burning calories/kilojoules or weight control. The Structured Interview for Anorexic and Bulimic Disorders (SIAB) from DSM-IV and ICD-10 [59] was used in other studies to separate excessive from non-excessive exercisers, through the endorsement of any of the following categories of exercise behaviour: 1) severe interference with important activities; 2) exercising more than 3 hours/day and distress if unable to exercise; 3) frequent exercise at inappropriate times and places; and 4) exercising despite illness, injury or medical complications. Other measures were questionnaires including the Commitment to Exercise Scale (CES: [55]) which assesses the obligatory pathological aspects of exercise and the Compulsive Exercise Test (CET: [32]) which assesses avoidance and rule-driven behavior, weight control exercise, lack of exercise enjoyment, mood improvement, guilt, negative and positive reinforcement of exercise, and behavioural rigidity.

Other assessment protocol for excessive exercise included questions regarding duration, frequency and intensity of exercise per week [2,21,30] and questions of lifetime exercise status.

OCD symptomatology was measured using different self-report questionnaires. The OBQ-44 assessed constructs of inflated responsibility/threat estimation, perfectionism/tolerance of uncertainty, and importance/control of thoughts [61]. The Obsessive Compulsive Inventory-Revised [62] was utilised to assess the distress associated with symptoms of OCD, such as checking, washing, obsessing and ordering. The Padua Inventory [49], Yale-Brown Obsessive Compulsive Scale [70] and the Maudsley Obsessive-Compulsive Inventory [53] measured similar constructs to the OCI-R. A number of other studies used the Symptom Checklist-90-R [66] to measure obsessive-compulsive symptoms.

OCPD traits were measured through a number of methods. The EATATE interview [43] was included in one study to assess for obsessive-compulsive traits in childhood (such as perfectionism, drive for order and symmetry, and excessive doubt). Two other studies used an inventory designed to assess the "obsessional" personality type derived from psychoanalytic theory as a measure of obsessive-compulsive personality traits [52], and two studies used the Multidimensional Perfectionism Scale [54] to measure perfectionism, demonstrated to be one of the main temperamental characteristics of AN [72].

Relationship between excessive exercise and OCD symptomatology

Davis and Kaptein [38] demonstrated that patients who were identified as excessive exercisers showed higher number of obsessive-compulsive symptoms ($p = .007$) than non-excessive exercisers, unaffected by dietary status. Both excessive exercisers and non-excessive exercisers demonstrated a reduction in OCD symptoms between admission and discharge ($p < .001$). There was an interaction trend demonstrating that, after re-feeding, OC symptoms decreased less in the excessive exercisers group. It was also noted that patients who presented with excessive exercise reported a higher number of obsessive compulsive symptoms on the Maudsley Obsessive Compulsive Inventory (at admission and discharge) than a group of patients diagnosed with OCD [73].

Similar findings were demonstrated in studies by Davis et al. [2,39] in which AN patients who exercised excessively reported more obligatory and pathological attitudes towards exercise ($p < .01$). Obsessive-compulsiveness was positively related to level of activity in AN patients ($p < .01$) and exercising participants also demonstrated higher OC symptomatology than non-exercisers ($p = .02$).

Naylor et al. [41] concluded that women with AN who had higher levels of beliefs of exercise behaviour also had higher levels of obsessive beliefs ($p < .01$), obsessive-compulsive behaviours ($p < .01$), as well as higher eating disorder psychopathology ($p < .01$). Specifically, the Checking subscale from the OCI-R contributed uniquely and significantly to the overall model explaining weight control exercise, signifying that these obsessive beliefs and behaviours predict the variance in exercise for purpose of weight control, after controlling for eating

Table 2 Characteristics, outcome measures and results of included studies

Authors (Year) (Country)	*Study design*	*Sample size/characteristic*	*Focus of study*	*Study schedule*
Anderluh et al. (2009) [35] **(Slovenia/UK)**	Cross-sectional study using clinical sample and retrospective reports	N = 97 female patients. ANR = 35, ANBP = 32, BN = 30. Mean current BMI for AN across subtypes = 16.7. Mean age of AN patients = 27.75 years.	Aimed to define an eating disorders (ED) phenotype by retrospectively assessing lifetime ED symptoms to examine a lifetime pattern of illness.	Initial screening diagnosis by experienced clinician in inpatient service. Participants interviewed by trained researcher. Demographic information collected, weight and height measured.
Bewell-Weiss & Carter (2010) (Canada) [36]	Cross-sectional design using clinical sample	N = 153 (148 female) first-admission inpatients with AN. Mean age = 26.0 years. Mean BMI = 15.0 kg/m^2.	Aimed to amalgamate findings into a comprehensive regression model of predictors of excessive exercise in patients with AN.	All patients diagnosed by experienced clinician, with EDE. Exercise behaviour classified as excessive (34% of total N)-endorsed obligatory exercise, at least one hour daily, six days per week, for >1 month.
Davis & Claridge (1998) (Canada/UK) [37]	Cross-sectional design using clinical sample	83 female patients, AN = 34, BN = 49, Mean age = 28.1 years. Only patients without a history of another ED classification were included in the study.	Aimed to determine whether patients with eating disorders display addictive and OC personality characteristics relevant to weight preoccupation and excessive exercising.	Participants completed questionnaires and interview was conducted at time of admission to program.
Davis & Kaptein (2006) (Canada) [38]	Prospective design using clinical sample	50 inpatients-ANR. Mean age = 25.4 years. Mean BMI at admission = 14.05. BMI at discharge =19.6.	Aimed to determine whether AN patients represented a phenotype linked with OCD.	Completed questionnaires within first week of admission. Exercise interview conducted shortly after. Follow-up questionnaires were completed as soon as they attained target weight, determined by clinical team.
Davis et al. (1998) (Canada) [2]	Quasi-experimental design using clinical sample	Clinical sample (inpatient and outpatients) classified by DSM-III-R (1987) criteria. AN-Restrictor N =26; AN with bulimia = N = 16. EDNOS with low body weight N = 11. Mean AN BMI = 16.5. Classified as high level exercisers (N = 22, mean age = 27.1) or moderate/non exercisers (N = 31, mean age = 28.8).	Explored relationships between exercise levels, Obsessive Compulsive symptomatology, and restricted eating in AN. Discussed in relation to models of biological mechanisms in AN.	Questionnaires completed, physical activity interview for exercise classification. Height and weight measured after interview.
Davis et al. (1995) (Canada) [39]	Cross-sectional study using clinical and non-clinical sample	Clinical sample; Inpatients with AN, or had met criteria within past year for AN (N = 46, Mean age = 24.2, SD = 4.7). Non-clinical samples: 2 samples of women (n = 88, Mean age = 23.3, SD = 3.8 and n = 40, Mean age =24.7, SD = 3.2)	Aimed to investigate relationship between obsessive-compulsiveness and psychological and behavioural aspects of exercise in women with AN	Clinical sample tested within first 5 or 6 weeks of hospital admission, through questionnaires and interview.
Holtkamp et al. (2004) (Germany) [40]	Cross-sectional study using clinical sample	30 female adolescent inpatients with AN. Mean age = 14.6 years. Mean BMI = 14.4 kg/m^2.	Examined relationships between restricted diet, increased physical activity and psychopathology in acute stage of AN.	All patients diagnosed by experienced clinician, AN subtype diagnosed by trained interviewer blind to study hypothesis within three days of admission.
Naylor et al. (2011) (UK) [41]	Cross-sectional study comparing clinical and non-clinical samples	Clinical sample recruited from 4 eating disorder services: AN =30; BN = 24; EDNOS = 10. Mean BMI = 19.23, Mean age =29.98. Non-clinical university student sample: mean BMI = 20.86, Mean age = 20.32.	Aimed to explore exercise beliefs, obsessive beliefs and obsessive compulsive behaviours to understand the role of excessive exercise in eating disorders.	Clinical participants assessed and diagnosed by experienced clinicians using semi-structured interview, permission granted to gather diagnoses, BMI from medical file. Nonclinical sample reported height and weight.
Penas-Lledo et al. (2002) (Spain) [31]	Cross-sectional design using retrospective case notes from inpatient service	ANR patients = 35; ANBP patients = 28. BN patients = 61. Mean age = 20.25 years. Mean AN BMI = 16.9	Examined whether physical exercise is related to different aspects of psychopathology and if this association is different between diagnoses.	Data collected routinely by clinicians blind to the hypotheses. Participants coded as excessive exercisers if exercised at least 5x week (>1 hr per session), with aim to burn up calories.
Shroff et al. (2006) [42] **USA**	Cross-sectional design using clinical sample, and relatives with history of eating disorder.	AN probands and biological relatives who met lifetime diagnosis of AN, N = 431. BN probands and biological affected relatives, N = 750. AN Trios study- probands and parents, N = 749. Resulting sample size = 1857.	Explored features associated with excessive exercise across subtypes of eating disorders.	Participants from multi-site international Price Foundation Genetic study. Probands and relatives assessed for psychological and personality features that may underlie vulnerability to eating disorders.

Table 3 Outcome measures and results of included studies

Authors (Year) (Country)	*Outcomes*	*Quality index assessment*	*Results relating to OCD*	*Results relating to OCPD*	*Limitations*
Anderluh et al. (2009) (Slovenia/UK) [35]	EATATE[1] to assess diagnosis, screen for lifetime obsessive compulsive disorder and eating disorder diagnosis using ICD-10 criteria; as well as obsessive compulsive traits in childhood.	9	Groups did not differ in lifetime duration of excessive exercising. No differences between groups in frequency of current or lifetime OCD.	No differences between groups in frequency of current OCPD. Children who were rule bound/cautious exercised excessively later in life ($p < .005$, $p < .02$).	Retrospective assessment subject to memory biases, although anchor points were used. Data from informants could have assisted with this. Participants recruited from secondary and tertiary treatment centre.
Bewell-Weiss & Carter (2010) (Canada) [36]	EDE[2]; EDE-Q; BSI for anxiety; BDI-II for depression; RSES for self-esteem; Padua Inventory for obsessive compulsive symptoms; EDI for eating disorder attitudes and behaviours.	11	Overall model significant ($p < .05$) explained 31% of variance in exercise status. Restraint, self esteem and depression positively associated with exercise ($p < .05$), OC symptomatology negatively associated with exercise status ($p = .038$).	NA	Need to replicate findings with other measures. Study of factors associated with specific definition of exercise. Cross-sectional nature could not demonstrate direction of associations. No measure of OCPD.
Davis & Claridge (1998) (Canada/UK) [37]	EPQR[3] for addictiveness; obsessive-compulsive personality subscales; Drive for thinness for weight preoccupation; Interview to determine lifetime and current exercise status- classified as excessive or non-excessive exercisers.	11	NA	Both addictiveness and obsessive-compulsiveness were positively associated with over-exercising (both currently and historically, $p < .05$ and $p < .01$ respectively).	Patients were specifically chosen to represent the two diagnoses, although commonly both AN and BN features co-occur in clinical syndromes and in personality structure of patients.
Davis & Kaptein (2006) (Canada) [38]	Interview to determine lifetime and current exercise status (excessive or non-excessive); MOCI[4] to assess for OCD symptomatology; obsessive-compulsive personality subscales; BMI.	11	Excessive exercisers showed higher intensity/number of OCD symptoms than non-excessive patients ($p = .007$). There was a decline in symptom severity between admission and discharge ($p < .001$).	Excessive exercisers demonstrated greater OC personality traits than non-excessive patients ($p = .03$). There was no significant decline in OC personality traits between admission and discharge.	Self-report recall data was used in this study. Indirect historical data is necessary, on account of low prevalence of AN-R. Difficulties with prospective designs.
Davis et al. (1998) (Canada) [2]	MOCI[5] -symptoms of OCD; Obsessive Compulsive Personality subscales; MPS for perfectionism; CES for commitment to exercise; EDI: weight preoccupation; BES for body image; JFFIS for self-esteem; BMI.	11	Exercisers scored significantly higher than non-exercisers on OC symptomatology, ($p = .02$). Exercisers also reported more obligatory and pathological attitudes to exercise ($p < 0.01$).	Exercisers scored significantly higher than non-exercisers on OC personality characteristics ($p < .05$), and self-oriented perfectionism ($p < .05$).	No information as to whether exercise and obsessionality influence prognosis. Obsessionality data obtained solely from self-report data, not structured diagnostic interview.
Davis et al. (1995) (Canada) [39]	SCL-90[6] to measure obsessive-compulsiveness; Drive for thinness to measure weight preoccupation; CES to measure commitment to exercise; interview to assess for physical activity.	12	Obsessive-compulsiveness significantly positively related to level of activity among AN patients ($p < .01$), and obligatory and pathological aspects of exercise were related to weight preoccupation ($p < .01$).	NA	Proposed activity-based anorexia model explains AN development only for some individuals. Does not take into account motivational factors, differences in selecting forms of exercise and reasons for exercising. No OCPD measure.
Holtkamp et al. (2004) (Germany) [40]	SIAB[7] to assess AN subtype; SCL-90-R to assess for anxiety, depression and obsessive-compulsiveness.	11	Obsessive-compulsiveness was not associated with physical activity levels ($r = -.072$, $p = .705$). Regression model based on BMI, food restriction, subtype, anxiety, depression and obsessive-compulsiveness (OC) explained 64% of variance in model, OC was not a significant contributor.	NA	Small sample size; data on food restriction were answered retrospectively; need more detailed measure of OCD symptoms; need to examine OCPD symptoms; SCL-90-R only validated for people 14 years and older.

Table 3 Outcome measures and results of included studies *(Continued)*

Naylor et al. (2011) (UK) [41]	Exercise Frequency; CET[8] to measure beliefs about exercise; OBQ-44 to assess OCD constructs; OCI-R to assess distress associated with OCD symptoms; EDE-Q.	12	Clinical: women with higher exercise beliefs had higher levels of obsessive beliefs and obsessive compulsive behaviours ($p < 0.01$). OBQ and OCI-R accounted for significant increase in variance of weight control exercise explained.	NA	Cross-sectional design of study does not show direction of variables; rather just associations. Use of Self-report measures risks of socially desirable responses. Student samples are arguably unrepresentative of general population, could use other control groups.
Penas-Lledo et al. (2002) (Spain) [31]	EAT-40[9]: overall level of eating pathology. BITE: bulimic attitudes and behaviours. SCL-90-R: current psychological symptoms BMI.	11	AN patients who exercised had higher levels of eating pathology (EAT; $p < .01$) Exercisers had higher levels of anxiety and depression on SCL-90-R ($p < .01$), but not OCD symptoms ($p > .05$).	NA	Problems in definition of excessive exercise used to classify groups; require different measures to examine OCD symptoms in more detail; no measurement of OCPD symptoms
Shroff et al. (2006) (USA) [42]	Clinical variables: ED duration, current/ minimum/maximum BMI obtained; SIAB; SCID for diagnosis; TCI for temperament; MPS for perfectionism; STAI for anxiety; Y-BOCS for OC symptoms; YBC-EDS; excessive exercise classification from SIAB.	13	Excessive exercise was associated with greater severity of ED symptoms, worst ritual, preoccupation and worst motivation to change in YBC-EDS. Also associated with higher obsessions and compulsions (YBOCS) ($p < .001$)	Excessive exercise was associated with all perfectionist traits ($p < .001$), as measured by MPS.	Exercise group determined by retrospective reports of exercise behaviour. Exercise assessment not comprehensive. Unable to determine association between duration of excessive exercise and other ED behaviours.

[1] *EATATE* EATATE Lifetime Diagnostic Interview [43].
[2] *EDE* Eating Disorder Examination [44]; *EDE-Q* Eating Disorder Examination-Questionnaire [45]; *BSI* Brief Symptom Inventory [46]; *BDI-II* Beck Depression Inventory [47].
RSES Rosenberg Self-Esteem Scale [48] Padua [49] *EDI* Eating Disorder Inventory [50].
[3] Eysenck Personality Questionnaire-Revised [51];Obsessive-compulsive personality subscales [52]; Subscale from the Eating Disorder Inventory [50]; exercise interview as used previously by [21,30].
[4] *MOCI* Maudsley Obsessive-Compulsive Inventory [53]; personality subscales [52].
[5] *MOCI* Maudsley Obsessive-Compulsive Inventory [53]; personality subscales [52]; *MPS* Multidimensional Perfectionism Scale [54]; *CES* Commitment to Exercise Scale [55]; *EDI* Eating Disorder Inventory [50]; *BES* Body Esteem Scale [56]; *JFIS* Janis-Field Feelings of Inadequacy Scale [57].
[6] *SCL-90* Symptom Checklist-90 [58]; *Drive for thinness* from EDI [50]; CES [55].
[7] *SIAB* Structured Interview of Anorexia and Bulimia Nervosa [59]; SCL-90-R [60].
[8] *CET* Compulsive Exercise Test [32]; *OBQ-44* Obsessive Beliefs Questionnaire-44 [61] *OCI-R* Obsessive Compulsive Inventory-Revised [62]; *EDE-Q* Eating Disorder Examination-Questionnaire [63].
[9] *EAT-40* Eating Attitudes Test [64]; *BITE* Bulimic Investigatory Test [65]; SCL-90-R [66]; *SIAB* Structured Interview for Anorexia and Bulimia Nervosa [59]; SCID [67]; *TCI* Temperament and Character Inventory [68]; Frost MPS [54]; STAI [69] Y-BOCS [70] YBC-EDS [71].

disorder psychopathology. Furthermore, Shroff et al. [42] reported that excessive exercise was associated with higher frequency and intensity of rituals and preoccupations ($p < .001$), and higher frequency of obsessions and compulsions ($p < .001$), when compared with AN patients who completed no or regular exercise.

However, Anderluh et al. [35] found no differences between groups in frequency of current or lifetime OCD. Bewell-Weiss & Carter [36] demonstrated that although self-esteem and depressive symptomatology were positively associated with exercise, obsessive compulsive symptomatology was negatively associated with exercise status ($p = .038$). Penas-Lledo et al. [31] found that OCD symptoms were not significantly higher in patients who exercised excessively when compared with those who did not ($p > .05$). Finally, Holtkamp et al. [40] concluded that obsessive-compulsiveness was not associated with physical activity levels ($p = .705$) and that obsessive-compulsiveness was not a significant contributor in the regression model predicting physical activity with other factors such as BMI, level of food restriction, depression and anxiety.

Relationship between excessive exercise and OCPD traits

Davis and Kaptein [38] demonstrated that patients who were excessive exercisers showed a higher number of obsessive-compulsive personality traits, both currently and historically throughout their disorder ($p = .03$) than non excessive exercisers, and this was unaffected by dietary status.

Davis et al. [2] showed that excessive exercisers had higher OC personality characteristics ($p < .05$) and levels of self-oriented perfectionism ($p < .05$) than non-excessive exercisers. Anderluh et al. [35] reported that patients with AN who exercised excessively had a higher prevalence of OCPD traits during childhood such as being rule bound ($p < .005$) and cautious ($p < .02$), however they did not find any significant differences in current OCPD comorbidity ($p > .05$).

Davis and Claridge [37] demonstrated that obsessive-compulsive personality traits were positively associated with over-exercising, both in current excessive exercising ($p < .05$) and historically throughout the eating disorder ($p < .01$). Furthermore, Shroff et al. [42] reported that excessive exercise was associated with significantly greater perfectionism ($p < .001$), measuring factors such as concern over mistakes, personal standards, organisation and parental criticism.

Discussion

The aims of this systematic review were to critically examine evidence as to whether OCPD traits and/or OCD are associated with excessive exercise in patients with AN, and to determine the nature of relationships between these constructs. The results of the systematic review indicated a positive relationship between excessive exercise and obsessive-compulsive personality traits. However, the relationship between OCD and excessive exercise in AN patients is less clear with studies producing varying results.

Davis et al. [39] proposed a theoretical model of the relationship between starvation, physical activity and obsessive-compulsiveness in the development of eating disorders for some patients. This model works on the understanding that significantly reduced dietary intake and increased physical activity, combined with OCD features, create a mutually reinforcing, destructive mechanism which may play an integral role in the development and maintenance of an eating disorder [39]. The results of this review also seem consistent with the theory of "activity anorexia" [23], providing preliminary evidence for this phenomenon in human samples. Results have also supported the notion that high level exercising and reduced dietary intake alter the functioning of 5-HT with increased OCD symptomatology [2], creating a cycle whereby the individual undertakes an even higher level of physical activity and decreases their dietary intake as their obsessions increase [39].

Furthermore, the findings of Naylor et al. [41] are consistent with research examining the reduction in quality of life for these patients [74] and descriptions of their exercise being "out of control" [39]. Having obsessive beliefs and compulsions was a significant predictor in the regression model for exercise beliefs, after controlling for BMI and eating disorder psychopathology [41]. Such findings are consistent with the premise that obsessionality plays a causal role in the development and maintenance of excessive exercise [38].

Bewell-Weiss and Carter [36] reported a negative relationship between OCD symptomatology and excessive exercise. The researchers concluded that it may have been that their regression model was more comprehensive than those used in previous studies, or that obsessive-compulsive symptomatology had shared variance with another variable that had not been explored with previous studies [36]. Additionally, they used different OCD measures than those used in other studies [36]. Penas-Lledo et al. [31] found a trend only for increased obsessive compulsive symptomatology in exercising patients using the SCL-90-R. Finally, Hotlkamp et al. [40] found no direct relationship between obsessive-compulsiveness and levels of physical activity, also assessed using the SCL-90-R. It may be that this measure is not as sensitive as other measures, or that OCD features affect cognitions or beliefs about exercise [40].

Davis et al. [2] speculated that it could be that greater obsessive-compulsive personality traits are exacerbated by the combination of starvation and high level exercise, or that these patients choose to combine dietary restraint with excessive exercise. It may be the case that patients who have obsessive tendencies are more likely to undertake exercise as an additional method to prevent weight gain (on top of restricted diet, purging behaviour) or to neutralise fears of changes in their body weight and shape [75]. Alternatively, patients may be using exercise to alleviate or reduce anxiety [76], or as a means of neutralising predominant weight or food related obsessions [40].

Anderluh et al. [35] found that participants with childhood traits of rigidity, extreme cautiousness and perfectionism underwent more severe food restriction and higher levels of excessive exercise, and experienced longer periods of underweight status. Their research identified the possibility of homogenous phenotypes of AN and demonstrates that premorbid obsessive-compulsive personality traits in childhood may influence the course of the eating disorder later in life, potentially contributing to a more severe form of restricting AN, which could be extremely resistant to treatment [38].

There are a number of limitations that were evident in the reviewed literature. The number of studies examined in the review (10) is small, and results must be interpreted with some caution as some of the studies did not support the association between OCD and excessive exercise. A number of the reviewed studies did not clearly differentiate between OCD and OCPD constructs in their presentation of results. Nine different types of measures were employed across the studies to assess OCPD traits and OCD symptomatology, many of these being self-report questionnaires, which may increase the incidence of socially desirable response styles. Others involved expert clinical assessment in the form of an interview (for example, the EATATE interview in Anderluh et al. [35]). These various instruments assess different constructs, and some measures may have provided more detailed information, both of which may have biased the results. In one study, the use of the SCL-90 may have been inappropriate, as it had been normed for participants aged 14 years and older, yet a proportion of their sample were aged between 13 and 14 years. It would thus be beneficial for future studies to utilise the most current and comprehensive assessment tools in the field to enable more reliable inter-study comparisons.

Denial commonly occurs in anorexia nervosa, and subjective measures may have underestimated the amount of physical activity completed by patients. Such underestimation may have led to significant bias and consequently inaccuracy of data regarding the extent of exercise, and its relationships with coexisting OCD and/or OCPD. This potential room for bias has led to the utilisation of more objective means of assessing for physical activity in patients with AN, for example accelerometers [77,78]. Yet no study included in the review used such devices. Numerous measures of exercise were utilised across studies, reflecting both the variety of measures available, and the time period over which the studies were undertaken (1995–2011). However, there is also a pervasive issue in this field regarding the lack of consensus on what defines excessive exercise, how it should be measured and how it should be managed in patients with AN [79].

There are also a number of limitations in regards to participants utilised in the studies. The small sample size of Holtkamp et al. [40] affected their capability to generalise their results, whilst the use of informants may have been beneficial for Anderluh et al. [35] to confirm retrospective data provided by participants and to limit memory bias effects. Participants across studies who were inpatients were not exercising at the time of completing study assessments and questionnaires, and it is unknown what effect this may have had on response style. Other participants (for example outpatients) would not have such intense restrictions. The research reviewed also did not take into account other factors which may be important in the study of obsessive-compulsive symptomatology with excessive exercisers, such as motivational factors and specific reasons for exercising (other than the use of CET in Naylor et al., [41]). Finally, across studies, the patients were recruited mostly from secondary and tertiary referral services, i.e. inpatient and outpatient eating disorder services. Thus, the findings from the review cannot be generalised to people with AN who are currently not seeking treatment, or whose eating disorder pathology is not as severe as those patients in hospital treatment.

As the vast majority of the studies employed a cross-sectional design, only relationships between variables could be determined, and there can be no demonstration of the direction of such associations. Acute starvation syndrome and severity of eating disorder psychopathology both have significant impact upon level of obsessive-compulsive symptoms and exercise [17]. There was also no information about how obsessionality might affect prognosis and treatment outcome for AN patients who exercise excessively.

Whilst this review has focused on the relationships between OCPD traits and/or OCD symptomatology with excessive exercise in patients with AN, it would be remiss not to mention the significant relationships which excessive exercise shares with other psychopathologies, which have important implications for treatment. Studies included in the review demonstrated that AN patients who exercised excessively demonstrated lower minimum BMI and lower novelty seeking, but higher harm avoidance, persistence and cooperativeness [42]. In other studies, these patients demonstrated higher levels of anxiety and food restriction [40]; higher levels of depression, self-esteem and dietary restraint [36]; higher addictive personality traits [37]; higher weight preoccupation [39]; and higher levels of bulimic and eating disorder psychopathology [31].

Conclusions

From the research reviewed, it appears that there is a positive association between obsessive- compulsive personality traits in patients with AN who excessively exercise, yet the relationship with obsessive-compulsive disorder is less clear. Although it is known that excessive exercise is associated with poor treatment outcome in AN [28,29] the effects of obsessionality on treatment outcome are not yet known. Results of this paper indicate that obsessive-compulsive symptomatology and/or obsessive-compulsive personality traits contribute greater complexity to individual cases and may make these patients more resistant to treatment. Results support integrated interventions addressing the role of driven exercise in the context of obsessionality and obsessive compulsive symptoms where present, providing therapeutic interventions to alleviate emotional distress [31] and addressing characteristics such as perfectionism and behavioural rigidity [80]. The Loughborough Eating Disorders Activity Programme (LEAP) is an exemplar in this regard [81]. It is a manualised intervention which addresses driven exercise behaviours and beliefs using psycho-education and specific cognitive behavioural techniques to manage unhelpful beliefs and attitudes towards exercise, negative affective and compulsivity. Finally, future research into the relationship between driven exercise and obsessionality should utilise the most comprehensive and reliable clinical assessment tools, and address prognostic factors, treatment factors and specific interventions for patients with OCPD and/or OCD and driven exercise.

Competing interests

The authors declare that they have no competing interests.

Authors' contributions

SY undertook the systematic review and with PH prepared this manuscript for journal submission. PH, ST and PR assisted with the editing of the manuscript and data interpretation. All authors read and approved the final manuscript.

Authors' information

SY submitted an alternate version of this manuscript as a requirement for the Doctor of Clinical Psychology/Master of Science thesis at University of Sydney. She is supervised by ST, PH and PR. PH, ST and PR are conducting a randomised controlled trial and evaluation of the Loughborough Eating Disorders Activity Programme (LEAP) referenced in this paper.

Acknowledgments

SY would like to acknowledge and sincerely thank PH, ST and PR for their assistance in preparing this manuscript, and for their supervision of her Master of Science thesis.

Author details

[1]Clinical Psychology Unit, Mackie Building K01, School of Psychology, University of Sydney, Sydney, NSW 2006, Australia. [2]School of Medicine, University of Western Sydney, Locked Bag 1797, Penrith, NSW 2751, Australia. [3]School of Medicine, James Cook University, Townsville, North Queensland, Australia.

References

1. Touyz S: *What kind of illness is anorexia nervosa? A clinical update.* The Australian Psychological Society; 2011. Accessed online via http://www.psychology.org.au; April, 2012.
2. Davis C, Kaptein S, Kaplan AS, Olmsted MP, Woodside DB: **Obsessionality in anorexia nervosa: the moderating influence of exercise.** *Psychosom Med* 1998, **60**:192–197.
3. Rothenberg A: **Eating disorder as a modern obsessive-compulsive syndrome.** *Psychiatry* 1986, **49**:45–53.
4. Jordan J, Joyce PR, Carter FA, Horn J, McIntosh VW, Luty SE, McKenzie JM, Mulder RT, Bulik CM: **Anxiety and psychoactive substance use disorder comorbidity in anorexia nervosa or depression.** *Int J Eat Disord* 2003, **34**:211–219.
5. O'Brien KM, Vincent NK: **Psychiatric comorbidity in anorexia and bulimia nervosa: nature, prevalence, and causal relationships.** *Clin Psychol Rev* 2003, **23**:57–74.
6. Jacobi C, Haywood C, de Zwaan M, Kraemer HC, Agras WS: **Coming to terms with risk factors for eating disorders: application of risk terminology and suggestions for a general taxonomy.** *Psychol Bull* 2004, **130**:19–65.
7. Halmi KA, Sunday SR, Klump KL, Strober M, Leckman JF, Fichter M, Kaplan A, Woodside B, Treasure J, Berrettini WH, Shabboat MA, Bulik CM, Kaye W: **Obsessions and compulsions in anorexia nervosa subtypes.** *Int J Eat Disord* 2003, **33**:308–319.
8. Bastiani AM, Altemus M, Pigott T, Rubenstein C, Weltzin TE, Kaye W: **Comparison of obsession and compulsion in patients with anorexia nervosa and obsessive–compulsive disorder.** *Biol Psychiatry* 1996, **39**:966–969.
9. Hasler G, LaSalle-Ricci VH, Ronquillo JG, Crawley SA, Cochran LW, Kazuba D, Greenberg BD, Murphy DL: **Obsessive–compulsive disorder symptom dimensions show specific relationships to psychiatric comorbidity.** *Psychiatry Res* 2005, **135**:121–132.
10. Matsunaga H, Kaye WH, McConaha C, Plotnicov K, Pollice C, Rao R: **Personality disorders among subjects recovered from eating disorders.** *Int J Eat Disord* 1999, **27**:353–357.
11. Jarry JL, Vaccarino FJ: **Eating disorder and obsessive-compulsive disorder: neurochemical and phenomenological commonalities.** *J Psychiatry Neurosci* 1996, **21**:36–48.
12. Gibbs NA, Oltmanns TF: **The relation between obsessive–compulsive personality traits and subtypes of compulsive behavior.** *J Anxiety Disord* 1995, **9**:397–410.
13. Rosen KV, Tallis F: **Investigation into the relationship between personality traits and OCD.** *Behav Res Ther* 1995, **33**:445–450.
14. Lilenfeld LR, Kaye WH, Greeno CG, Merikangas KR, Plotnicov K, Pollice C, Rao R, Strober M, Bulik CM, Nagy L: **A controlled family study of anorexia nervosa and bulimia nervosa: psychiatric disorders in first-degree relatives and effects of proband comorbidity.** *Arch Gen Psychiatry* 1998, **55**:603–610.
15. Hsu LKG, Kaye W, Weltzin T: **Are the eating disorders related to obsessive compulsive disorder?** *Int J Eat Disord* 1993, **14**:305–318.
16. Kaye WH, Weltzin TE, Hsu LKG, Bulik C: **An open trial of fluoxetine in patients with anorexia nervosa.** *J Clin Psychiatry* 1991, **52**:464–471.
17. Keys A: *The biology of human starvation.* Minneapolis: University of Minnesota Press; 1950.
18. Strober M: **Personality and symptomatological features in young, nonchronic anorexia nervosa patients.** *J Psychosom Res* 1980, **24**:353–359.
19. Casper R: **Behavioral activation and lack of concern, core symptoms of anorexia nervosa?** *Int J Eat Disord* 1998, **24**:381–393.
20. Davis C: **Eating disorders and hyperactivity: a psychobiological perspective. [Review].** *Can J Psychiatry* 1997, **42**:168–175.
21. Davis C, Kennedy SH, Ralevski E, Dionne M: **The role of physical activity in the development and maintenance of eating disorders.** *Psychol Med* 1994, **24**:957–967.

22. Davis C, Katzman DK, Kaptein S, Kirsh C, Brewer H, Kalmbach K, *et al:* **The prevalence of high-level exercise** in the eating disorders: etiological **implications.** *Compr Psychiatry* 1997, **38:**321–326.
23. Epling WF, Pierce WD, Stefan L: **A theory of activity based anorexia.** *Int J Eat Disord* 1983, **3:**7–46.
24. Boyd C, Abraham S, Luscombe G: **Exercise behaviours and feelings in eating disorder and non-eating disorder groups.** *Eur Eat Disord Rev* 2007, **15:**112–118.
25. Hausenblas HA, Cook BJ, Chittester NI: **Can exercise treat eating disorders?** *Exerc Sport Sci Rev* 2008, **36:**43–47.
26. Bamber D, Cockerill IM, Rodger S, Carroll D: **"It's exercise or nothing": a qualitative analysis of exercise dependence.** *Br J Sports Med* 2000, **34:**423–430.
27. Kaye WH, Gwirtsman HE, Obarzanek E, George DT: **Relative importance of calorie intake needed to gain weight and level of physical activity in anorexia nervosa.** *Am J Clin Nutr* 1998, **47:**989–994.
28. Dalle Grave R, Calugi S, Marchesini G: **Compulsive exercise to control shape or weight in eating disorders: prevalence, associated features and treatment outcome.** *Compr Psychiatry* 2008, **49:**346–352.
29. Carter JC, Blackmore E, Sutander-Pinnock K, Woodside DB: **Relapse in anorexia nervosa: a survival analysis.** *Psychol Med* 2004, **34:**671–679.
30. Brewerton TD, Stellefson EJ, Hibbs N, Hodges EL, Cochrane CE: **Comparison of eating disorder patients with and without compulsive exercising.** *Int J Eat Disord* 1995, **17:**413–416.
31. Penas-Lledo E, Vaz Leal FJ, Waller G: **Excessive exercise in anorexia nervosa and bulimia nervosa: relations to eating characteristics and general psychopathology.** *Int J Eat Disord* 2002, **31:**370–375.
32. Taranis L, Meyer C, Touyz S: **Disordered Eating and Exercise: Development and Preliminary Validation of the Compulsive Exercise Test (CET).** *Eur Eat Disorders Rev* 2011, **19:**256–268.
33. Downs SH, Black N: **The feasibility of creating a checklist for the assessment of the methodological quality both of randomized and non-randomised studies of health care interventions.** *J Epidemiol Community Health* 1998, **52:**377–384.
34. Ferro MA, Speechley KN: **Depressive symptoms among mothers of children with epilepsy: a review of prevalence, associated factors, and impact on children.** *Epilepsia* 2009, **50:**2344–2354.
35. Anderluh M, Tchanturia K, Rabe- Hesketh S, Collier D, Treasure J: **Lifetime course of eating disorders: design and validity testing of a new strategy to define the eating disorders phenotype.** *Psychol Med* 2009, **39:**105–114.
36. Bewell-Weiss CV, Carter JC: **Predictors of excessive exercise in anorexia nervosa.** *Compr Psychiatry* 2010, **51:**566–571.
37. Davis C, Claridge G: **The eating disorders as addiction: a psychobiological perspective.** *Addict Behav* 1998, **23:**463–475.
38. Davis C, Kaptein S: **Anorexia nervosa with excessive exercise: a phenotype with close links to obsessive-compulsive disorder.** *Psychiatry Res* 2006, **142:**209–217.
39. Davis C, Kennedy SH, Ralevski E, Dionne M, Brewer H, Neitzert C, Ratusny D: **Obsessive compulsiveness and physical activity in anorexia nervosa and high-level exercising.** *J Psychosom Res* 1995, **39:**967–976.
40. Holtkamp K, Hebebrand J, Herpertz-Dahlmann B: **The contribution of anxiety and food restriction on physical activity levels in acute anorexia nervosa.** *Int J Eat Disord* 2004, **36:**163–171.
41. Naylor H, Mountford V, Brown G: **Beliefs about excessive exercise in eating disorders: the role of obsessions and compulsions.** *Eur Eat Disord Rev* 2011, **19:**226–236.
42. Shroff H, Reba L, Thornton LM, Tozzi F, Klump KL, Berrettini WH, *et al:* **Features associated with excessive exercise in women with eating disorders.** *Int J Eat Disord* 2006, **39:**454–461.
43. Anderluh MB, Tchanturia K, Rabe-Hesketh S, Treasure J: **Childhood obsessive-compulsive personality traits in adult women with eating disorders: defining a broader eating disorder phenotype.** *Am J Psychiatry* 2003, **160:**242–247.
44. Fairburn CG, Cooper Z: **The eating disorders examination.** In *Binge eating: nature, assessment, and treatment.* 12th edition. Edited by Fairburn CG, Wilson GT. New York: The Guilford Press; 1993:317–360.
45. Fairburn CG, Beglin SJ: **Assessment of eating disorders: interview or self report questionnaire?** *Int J Eat Disord* 1994, **16:**363–370.
46. Derogatis LR: *Brief Symptom Inventory: administration, scoring, and procedures manual.* Minneapolis: National Computer Systems; 1993.
47. Beck AT, Steer RA, Brown GK: *Beck depression inventory manual.* 2nd edition. New York: Guilford Press; 1996.
48. Rosenberg M: *Conceiving the self.* New York: Basic Books; 1979.
49. Van Oppen P, Hoekstra RJ, Emmelkamp PMG: **The structure of obsessive-compulsive symptoms.** *Behav Res Ther* 1995, **33:**15–23.
50. Garner DM, Olmsted MP: *Eating disorder inventory manual.* Florida: Psychological Assessment Resources; 1984.
51. Eysenck HJ, Eysenck SBG: *Manual of the Eysenck personality scales.* London: Hodder & Stoughton; 1991.
52. Lazare A, Klerman GL, Armour DJ: **Oral, obsessive and hysterical personality patterns.** *J Psychiatry Res* 1970, **7:**275–290.
53. Hodgson RJ, Rachman S: **Obsessional-compulsive complaints.** *Behav Res Ther* 1977, **15:**389–395.
54. Frost R, Marten P, Lahart C, Rosenblate R: **The dimensions of perfectionism.** *Cogn Ther Res* 1990, **14:**449–468.
55. Davis C, Brewer H, Ratusny D: **Behavioral frequency and psychological commitment: necessary concepts in the study of excessive exercising.** *J Behav Med* 1993, **16:**611–628.
56. Franzoi SL, Shields SA: **The body esteem scale: multidimensional structure and sex differences in a college population.** *J Personality Assess* 1984, **48:**173–178.
57. Janis IL, Field PB: **A behavioral assessment of persuasibility: consistency of individual differences.** In *Personality and persuasibility.* Edited by Jovland CI, Janis IL. New Haven: Yale University Press; 1959:29–54.
58. Derogatis LR, Rickels K, Rock AF: **The SCL-90 and the MMPI: a step in the validation of a new self-report scale.** *Br J Psychiatry* 1976, 128:280–289. 7.
59. Fichter MM, Herpertz S, Quadflieg N, Herpertz-Dahlmann B: **Structured interview for anorexic and bulimic disorders for DSM-IV and ICD-10 (3rd Rev. ed.).** *Int J Eat Disord* 1998, **24:**227–249.
60. Schmitz N, Hartkamp N, Kiuse J, Franke GH, Reister G, Tress W: **The symptom check-list-90-R (SCL-90-R): a german validation study.** *Qual Life Res* 2000, **9:**185–193.
61. Obsessive Compulsive Cognitions Working Group: **Psychometric validation of the obsessive belief questionnaire and interpretation of intrusions inventory– part 2: Factor analyses and testing of a brief version.** *Behav Res Ther* 2005, **43:**1527–1542.
62. Foa EB, Huppert JD, Leiberg S, Langner R, Kichic R, Hajcak G, *et al:* **The obsessive-compulsive inventory: development and validation of a short version.** *Psychol Assess* 2002, **14:**485–496.
63. Fairburn CG, Beglin SJ: **Eating disorder examination questionnaire-6.** In *Cognitive behaviour therapy and eating disorders.* Edited by Fairburn CG. New York: Guilford Press; 2008:309–313.
64. Garner DM, Garfinkel PE: **The eating attitudes test: an index of the symptoms of anorexia nervosa.** *Psychological Med* 1979, **9:**273–279.
65. Henderson M, Freeman CPL: **A self-rating scale for bulimia- the BITE.** *Br JPsychiatry* 1987, **150:**18–24.
66. Derogatis LR: *The SCL-90-R Administration, scoring and procedures: Manual-II for the Revised version (2nd Ed.).* Towson: Clinical Psychometric Research; 1983.
67. First M, Spitzer R, Gibbon M, Williams J: *Structured clinical interview for DSM-IV axis I disorders, research version, patient edition.* New York: Biometrics Research, New York State Psychiatric Institute; 1996.
68. Cloninger CR, Przybeck TR, Svrakic DM, Wetzel RD: *The temperament and character inventory (TCI): a guide to its development and use.* St. Louis, MO: Center for Psychobiology of Personality, Washington University; 1994.
69. Spielberger C, Gorsuch R, Luchene R: *The state-trait anxiety inventory: test manual for form X.* Palo Alto, CA: Consulting Psychologists Press; 1970.
70. Goodman W, Price L, Rasmussen S, Mazure C, Fleischmann R, Hill C, *et al:* **The Yale–brown obsessive-compulsive scale (YBOCS): it's development, use, and reliability.** *Arch Gen Psychiatry* 1989, **46:**1006–1011.
71. Sunday SR, Halmi KA, Einhorn A: **The Yale–brown–Cornell eating disorder scale: a new scale to assess eating disorder symptomatology.** *Int J Eat Dis* 1995, **18:**237–245.
72. Cassin SE, von Ranson KM: **Personality and eating disorders: a decade in review.** *Clin Psychol Rev* 2005, **25:**895–916.
73. Richter MA, Cox BJ, Direnfeld DM: **A comparison of three assessment instruments for obsessive–compulsive symptoms.** *J Behav Ther J Exp Psychol* 1994, **25:**143–147.
74. Mond JM, Hay PJ, Rodgers B, Owen C: **An update on the definition of "excessive exercise" in eating disorders research.** *Int J Eat Disord* 2006, **39:**147–153.
75. Davis C, Blackmore E, Katzman DK, Fox J: **Female adolescents with Anorexia nervosa and their parents: a case control study of exercise attitudes and behaviors.** *Psychol Med* 2005, **35:**377–386.
76. Geller J, Cockell SJ, Goldner EM: **Inhibited expression of negative emotions and the interpersonal orientations in anorexia nervosa.** *Int J Eat Disord* 2000, **28:**8–19.

77. Harris AM, Mcalpine DE, Shirbhate R, Manohar CU, Levine JA: **Measurement of daily activity in restrictive type anorexia nervosa.** *Int J Eat Disord* 2008, **41**:280–283.
78. Westerterp KR: **Assessment of physical activity: a critical appraisal.** *Eur J Appl Physiol* 2009, **105**:823–828.
79. Meyer C: **Excessive exercise in the eating disorders: a need for less activity from patients and more from researchers.** *Eur Eat Disord Rev* 2008, **16**:81–83.
80. Crane AM, Roberts ME, Treasure J: **Are obsessive-compulsive personality traits associated with a poor outcome in anorexia nervosa? A systematic review of randomized controlled trials and naturalistic outcome studies.** *Int J Eat Disord* 2007, **40**:581–588.
81. **The Loughborough eating disorders activity programme (LEAP) manual.** http://store.lboro.ac.uk/browse/department.asp?compid=1&modid=1&deptid=233.

Personality Assessment Inventory profiles of university students with eating disorders

Michael Wm MacGregor* and Paige Lamborn

Abstract

Background: Eating disorders are complex disorders that involve medical and psychological symptoms. Understanding the psychological factors associated with different eating disorders is important for assessment, diagnosis, and treatment.

Methods: This study sought to determine on which of the 22 Personality Assessment Inventory (PAI) scales patients with anorexia nervosa, bulimia nervosa, and eating disorder not otherwise specified (EDNOS) differed, and whether the PAI can be used to classify eating disorder subtypes. Because we were interested in both whether the PAI could be used to differentiate eating disorder subtypes from each other, as well as from other disorders, we also included a group of patients with major depression.

Results: The three eating disorder groups did differ significantly from each other, and from the patients with depression, on a number of the PAI scales. Only two PAI scales (Anxiety and Depression), however, exceeded a T-score of 70 for the patients with anorexia nervosa, no scales exceeded a T-score of 70 for the patients with bulimia nervosa or EDNOS, and only two exceeded a T-score of 70 for the patients with depression (Depression and Suicide). A discriminant function analysis revealed an overall correct classification between the groups of 81.6%.

Conclusions: The PAI helps to understand the psychological factors associated with eating disorders and can be used to assist with assessment. Continued investigation using the PAI in an eating disordered population is supported.

Keywords: Personality Assessment Inventory, PAI, Eating disorders, Anorexia nervosa, Bulimia nervosa, Assessment

Background

The Personality Assessment Inventory (PAI) is a widely available assessment tool that has been used across different settings with different populations [1-8]. To date, however, there has been little research on using the PAI in an eating disordered population. The generalizability of the PAI to disordered eating populations and its utility in terms of aiding diagnosis and understanding of symptoms is important for the ongoing psychometric evaluation of the PAI. It is also necessary if the PAI is to be used with those suffering from eating disorder symptoms. PAI data can additionally contribute to a more full understanding of eating disorder patients and their treatment considerations. We sought to determine 1) on which of the 22 PAI scales patients with eating disorder subtypes differed from each other, and 2) whether the PAI can differentiate among patients with different eating disorder subtypes, and 3) whether it can distinguish between patients with eating disorders and patients with depression. This later group was chosen for inclusion because it is characterized by features that are similar to those found in eating disorders such as loss of weight, feelings of worthlessness, and guilt. Thus, being able to differentiate eating disorder from this comparison group would add to the PAIs discriminant validity. The PAI has the potential to meaningfully differentiate between eating disorder groups and help better understand the nature of the differences between the groups.

The Diagnostic and Statistical Manual of Mental Disorders (4th edition; *DSM-IV*) [9] identifies three types of eating disorders: Anorexia nervosa, bulimia nervosa, and eating disorder not otherwise specified (EDNOS). Both anorexia nervosa and bulimia nervosa are also found in the new *DSM-5*, although a new diagnosis of binge-eating disorder has been added to aid in diagnosis [10-14]. Patients with anorexia nervosa refuse to maintain a minimally normal body weight, have an intense fear of gaining weight or becoming fat, and have a disturbed view

* Correspondence: michael.macgregor@usask.ca
University of Saskatchewan, Saskatoon, Saskatchewan, Canada

of their weight or body shape [13,15,16]. These patients may have an almost delusional view of their bodies, an inability to identify feelings and needs, and a sense of ineffectiveness often accompanied by perfectionism [17-22]. The *DSM-IV* and the new *DSM-5* criteria for bulimia nervosa include recurrent episodes of binge eating and inappropriate compensatory behavior in order to prevent weight gain, and self-evaluation that is unduly influenced by body shape and weight [16,23,24]. Unlike patients with anorexia nervosa, patients with bulimia nervosa are not underweight. Compared to patients with anorexia nervosa, patients with bulimia nervosa are usually less enmeshed with their family, less perfectionistic, less resistant to treatment, more impulsive, and more likely to use alcohol [15,16,25,26]. Finally, EDNOS (in the DSM-IV) and unspecified feeding or eating disorder (in the *DSM-5*) refer to as an eating disorder that does not meet the criteria for any specific eating disorder. This category is much more heterogeneous than the other two. It includes a wider range of disorders related to eating and a diverse set of medical complications.

Many studies have attempted to differentiate among eating disorder subtypes on the basis of psychopathology [27-30]. These investigations have sought: 1) to determine the utility of personality and psychopathology measures as diagnostic and/or classification instruments, 2) to evaluate the psychometrics of these tests when generalized to different populations, and 3) to elucidate the personality and psychopathology differences among eating disorder subtypes. This latter point is particularly important as different eating disorders share some similar diagnostic features (e.g., concern about weight). Wildes and Marcus argue in favour of considering psychopathology and other associated features when classifying eating disorders and using the information when making diagnosis [30]. Personality and psychopathology instruments such as the PAI are often routinely administered at intake to all patients seeking treatment [31]. Thus, investigating the applicability of such widely used instruments beyond the samples in which they were originally developed is important to ensure an accurate understanding of their psychometric properties and validity. If such an instrument can help identify or aid in the understanding of eating disorders, this may benefit clinicians, patients, and researchers. Information from the PAI may also aid in treatment planning and case conceptualization. Given the medical sequelae associated with eating disorders timely identification, easy assessment, and more complete conceptualization has the potential to improve outcomes and reduce health care costs [32-36].

Several models of eating disorders implicate personality characteristics in the emergence of symptoms and onset of the eating disorder [36-38]. Despite sharing some similar diagnostic features, patients with anorexia nervosa differ from patients with bulimia nervosa in personality characteristics (e.g., perfectionism, obsessions), and both groups differ from non-eating disordered persons [15,16]. One measure of personality that has been used to better understand eating disorders is the PAI. To date, however, there has only been one published study that has assessed the applicability of the PAI to an eating disordered sample [3]. The authors found, in general, that patients with a binge eating disorder (BED) displayed less distress and less impairment than patients with anorexia nervosa (both restricting and binge-purge type) or bulimia nervosa. They also found that the two anorexia nervosa groups and the bulimia nervosa group had significantly higher scores than the BED group on the Infrequency, Anxiety, and Schizophrenia scales of the PAI. Further, the binge-purge anorexia nervosa group and the bulimia nervosa group had significantly more elevated scores than the BED group on the Negative Impression, Somatic Complaints, Anxiety Related Disorders, Depression, and Suicidal Ideation scales of the PAI. Finally, the authors found that patients with binge-purge anorexia nervosa and bulimia nervosa had significantly high scores than the BED group on the PAI Borderline Features scale, and that those with bulimia nervosa had significantly more elevated scores than those with restricting anorexia nervosa on the PAI Borderline Features scale. Tasca and colleagues concluded that the BED group generally had lower scores than some or all of the other groups, and that for the most part the patients with restricting anorexia nervosa were not different from the bulimic or the patients with binge-purge anorexia nervosa [3]. These results suggest that there may be some differences on the PAI scales between different eating disorder groups, although perhaps not between patients with anorexia nervosa and bulimia nervosa. The study by Tasca and colleagues did not address the utility of the PAI in classifying eating disorder subtypes. Further, it used a sample in which groups were not matched for age: the BED group was significantly older than the other groups, and the patients with bulimia nervosa were older than the patients with restricting anorexia nervosa [3]. The age differences were not statistically controlled for and need to be investigated further given that a number of the significant differences on the 22 PAI scales were found between the BED group and the other eating disordered groups.

The present study investigated the relation between eating disorders and the PAI scales in a sample of female college students. We sought to determine which of the 22 PAI scales would be different among patients with differing eating disorder subtypes. We also wanted to determine whether the PAI can differentiate patients with eating disorder subtypes from each other, as well as from patients with depression.

Based on previous research looking at personality differences among eating disorder groups and the study by Tasca we made three hypotheses. 1) All three eating disorder groups would have specific elevations on the PAI scales related to Anxiety, Depression, and Borderline Features (as a marker of negative relationships and identity problems). 2) Patients with anorexia nervosa would have significantly higher scores than the patients with bulimia nervosa or EDNOS on the PAI scales related to Anxiety, Depression, and Treatment Rejection. 3) PAI scales would be able to differentiate among the eating disorder subtypes, and between the eating disorder groups and patients with depression.

Methods

Participants

Two hundred and ninety-three female students from a large southeastern American university participated in this study. All participants were enrolled as full-time students and had presented to the university's Counseling and Psychological Services center for assessment and/or treatment between 1997 and 2000. A group of patients with major depressive disorder was included for comparison purposes because of the high prevalence of depressive symptoms among patients with eating disorders. Participants met *DSM-IV* criteria for either anorexia nervosa ($n = 49$), bulimia nervosa ($n = 44$), EDNOS ($n = 55$)[a], or major depressive disorder ($n = 145$). Participants did not have any co-morbid diagnoses. Participants' ages ranged from 17 to 52 years of age, and there were no significant age differences among the groups.

Measures

Personality Assessment Inventory

The PAI [2,39] is a self-report inventory consisting of 344 statements that participants rate on a four point Likert scale. When scored, the PAI consists of 22 non-overlapping scales: Four validity scales, eleven clinical scales, five treatment scales, and two interpersonal scales. The four validity scales include Inconsistency, Infrequency, Negative Impression, and Positive Impression. The eleven clinical scales include Somatic Complaints, Anxiety, Anxiety Related Disorders, Depression, Mania, Paranoia, Schizophrenia, Borderline Features, Antisocial Features, Alcohol Problems, and Drug Problems. The five treatment scales consist of Aggression, Suicidal Ideation, Stress, Nonsupport, and Treatment Rejection. Finally, the two interpersonal scales consist of Dominance and Warmth.

The PAI has good internal consistency and test-retest reliability [40,41]. For example, previous studies have found median alphas of 0.86 and 0.82 for the 22 scales for clinical and college samples, respectively. The median alpha for the 22 scales in this study was 0.85.

Psychiatric diagnosis

Psychiatric diagnoses were derived through a two-part process. First, participants underwent a 1.5-hour unstructured clinical intake interview. During this interview, information was obtained relating to the participant's presenting complaint, psychiatric and medical history, somatic functioning, substance use, developmental, social, and family history, mental status, and suicide and homicide risk. All interviews were conducted by a mental health professional (i.e., a psychologist, psychiatrist, social worker, psychiatric resident, or psychology intern). Based on this interview, initial tentative *DSM-IV* Axis I and II psychiatric diagnoses were determined for each participant. Second, information from the intake interview was presented at a team meeting for discussion. Team meetings consisted of at least one psychologist, one psychiatrist, one social worker, and one psychology intern. The team discussed these intake interviews and diagnoses until the team reached consensus about the diagnoses. When there was doubt as to the appropriate diagnosis, a second interview was conducted to gather follow-up information, and this information was presented at a second team meeting for further discussion. The PAI scores were not used by the mental health professionals or the teams to make diagnoses.

Procedures

Participants first completed the PAI and then met with the mental health profession who conducted the intake interview. Data collection and analysis was approved by the appropriate university ethics boards.

Data collection was approved by the Institutional Review Board for Social and Behavioural Sciences.

Results

Multivariate analysis of variance (MANOVA) was conducted to determine if the 22 PAI scales differed among the four groups (patients with anorexia nervosa, bulimia nervosa, EDNOS, and depression) as a combined dependent variable. A significant difference was found between the four groups on the combined PAI scales, F (66, 293) = 12.02, $p < .001$, $h_p{}^2 = .50$. Analyses of variance (ANOVA) on each of the 22 scales were conducted as follow-up tests to the MANOVA. The Bonferroni method was used to control for Type I error across all the tests. Table 1 contains the mean T-scores, standard deviations, F values, and partial eta squared values for the univariate ANOVAs for the four groups on each of the 22 scales.

Patients with anorexia nervosa had significantly higher scores than patients with bulimia nervosa on 8 scales (Somatic Complaints, Anxiety, Depression, Borderline Features, Suicide, Stress, Nonsupport, and Treatment

Table 1 Mean T-score values (standard deviations) and F values for univariate tests for differences between patients with anorexia nervosa, bulimia nervosa, those with an eating disorder NOS, and those with major depressive disorder

	Anorexia nervosa (N = 49)	Bulimia nervosa (N = 44)	Eating disorder NOS (N = 55)	Depression (N = 145)	F value[a]	Sig.	Partial eta squared
Inc	51.5 (06.9)	52.3 (08.1)	51.6 (08.5)	52.8 (07.1)	00.6	.632	.006
Inf	51.0 (06.9)	55.3 (10.2)	51.4 (08.7)	51.9 (09.0)	02.3	.075	.024
Nim	54.9 (15.0)a	50.9 (10.4)b	52.4 (08.0)c	64.0 (11.2)abc	24.9	.000	.205
Pim	47.0 (11.5)a	46.6 (09.1)b	44.8 (10.9)c	36.7 (09.0)abc	22.5	.000	.190
Som	65.8 (09.6)ab	55.7 (07.1)ac	51.5 (08.7)bd	62.3 (09.0)cd	30.9	.000	.243
Anx	71.3 (12.9)ab	64.5 (08.2)ac	57.5 (10.6)bcd	69.4 (10.9)d	19.9	.000	.171
Ard	66.3 (13.8)a	60.1 (10.0)b	53.6 (11.6)abc	64.5 (11.5)c	14.1	.000	.127
Dep	72.0 (15.0)ab	65.6 (13.1)acd	57.7 (13.0)bce	74.7 (05.3)de	38.3	.000	.284
Man	52.3 (10.8)	50.1 (10.8)	51.9 (09.9)	50.1 (09.6)	00.9	.429	.010
Par	48.2 (09.9)a	46.9 (11.4)b	49.7 (09.8)c	55.7 (10.4)abc	12.9	.000	.118
Scz	64.8 (13.1)ab	67.0 (08.7)cd	52.3 (10.4)ace	60.0 (11.5)bde	19.3	.000	.167
Bor	63.5 (13.8)a	55.3 (12.6)ab	59.4 (12.8)c	65.5 (08.6)bc	11.4	.000	.106
Ant	48.8 (07.5)	50.9 (09.3)	50.1 (06.5)	50.4 (09.5)	00.5	.652	.006
Alc	46.2 (10.5)a	49.7 (11.2)b	49.9 (09.3)c	55.2 (10.0)abc	11.6	.000	.108
Drg	46.6 (07.0)a	53.7 (09.4)abc	48.5 (10.6)b	48.7 (08.5)c	05.4	.001	.053
Agg	44.8 (08.6)a	46.6 (12.8)b	47.3 (10.8)c	55.0 (11.3)abc	15.6	.000	.140
Sui	66.9 (14.7)ab	55.5 (09.7)ac	54.5 (12.3)bd	70.8 (17.2)cd	22.4	.000	.189
Str	58.8 (08.5)ab	51.8 (10.3)ac	53.7 (11.2)d	68.5 (11.2)bcd	44.0	.000	.314
Non	54.4 (13.3)a	47.7 (09.4)ab	51.6 (10.7)c	59.2 (12.0)bc	13.6	.000	.124
Rxr	43.5 (12.6)ab	34.6 (08.8)ac	40.8 (11.7)cd	34.3 (08.7)bd	13.6	.000	.124
Dom	49.2 (11.4)ab	56.5 (11.7)acd	49.0 (11.3)ce	43.6 (11.9)bde	14.8	.000	.133
Wrm	52.8 (10.8)a	55.0 (11.4)b	51.2 (10.3)c	45.9 (10.9)abc	11.1	.000	.104

Notes: Means that share a similar subscript differ from each other by at least the $p < .05$ level.
NOS = Not otherwise specified; *Inc* = Inconsistency; *Inf* = Infrequency; *Nim* = Negative Impression; *Pim* = Positive Impression; *Som* = Somatic Complaints; *Anx* = Anxiety; *Ard* = Anxiety Related Disorders; *Dep* = Depression; *Man* = Mania; *Par* = Paranoia; *Scz* = Schizophrenia; *Bor* = Borderline Features; *Ant* = Antisocial Features; *Alc* = Alcohol Problems; *Drg* = Drug Problems; *Agg* = Aggression; *Sui* = Suicidal Ideation; *Str* = Stress; *Non* = Nonsupport; *Rxr* = Treatment Rejection; *Dom* = Dominance; *Wrm* = Warmth.
[a]Univariate ANOVAs were conducted using Bonferroni's correction.

Rejection) and significantly lower scores on two scales (Drug Problems and Dominance). They had significantly higher scores than patients with EDNOS on 6 scales (Somatic Complains, Anxiety, Anxiety Related Disorders, Depression, Schizophrenia, and Suicide). Finally, patients with anorexia nervosa had significantly higher scores than patients with depression on five scales (Positive Impression, Schizophrenia, Treatment Rejection, Dominance, and Warmth) and significantly lower scores on five scales (Negative Impression, Paranoia, Alcohol Problems, Aggression, and Stress).

Patients with bulimia nervosa had significantly higher scores than patients with EDNOS on 6 scales (Anxiety, Anxiety Related Disorders, Depression, Schizophrenia, Drug Problems, and Dominance) and significantly lower scores on one scale (Treatment Rejection). Patients with bulimia nervosa also had significantly higher scores than patients with depression on five scales (Positive Impression, Schizophrenia, Drug Problems, Dominance, and Warmth) and significantly lower scores on 10 scales (Negative Impression, Somatic Complaints, Depression, Paranoia, Borderline Features, Alcohol Problems, Aggression, Suicide, Stress, and Nonsupport).

Finally, EDNOS had significantly higher scores than patients with depression on four scales (Positive Impression, Treatment Rejection, Dominance, and Warmth) and significantly lower scores on 13 scales (Negative Impression, Somatic Complaints, Anxiety, Anxiety Related Disorders, Depression, Paranoia, Schizophrenia, Borderline Features, Alcohol Problems, Aggression, Suicide, Stress, and Nonsupport).

Discriminant function analysis

A discriminant function analysis was conducted to determine whether the four groups could be differentiated on the basis of their scores on the 22 PAI scales. The discriminant function was significant, $\chi 2$ (66) = 573.28, p = .001, and accounted for 54% of the between group variability. The percentage correct cross-validation classification for patients with anorexia nervosa, bulimia nervosa, EDNOS, and depression was 69.4%, 77.3%, 74.5%, and 89.7% respectively. Overall, 81.6% of cases were correctly classified. The PAI profiles for each of the four groups are presented in Figure 1.

Discussion

Results suggest that patients with anorexia nervosa, bulimia nervosa, and EDNOS differ significantly from each other, as well as from patients with depression, on a number of PAI scales. An examination of the overall MANOVA effect size revealed that a significant 50% of the variability in diagnoses was accounted for by the PAI scales, indicative of a medium to large effect size [42]. Consistent with previous research, we found that the three eating disorder groups evidenced elevations indicative of or consistent with psychopathology across a number of dimensions. For example, as can be seen in Figure 1, the patients with anorexia nervosa were most elevated on Anxiety, Depression, and Suicide. In our study, as in previous research [43], not all elevations reached clinical significance (i.e., a T-score of 70 or greater) [39]. For example, only 2 PAI scales (Anxiety and Depression) exceeded a T-score of 70 for the patients with anorexia nervosa, no scales exceeded a T-score of 70 for the bulimia nervosa or EDNOS group, and only two exceeded a T-score of 70 for the patients with depression (Depression and Suicide). It is also interesting to note that although there were a number of statistically significant differences among the eating disorder groups and the patients with depression, several of these differences were not clinically significant (e.g., Paranoia). From the results it would appear that there are a number of similar features shared between patients with anorexia nervosa and patients with depression (e.g., high levels of depression). This finding supports previous research which has found similar results [44-46].

Based on previous research we hypothesized that all three eating disorder groups would show elevated scores on the Anxiety, Depression, and Borderline Features scales. This hypothesis was only partially supported. For example, the patients with anorexia nervosa and bulimia nervosa demonstrated clinically significant elevations on the Anxiety and Depression scales, consistent with the presence of stress and worry, while the EDNOS group did not evidence elevations associated with anxiety or depression. Although a number of statistically significant differences were found among our groups, not all of these differences exceeded a T-score of 70. This has been reported by others such as Vitousek and Manke who found that not all statistical elevations found on personality measures between eating disorder groups are large enough to reach clinical significance and interpretation even though they may be able to differentiate between groups [47].

Patients with anorexia nervosa had significantly higher scores than patients with bulimia nervosa and EDNOS on the Anxiety scale. This is consistent with previous research which has also found patients with anorexia nervosa to be elevated on measures of anxiety [47-49]. For the Anxiety Related Disorders scale, which assesses

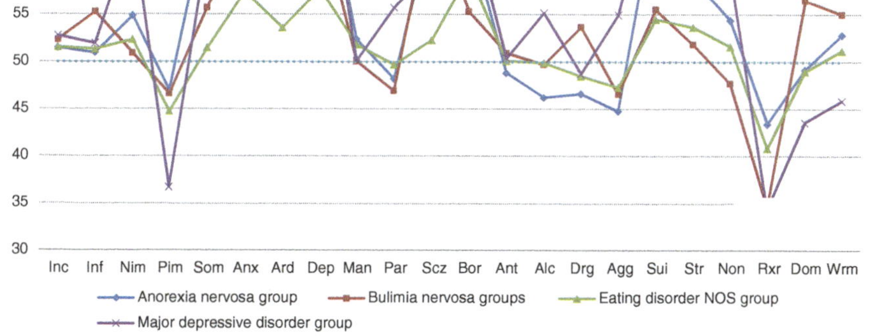

Figure 1 PAI profiles for patients with anorexic, bulimic, eating disorder NOS, and depression.

features such as obsessions and compulsions, patients with anorexia nervosa had significantly higher scores than patients with EDNOS, but they did not differ from the bulimia nervosa group. As Vitousek and Manke reported, obsessional features are often found in patients with anorexia nervosa and are often exacerbated by the medical sequelae of restricting behavior [47,50]. As such, the significant elevation for patients with anorexia nervosa is consistent with previous literature, although it was surprising that the patients with anorexia nervosa did not have significantly higher scores on this scale than the patients with bulimia nervosa. Perhaps if the patients with anorexia nervosa had presented with more severe symptoms, this difference would reach significance. The present sample consisted of participants who were out-patients so their symptom severity was also less than that found in inpatients.

Our hypothesis that the patients with anorexia nervosa would show the largest elevations on the Depression scale was supported. The effect size for Depression was the second largest effect size found, accounting for approximately 28% of the between group variability ($h_p^2 = .284$). Patients with anorexia nervosa had significantly higher Depression scores than patients with bulimia nervosa and EDNOS. This is one of only two PAI scales for patients with anorexia nervosa that exceeded a T-score of 70, and this is consistent with previous research [3]. Depression is also one of the most consistent findings associated with anorexia nervosa in studies using other measures of personality [29,51,52], and the psychological effects of starvation closely mimic depressive symptoms [37,53].

We hypothesized that all three groups would display elevations on the Borderline Features scale of the PAI. All three eating disorder groups had T-scores greater than 50, however, only the patients with anorexia nervosa and depression had scores above a T-score of 59 and therefore interpretable as above normal limits. Patients with anorexia nervosa had significantly higher scores on this scale than patients with bulimia nervosa. A central feature of anorexia nervosa is confusion over identity [18,54,55]. For example, as children, patients with anorexia nervosa tend to have been denied the opportunity to determine their own fate and were expected to perform according to familial expectations [37]. In a sense, they have an identity that is defined by others rather than by themselves [16,18,56]. This is consistent with the elevations on Borderline Features scale seen in the patients with anorexia nervosa in the current research, although it is important to note that the T-score was below 70 (i.e., below clinical significance). Other researchers [47,57] have found borderline personality disorder to be associated with bulimia nervosa. This would suggest that patients with bulimia nervosa should also have elevations on the Borderline Features scale of the PAI. Our findings may reflect that the Borderline Features scale is not a measure of borderline personality disorder *per se*. The scale only assesses borderline personality characteristics such as affect instability, unstable interpersonal relationships, and anger. It may be that patients with bulimia nervosa would score higher on a scale specifically assessing borderline personality disorder than they would score on a scale that assesses a few associated features that are also shared by other disorders. This speculation also remains to be further investigated.

Of the three eating disorder groups, we hypothesized that the patients with anorexia nervosa would have the highest score on the Treatment Rejection scale. This hypothesis was supported. The patients with anorexia nervosa had significantly higher scores than the bulimics and patients with depression, however, all scores were in the range indicative of little resistance to treatment (See Figure 1). Our findings may reflect the fact that the participants in this study had already sought, or were in the process of seeking, treatment for their eating disorder. It may be that in a different sample (e.g., one that included patients reluctantly seeking treatment or hospitalized patients) greater differences among the groups would emerge on this scale.

Additional findings

In terms of the clinical scales, the patients with anorexia nervosa and depression had higher scores than the patients with bulimia nervosa and EDNOS on the Somatic Complaints scale. This is consistent with the literature, given the severity of anorexia nervosa and the medical sequelae that accompany it [33,58]. The elevation for the patients with depression is also consistent with the physiological symptoms of major depression [59-62]. The effect size for the Somatic Complaints scale revealed that this variable accounted for approximately 24% of the between group variability, $h_p^2 = .243$, the third largest effect size found in this study.

Both the patients with anorexia nervosa and bulimia nervosa had significant elevations on the Schizophrenia scale, and were higher than those of patients with EDNOS and depression. The Schizophrenia scale assesses psychotic experiences, social detachment, and thought disorder. As identified by Bruch [17] and others [13], patients with anorexia nervosa have distorted views of their bodies than can be thought of as a delusionality of appearance [63]. Schmidt, Tiller, and Morgan report that patients with anorexia nervosa are shy, avoidant, socially detached, and never feel close to others [64]. These features may explain the elevations on the Schizophrenia scale. It is important to explore further how social detachment or perceptual distortions around body image may be captured by this scale or other measures that assess similar constructs.

The patients with anorexia nervosa and depression had higher scores than the other two eating disorder groups on the Suicide scale. The patients with anorexia nervosa approached a T-score of 70 and the patients with depression just exceeded a T-score of 70. The Suicide scale includes questions related to hopelessness, suicidal ideation, and previous suicide attempts. The significant elevation for the patients with anorexia nervosa may represent feelings of hopelessness associated with the more severe nature of the anorexia nervosa compared to bulimia nervosa or EDNOS. The elevation for the patients with depression is consistent with the symptoms of depression [15,29,43,60,65,66].

On the Stress scale the patients with anorexia nervosa had significantly higher scores than the patients with bulimia nervosa, and all three eating disorder groups had significantly lower scores than the patients with depression. An examination of the effect size revealed that the Stress scale accounted for approximately 31% of the between group variability, $h_p^2 = .314$, the largest effect size found in this study. Results suggest that patients with anorexia nervosa may be experiencing more stress than patients with bulimia nervosa, but that relative to patients with depression their stress levels are considerably lower. This may reflect the ego-syntonic nature of anorexic symptoms relative to ego-dystonic nature of depressive symptoms, the desire to lose weight even though underweight, and the distorted and unrealistic view of their bodies [15,17,67-69]. In terms of interpretation, however, only the patients with depression had a T-score that represented a 'moderate degree of stress' according to Morey [2].

When we looked at the discriminant ability of the PAI, we found that the 22 scales on the PAI could distinguish among the groups. The PAI scales were least successful in identifying patients with anorexia nervosa (69.4%) and most successful in identifying patients with depression (89.7%). This suggests that the PAI may be helpful in identifying and/or classifying eating disorders when a discriminant function analysis is employed; although it is important to remember that approximately 30% of the anorexia nervosa cases were not correctly classified. This must be considered when deciding on how to use the PAI. As a screening instrument that is routinely administered, the PAI may be helpful in alerting clinicians to the possible presence of an eating disorder. Future studies will need to investigate the utility of the PAI in terms of diagnosing and classifying eating disorders compared to other measures specifically designed to assess eating disorders. Future research should also explore in larger more representative samples how statistical differences on the PAI scales can be used clinically to identify patients with an eating disorder.

The PAI can also be used in a number of other ways beyond diagnosis. For example, two-point codes can be used to help identify treatment considerations [70]. In this study the anorexia nervosa group had elevations related to anxiety and depression. Patients with elevations such as these often have low energy and display passivity making it difficult to engage them in treatment. They are also at increased risk for suicide. This information is helpful in treatment planning and contributes to a better understanding of the person. Continued research relating to two- and three-point codes associated with eating disorders, and implications for treatment would likely be beneficial.

Not all the statistically significant differences among the eating disorder groups reached clinically significant levels (i.e., T-score > 70). This suggests that future studies may want to consider the presence of other forms of psychopathology in addition to the diagnosis of an eating disorder when studying this population. For example, comparing those with an eating disorder and borderline personality disorder (BPD) separately from those without BPD, and those with obsessive compulsive disorder separately from those without the comorbid diagnosis [30,71-74]. It may be that eating disorder symptoms present differently when there are comorbid diagnoses and this is why there have been inconsistent results relating psychopathology to eating disorders.

Conclusion

There are a number of strengths associated with this study. The first strength is that all the participants were clinical patients who met *DSM-IV* criteria for eating disorders or major depression. A second is the method by which the diagnoses were derived. Our use of a comprehensive intake interview, presented at a team meeting of mental health professionals, resulted in less chance for error in the diagnoses. The participants for this study were almost all young university students, a high risk population for eating disorders. Unlike the previous study using the PAI in an eating disordered sample, there were no age differences among our diagnostic groups [3]. Future studies, however, should study different samples and different ages, and assess the generalizability of the current results. This is particularly important given that some eating disorders (e.g., binge eating disorder) are more common in older adults [75,76]. For example, investigations need to assess the generalizability and utility of the PAI in community adults with eating disorders, in men, and in hospitalized patients. Finally, future studies should consider comparing patients with eating disorders not only to each other, but also to other diagnostic groups that share similar features. This study investigated whether the PAI could be used to differentiate eating disorder groups from each other and from a group of patients with depression, but there are many other diagnostic groups to consider. For example, give the high anxiety scores found in this study, it would be important to demonstrate that the PAI can be used to differentiate patients with an eating disorder diagnosis from those with co-morbid diagnoses of major depression and an anxiety disorder. This is particularly important if the PAI is going to continue to be used as a screening instrument. As well, future studies using larger and more representative samples should explore the possibility of identifying eating disorder clusters or profiles from the PAI to aid in the clinical interpretation of results, much as Morey has done in the standardization sample [2]. These results lend support to the continued use of the PAI and its potential to identify those with eating disorders.

Endnote

[a]Using the new *DSM-5* criteria a number of these participants would likely be diagnosed as having binge-eating disorder.

Competing interest

The authors declare that they have no competing interests.

Authors' contributions

MWmM is the primary investigator of this research. He designed the study and is the primary author of the manuscript. PL was the secondary author of the manuscript and assisted with the conceptualization and writing. Both authors read and approved the final manuscript.

Authors' information

Correspondence concerning this article should be addressed to Michael Wm. MacGregor, Ph.D., R.D.Psych., Department of Psychology, University of Saskatchewan, 9 Campus Drive, Saskatoon, Saskatchewan, S7N 5A5, Canada. E-mail: michael.macgregor@usask.ca. Telephone: (306) 966-2525. Facsimile: (306) 966-6630.

Acknowledgements

We would like to thank all the clinicians who helped with the assessment and diagnosis of the participants. We would also like to thank Sara Bartel, Krista Bloski, Jessica Campoli, and Darryl Quinlan for their comments and assistance on earlier drafts of this manuscript.

References

1. Bagby RM, Nicholson RA, Bacchiochi JR, Ryder AG, Bury AS: **The predictive capacity of the MMPI-2 and PAI validity scales and indexes to detect coached and uncoached feigning.** *J Pers Assess* 2002, **78:**69–86.
2. Morey LC: *Personality assessment inventory.* Odessa, FL: Psychological Assessment Resources; 1991.
3. Tasca GA, Wood TJ, Demidenko N, Bissada H: **Using the PAI with an eating disordered population: Scale characteristics, factor structure, and differences among diagnostic groups.** *J Pers Assess* 2002, **79:**337–356.
4. Slavin-Mulford J, Sinclair SJ, Stein M, Malone J, Bello I, Blais MA: **External validity of the personality assessment inventory (PAI) in a clinical sample.** *J Pers Assess* 2012, **94:**593–600.
5. Ansell EB, Kurtz JE, DeMoor RM, Markey PM: **Validity of the PAI interpersonal scales for measuring the dimensions of the interpersonal circumplex.** *J Pers Assess* 2011, **93:**33–39.
6. Gale SD, Hill SW: **Concurrent administration of the MMPI-2 and PAI in a sample of patients with epileptic or non-epileptic seizures: Implications for an inpatient epilepsy monitoring unit.** *Epilepsy Behav* 2012, **25:**181–184.
7. Blais MA, Hopwood CJ: **Personality focused assessment with the PAI.** In *Clinical applications of the Personality Assessment Inventory.* Edited by Blais MA, Baity MR, Hopwood CJ. New York, NY, US: Routledge/Taylor & Francis Group; US; 2010:195–209.
8. Hopwood CJ, Wright AGC, Krueger RF, Schade N, Markon KE, Morey LC: **DSM-5 pathological personality traits and the personality assessment inventory.** *Assessment* 2013, **20:**269–285.
9. American Psychiatric Association: *Diagnostic and statistical manual of mental disorders (4th ed.).* Washington, DC: Author; 1994.
10. Dooley-Hash S: **Review of developing an evidence-based classification of eating disorders: scientific findings for DSM-5.** *Eat Disord J Treat Prev* 2013, **21:**177–178.
11. American Psychiatric Association: *Diagnostic and statistical manual of mental disorders fifth edition; DSM-5.* Washington, DC: American Psychiatric Publishing; 2013.
12. Rushford N: **Fear of gaining weight: its validity as a visual analogue scale in anorexia nervosa.** *Eur Eat Disord Rev* 2006, **14:**104–110.
13. Hartmann AS, Thomas JJ, Wilson AC, Wilhelm S: **Insight impairment in body image disorders: Delusionality and overvalued ideas in anorexia nervosa versus body dysmorphic disorder.** *Psychiatry Res* 2013, **210**(3):1129–1135.
14. Keel PK, Brown TA, Holm-Denoma J, Bodell LP: **Comparison of DSM-IV versus proposed DSM-5 diagnostic criteria for eating disorders: Reduction of eating disorder not otherwise specified and validity.** *Int J Eat Disord* 2011, **44:**553–560.
15. Petrucelli J, Stuart C: *Hungers and compulsions: The psychodynamic treatment of eating disorders & addictions.* Northvale, NJ: Jason Aronson; 2001.
16. Johnson C: *Psychodynamic treatment of anorexia nervosa and bulimia.* New York: NY: The Guilford Press; 1991.
17. Bruch H: *Eating disorders: Obesity, anorexia, and the person within.* New York: Basic Books; 1973.
18. Gordon RA: *Eating disorders: Anatomy of a social epidemic.* Oxford: Blackwell Publishers; 2000.
19. Thorpe M, Nance M, Gilchrist P, Schutz J: **Symptoms of psychosis in a patient with anorexia nervosa.** *Aust N Z J Psychiatry* 2011, **45:**791.
20. Steinglass JE, Eisen JL, Attia E, Mayer L, Walsh BT: **Is anorexia nervosa a delusional disorder? An assessment of eating beliefs in anorexia nervosa.** *J Psychiatr Pract* 2007, **13:**65–71.
21. Nilsson K, Sundbom E, Hagglof B: **A longitudinal study of perfectionism in adolescent onset anorexia nervosa-restricting type.** *Eur Eat Disord Rev* 2008, **16:**386–394.
22. Sutandar-Pinnock K, Woodside DB, Carter JC, Olmsted MP, Kaplan AS: **Perfectionism in anorexia nervosa: A 6-24-month follow-up study.** *Int J Eat Disord* 2003, **33:**225–229.
23. Kerr JK, Skok RL, McLaughlin TF: **Characteristics common to females who exhibit anorexic or bulimic behaviour: a review of current literature.** *J Clin Psychol* 1991, **47**(6):846–853.
24. Hadigan CM, Walsh BT: **Body shape concerns in bulimia nervosa.** *Int J Eat Disord* 1991, **10:**323–331.
25. Anestis MD, Peterson CB, Bardone-Cone AM, Klein MH, Mitchell JE, Crosby RD, Wonderlich SA, Crow SJ, le Grange D, Jointer TE: **Affective lability and impulsivity in a clinical sample of women with bulimia nervosa: the role of affect in severely dysregulated behavior.** *Int J Eat Disord* 2009, **42:**259–266.
26. Kemps E, Wilsdon A: **Preliminary evidence for a role for impulsivity in cognitive disinhibition in bulimia nervosa.** *J Clin Exp Neuropsychol* 2010, **32:**515–521.
27. Cumella EJ, Wall AD, Ker-Almeida N: **MMPI-2 in the inpatient assessment of women with eating disorders.** *J Pers Assess* 2000, **75:**387–403.
28. Grilo CM, Masheb RM, Wilson GT: **A comparison of different methods for assessing the features of eating disorders in patients with binge eating disorder.** *J Consult Clin Psychol* 2001, **69:**317–322.
29. Pryor T, Wiederman MW: **Use of the MMPI-2 in the outpatient assessment of women with anorexia nervosa or bulimia nervosa.** *J Pers Assess* 1996, **66:**363–373.
30. Wildes JE, Marcus MD: **Alternative methods of classifying eating disorders: models incorporating comorbid psychopathology and associated features.** *Clin Psychol Rev* 2013, **33:**383–394.
31. Piotrowski C: **How popular is the personality assessment inventory in practice and training?** *Psychol Rep* 2000, **86:**65–66.

32. Garvin V, Striegel-Moore RH: **Health services research for eating disorders in the united states: A status report and call to action.** In *Eating disorders: Innovative directions in research and practice.* Edited by Striegel-Moore RH, Smolak L. Washington, DC: American Psychological Association; 2001:135–152.
33. Herzog DB, Copeland PM: **Eating disorders.** *N Engl J Med* 1985, **313:**295–303.
34. Maxmen JS, Ward NG: **Eating disorders.** In *Essential psychopathology and its treatment: Second edition, revised for the DSM-IV.* Edited by Maxmen JS, Ward NG. New York: W. W. Norton & Company; 1995:332–348.
35. Treasure J, Szmukler GI: **Medical complications of chronic anorexia nervosa.** In *Handbook of eating disorders: Theory, treatment, and research.* Edited by Szmukler G, Dare C, Treasure J. New York: Wiley; 1997:197–220.
36. Mas MB, Avargues Navarro ML, Lopez Jimenez AM, Perez IT, Del Rio Sanchez C, Perez San Gregorio MA: **Personality traits and eating disorders: Mediating effects of self-esteem and perfectionism.** *Int J Clin Health Psychol* 2011, **11:**205–227.
37. Halmi KA, Sunday SR, Strober M, Kaplan A, Woodside DB, Fichter M, Treasure J, Berrettini WH, Kaye WH: **Perfectionism in anorexia nervosa: variation by clinical subtype, obsessionality, and pathological eating behavior.** *Am J Psychiatry* 2000, **157:**1799–1805.
38. Steiner-Adair C: **New maps of development, new models of therapy: The psychology of women and the treatment of eating disorders.** In *Psychodynamic treatment of anorexia nervosa and bulimia.* Edited by Johnson C. New York: The Guilford Press; 1991:225–244.
39. Morey LC: **Interpretation.** In *Personality assessment inventory.* Odessa, Florida: Psychological Assessment Resources; 1991:11–46.
40. Boone D: **Internal consistency reliability of the personality assessment inventory with psychiatric inpatients.** *J Clin Psychol* 1998, **54:**839–843.
41. Boyle GJ, Lennon TJ: **Examination of the reliability and validity of the personality assessment inventory.** *J Psychopathol Behav Assess* 1994, **16:**173–187.
42. Cohen J: **A power primer.** *Quant Methods Psychol* 1992, **112**(1):155–159.
43. Norman DK, Herzog DB: **A follow-up study of 33 subdiagnostic eating disordered women.** *Int J Eat Disord* 1983, **14:**261–267.
44. Wade TD, Bulik CM, Neale M, Kendler KS: **Anorexia nervosa and major depression: shared genetic and environmental risk factors.** *Am J Psychiatry* 2000, **157:**469–471.
45. Bizeul C, Brun JM, Rigaud D: **Depression influences the EDI scores in anorexia nervosa patients.** *Eur Psychiatry* 2003, **18:**119–123.
46. Brockmeyer T, Bents H, Holtforth MG, Pfeiffer N, Herzog W, Friederich H: **Specific emotion regulation impairments in major depression and anorexia nervosa.** *Psychiatry Res* 2012, **200:**550–553.
47. Vitousek K, Manke F: **Personality variables and disorders in anorexia nervosa and bulimia nervosa.** *J Abnorm Psychol* 1994, **103:**137–147.
48. Hughes EK: **Comorbid depression and anxiety in childhood and adolescent anorexia nervosa: prevalence and implications for outcome.** *Clin Psychol* 2012, **16:**15–24.
49. Kaye WH, Bulik CM, Thornton L, Barbarich N, Masters K, Price Foundation Collaborative Group: **Comorbidity of anxiety disorders with anorexia and bulimia nervosa.** *Am J Psychiatry* 2004, **161:**2215–2221.
50. Halmi KA, Sunday SR, Klump KL, Strober M, Leckman JF, Fichter M, Kaplan A, Woodside B, Treasure J, Berrettini WH, Al Shabboat M, Bulik CM, Kaye WH: **Obsessions and compulsions in anorexia nervosa subtypes.** *Int J Eat Disord* 2003, **33:**308–319.
51. Lucka I: **Depression syndromes in patients suffering from anorexia nervosa.** *Psychiatr Pol* 2004, **38:**621–629.
52. Levy AB, Dixon KN: **The relationship between anorexia nervosa and depression: a reevaluation.** *Int J Eat Disord* 1985, **4:**389–405.
53. Laessle RG, Schweiger U, Pirke K: **Depression as a correlate of starvation in patients with eating disorders.** *Biol Psychiatry* 1988, **23:**719–725.
54. Winston AP: **Projection, introjection and identity in anorexia nervosa.** *British J Psychother* 2005, **21:**389–399.
55. Stein KF, Corte C: **Identity impairment and the eating disorders: content and organization of the self-concept in women with anorexia nervosa and bulimia nervosa.** *Eur Eat Disord Rev* 2007, **15:**58–69.
56. Bers SA, Besser A, Harpaz-Rotem I, Blatt SJ: **An empirical exploration of the dynamics of anorexia nervosa: representations of self, mother, and father.** *Psychoanal Psychol* 2013, **30:**188–209.
57. Perez IT, del Rio SC, Mas MB: **MCMI-II borderline personality disorder in anorexia and bulimia nervosa.** *Psicothema* 2008, **20:**138–143.
58. Erdur L, Kallenbach-Dermutz B, Lehmann V, Zimmermann-Viehoff F, Kopp W, Weber C, Deter H: **Somatic comorbidity in anorexia nervosa: first results of a 21-year follow-up study on female inpatients.** *Bio Psycho Soc Med* 2012, **6:**1–6. 6 Feb:Art 4-6.
59. Buchwald AM, Rudick-Davis D: **The symptoms of major depression.** *J Abnorm Psychol* 1993, **102:**197–205.
60. Frosch J: **The affective disorders.** In *Psychodynamic psychiatry: Theory and practice.* Madison CT: International Universities Press; 1990:363–374.
61. Gotlib IH, Lewinsohn PM, Seeley JR: **Symptoms versus a diagnosis of depression: differences in psychosocial functioning.** *J Consult Clin Psychol* 1995, **63:**90–100.
62. Chakraborty K, Avasthi A, Kumar S, Grover S: **Psychological and clinical correlates of functional somatic complaints in depression.** *Int J Soc Psychiatry* 2012, **58:**87–95.
63. Miotto P, Pollini B, Restaneo A, Favaretto G, Sisti D, Rocchi MBL, Preti A: **Symptoms of psychosis in anorexia and bulimia nervosa.** *Psychiatry Res* 2010, **175:**237–243.
64. Schmidt U, Tiller J, Morgan HG: **The social consequences of eating disorders.** In *Handbook of eating disorders: Theory, treatment, and research.* Edited by Szmukler G, Dare C, Treasure J. New York: Wiley; 1997:259–272.
65. Frosch J: **The neuroses.** In *Psychodynamic psychiatry: Theory and practice.* Madison CT: International Universities Press; 1990:293–362.
66. Hawton K, Comabella CCI, Haw C, Saunders K: **Risk factors for suicide in individuals with depression: a systematic review.** *J Affect Disord* 2013, **147:**17–28.
67. Andersen A: **Stories I, tell my parents: ask the dry cleaner.** *Eat Disord J Treat Prev* 2010, **18:**264–265.
68. Johnson CL, Sansone RA, Chewning M: **Good reasons why young women would develop anorexia nervosa: the adaptive context.** *Pediatr Ann* 1992, **21:**731–737.
69. Petrosky EM: **The relationship between the morbid response of the rorschach inkblot test and self-reported depressive symptomatology.** *J Proj Psychol Ment Health* 2005, **12:**87–98.
70. Morey LC: *Essentials of PAI assessment.* Hoboken, NJ: John Wiley & Sons; 2003.
71. Altman SE, Shankman SA: **What is the association between obsessive-compulsive disorder and eating disorders?** *Clin Psychol Rev* 2009, **29:**638–646.
72. Friedel RO: **Dopamine dysfunction in borderline personality disorder: a hypothesis.** *Neuropsychopharmacology* 2004, **29:**1029–1039.
73. Johnson C, Tobin DL, Dennis A: **Differences in treatment outcome between borderline and non-borderline bulimics at one-year follow-up.** *Int J Eat Disord* 1990, **9:**617–627.
74. Johnson C, Tobin DL, Enright A: **Prevalence and clinical characteristics of borderline patients in an eating-disordered population.** *J Clin Psychiatry* 1989, **50:**9–15.
75. Fisher M, Schneider M, Burns J, Symons H, Mandel FS: **Differences between adolescents and young adults at presentation to an eating disorders program.** *J Adolesc Health* 2001, **28:**222–227.
76. Hay P: **The epidemiology of eating disorder behaviours: an Australian community-based survey.** *Int J Eat Disord* 1988, **23:**371–382.

Alexithymia and eating disorders: a critical review of the literature

Matilda E Nowakowski[1*], Traci McFarlane[1,2] and Stephanie Cassin[1]

Abstract

Alexithymia is characterized by difficulties identifying feelings and differentiating between feelings and bodily sensations, difficulties communicating feelings, and a concrete cognitive style focused on the external environment. Individuals with eating disorders have elevated levels of alexithymia, particularly difficulties identifying and describing their feelings. A number of theoretical models have suggested that individuals with eating disorders may find emotions unacceptable and/or frightening and may use their eating disorder symptoms (i.e., restricting food intake, bingeing, and/or purging) as a way to avoid or cope with their feelings. The current critical review synthesizes the literature on alexithymia and eating disorders and examines alexithymia levels across eating disorders (i.e., anorexia nervosa, bulimia nervosa, and eating disorder not otherwise specified), the role of alexithymia in binge eating disorder, and the influence of alexithymia on the development of eating disorders as well as treatment outcome. The clinical implications of the research conducted to date and directions for future research are discussed.

Keywords: Alexithymia, Eating disorders, Emotion regulation

Alexithymia and eating disorders: a critical review

The concept of alexithymia was first identified by Sifneos [1], who described a set of characteristics observed in psychosomatic patients that included difficulties identifying feelings and differentiating between feelings and bodily sensations, difficulties communicating feelings, lack of fantasy, and a concrete cognitive style focused on the external environment.

The majority of studies focusing on eating disorders have found higher levels of alexithymia in individuals with eating disorders and disturbed eating compared to healthy controls [2-8]. When the individual characteristics of alexithymia are examined, individuals with eating disorders have specific deficits in identifying and communicating their feelings.

A number of theories have been proposed regarding the underlying role of emotions in eating disorders. It has been suggested that patients use maladaptive eating behaviors (e.g., bingeing, purging, dietary restriction) and excessive exercise as a way to avoid or cope with their emotions [9-11]. Specifically, an early childhood environment in which emotions are viewed as unacceptable or frightening leads to the development of the belief that emotions are bad and should not be experienced or expressed. These beliefs become activated each time that an emotion is experienced, which then leads to a secondary emotion (i.e., an emotion in response to another emotion) such as shame, guilt, or disgust about experiencing an emotion. These secondary emotions increase the patient's distress and decrease his/her coping abilities, thus leading to engagement in eating disorder behaviors in an attempt to avoid or cope with the emotion [12].

Although a robust body of literature illustrates that alexithymia levels, especially difficulties identifying and communicating feelings, are elevated in individuals with eating disorders, there remains much debate surrounding a number of issues, including: 1) whether alexithymia levels vary across eating disorder diagnoses; 2) whether alexithymia is a trait or state variable; and 3) whether current treatments for eating disorders effectively target alexithymia. To date, no review paper has synthesized the research on alexithymia in eating disorders. The purpose of the current paper is to synthesize the research addressing the aforementioned questions in order to increase

* Correspondence: mnowakowski@psych.ryerson.ca
[1]Department of Psychology, Ryerson University, 350 Victoria Street, Toronto, Ontario M5B 2K3, Canada
Full list of author information is available at the end of the article

theoretical knowledge of alexithymia and eating disorders and enhance clinical interventions.

Methods

A systematic review of the literature on alexithymia and eating disorders was conducted in September 2012 using PsycInfo. The following search terms were used in four literature searches: "alexithymia" and "anorexia nervosa", "bulimia nervosa", "eating disorders", or "binge eating disorder". The literature searches were limited to articles focusing on adolescents and adults that were published in peer-reviewed journals after January 1, 1988, and were written in English. We limited our search to articles published in 1988 or later as 1988 is the publication year of the first version of the Toronto Alexithymia Scale [13]. Our systematic review was limited to studies using the Toronto Alexithymia Scale, the most widely used and well-established measure of alexithymia, in order to facilitate comparisons across studies. This initial search identified 198 articles. The reference list of each article was subsequently examined for relevant articles that may have been omitted by PsycInfo, which resulted in 3 more articles being identified. After eliminating duplicates, 119 articles were identified. The article abstracts were then reviewed and coded for the following criteria: 1) one of the three versions of the Toronto Alexithymia Scale was used to assess alexithymia; 2) the study included clinical or non-clinical adolescent and/or adult participants with disturbed eating; 3) the study focused on identifying and/or explaining group differences in alexithymia levels; and 4) the study had a quantitative experimental design. Consistent with the continuum perspective of eating behaviors [14], studies including both clinical and non-clinical samples were included in the current review to provide a more complete picture of the research on alexithymia and disordered eating. This initial review of the abstracts resulted in 58 articles being excluded (5 did not use one of the versions of the TAS, 23 did not focus on eating disorders, 5 did not have a quantitative experimental design, and 27 did not address group differences or the role of alexithymia in eating disorders). After reviewing the full articles, two more articles were excluded as they did not use one of the three versions of the TAS to assess alexithymia levels. This resulted in 59 articles being included in the qualitative synthesis of the current review paper. The process of article selection is outlined in Figure 1.

Measurement of alexithymia

The Toronto Alexithymia Scale (TAS) is the most widely used self-report measure of alexithymia. It was originally developed by Bagby and colleagues in 1988 and has since undergone two revisions (TAS-R and TAS-20). The original version of the TAS consisted of 26 items that were reduced to 4 factors: 1) difficulties identifying feelings and differentiating between feelings and bodily sensations (e.g., "I have feelings that I can't quite identify"); 2) difficulties describing feelings (e.g., "People tell me to describe my feelings more"); 3) lack of fantasy (e.g., "I daydream rarely"); and 4) externally-oriented thinking

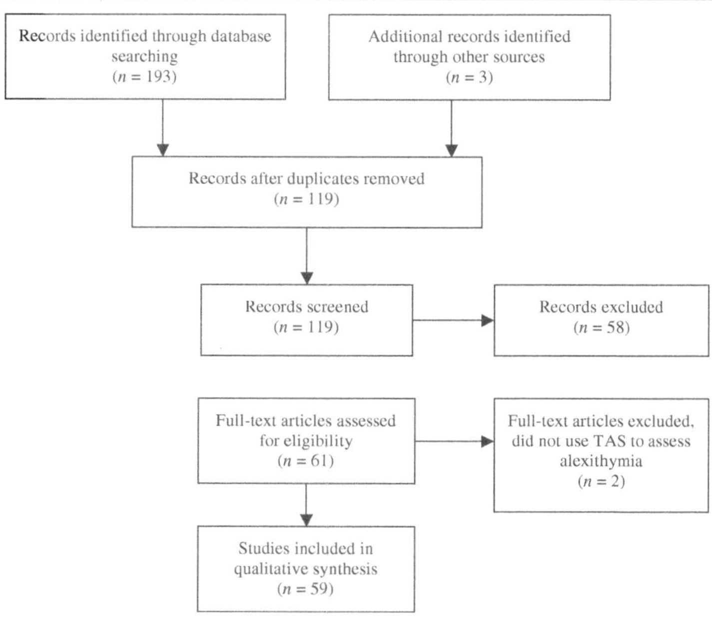

Figure 1 Diagram illustrating the process of selecting articles for the critical review.

(e.g., "Knowing the answers to problems is more important than knowing the reasons for the answers") [13]. The psychometric properties of the original TAS had a number of limitations, including susceptibility to social desirability response biases and low item-total correlations for the lack of fantasy factor, which lead to the creation of a 23-item revised version (TAS-R) [15]. However, the TAS-R [15] had an unstable factor structure such that the difficulties identifying and describing feelings factors collapsed into one single factor. As well, the majority of the lack of fantasy items still showed poor item-total correlations. As a result, in the second revision of the TAS (TAS-20) [16], the items for the lack of fantasy factor were eliminated and the items for the identifying and describing feelings factors were modified. The final scale consisted of 20 items and 3 factors: 1) difficulties identifying feelings and differentiating between feelings and bodily sensations (e.g., "I am often confused about what emotion I am feeling"); 2) difficulties describing feelings (e.g., "It is difficult for me to find the right words for my feelings"); and 3) externally-oriented thinking (e.g., "I prefer to just let things happen rather than to understand why they turned out that way"). Based on empirically determined cut-off scores, individuals who score 61 or higher on the TAS-20 are identified as alexithymic [16]. Therefore, alexithymia can be assessed on both a continuous and a categorical basis.

The majority of studies using patient and non-patient samples have replicated the 3-factor structure of the TAS-20 [16-20], although some studies using patient samples have found a 2-factor structure, with the difficulties identifying and difficulties describing feelings factors comprising a single factor [21,22]. The internal consistencies for the difficulties identifying feelings and difficulties describing feelings factors have been in the acceptable range across numerous studies [17-20]. In contrast, the internal consistency for the externally oriented thinking factor has been low [17-20]. Studies using non-clinical samples have demonstrated good test-retest reliability for all factors, although no studies have examined a time-span longer than 3 months [16,17,19]. Thus, although the TAS-20 appears to be a psychometrically sound measure, it is important to note its psychometric limitations, notably the low internal consistency for the externally oriented thinking factor and the absence of studies investigating its test-retest reliability in clinical samples.

Is alexithymia elevated in individuals with eating disorders compared to controls?

To date, 24 studies have investigated whether alexithymia is elevated in individuals with eating disorders using one of the three versions of the Toronto Alexithymia Scale. See Table 1 for a summary of the studies. Across studies, significantly more eating disorder patients are categorized as alexithymic compared to healthy community controls [4,5,8,23-34]. When examining alexithymia as a continuous measure, studies have shown that individuals with eating disorders have higher total alexithymia scores as well as higher scores on two out of three factors: 1) Difficulties identifying feelings and differentiating between feelings and bodily sensations, and 2) Difficulties describing feelings [2,4,5,24-28,30-43]. Studies have generally not reported differences between individuals with eating disorders and healthy community controls on externally oriented thinking (but see [30,42]), although this may be a reflection of the poor internal consistency for the externally oriented thinking factor. In sum, a robust body of research illustrates that individuals with eating disorders show specific deficits in identifying and describing affective states compared to healthy community controls.

Is alexithymia elevated in nonclinical samples with disturbed eating?

Studies conducted with nonclinical undergraduate samples have found that higher levels of eating disorder behaviors (e.g., bingeing, purging, dietary restriction, excessive exercise) are associated with higher scores on the difficulties identifying feelings and difficulties describing feelings factors of the TAS/TAS-R/TAS-20 [3,6,7,48-55]. In general, no relations have been found between eating disorder behaviors and the externally oriented thinking factor on the TAS/TAS-R/TAS-20. This pattern of results is consistent with the pattern found for clinical samples, providing further support that individuals with eating disturbances experience difficulties with identifying and communicating emotions.

Is the relation between alexithymia and eating disorders accounted for by general distress?

Clinical studies investigating the relation between eating disorder behaviors and alexithymia when controlling for general distress (i.e., anxiety and depression) have generated mixed results. Some studies have found that group differences on difficulties identifying and describing feelings disappear when general distress is controlled for [4,25,30,36,39]. For instance, using a female sample of 40 outpatients with DSM-IV eating disorders (i.e., AN-R, AN-B/P, and BN), 19 of who also had comorbid major depressive disorder, and a sample of 20 healthy control females, Gilboa-Schechtman and colleagues [36] found that patients with eating disorders reported significantly higher scores on the TAS-20 difficulties identifying and difficulties describing feelings factors compared to the healthy controls. However, group differences disappeared when analyses controlled for both depression and anxiety.

In contrast, other studies have found that individuals with eating disorders continue to exhibit elevated

Table 1 Studies investigating alexithymia in clinical samples of patients with anorexia nervosa, bulimia nervosa, and binge eating disorder

Authors	Year	Diagnostic Tool	Sample Characteristics	Alexithymia Measure	Results
Beales & Dolton	2000	EDI	Females, outpatient, 17–46 years old, AN-R (26), BN (29), recovered (24)	TAS-20	Alexithymic: BN (83%), AN-R (65%), recovered (33%)
Berthoz et al.	2007	MINI	Females, AN-R (50), AN-B/P (5), BN (20)	TAS-20	No group differences on TAS-20 scores
Bourke et al.	1992	DSM-III-R	Females, outpatient, AN-R (30), AN-B/P (18), HC (30)	TAS	Alexithymic: AN (77.1%), HC (6.7%); TAS Total: AN > HC
Bydlowski et al.	2005	DSM-IV	Females, outpatient, AN-R (18), AN-B/P (15), BN (37), HC (70)	TAS-20	Alexithymic: EDs (60%), HC (30%); TAS-20 Total: EDs > HC, no differences between EDs, group differences disappeared when controlling for depression but not when controlling for anxiety
Carano et al.	2006	DSM-IV	Males and females, outpatient, obese + BED (101)	TAS-20	Alexithymic: 39.6%
Corcos et al.	2000	DSM-IV	Males and females, outpatient, AN-R (21), AN-B/P (11), BN (32), HC (74)	TAS-20	TAS Total: EDs > HC, AN > BN, group differences between AN and BN disappeared when controlling for depression
Cochrane et al.	1993	DSM-III-R	Females, outpatient, AN (19), BN (52), AN + BN (18), EDNOS (25), HC (370)	TAS	TAS Total Score: EDs > HC, no differences between EDs
de Groot	1995	DSM-III-R	Females, day hospital program, BN (31), HC (female nurses; 20)	TAS	Alexithymic: BN (61.3%), HC (5%), TAS Total, DIF, DDF: BN > HC, group differences for TAS Total and DIF remained when controlling for depression
De Panfilis et al.	2003	DSM-IV	Females, outpatient, AN-R (4), AN-B/P (12), BN (20), BED (28), HC (68)	TAS-20	Alexithymic: EDs (14.4%), HC (1.6%); TAS-20 Total, DIF: EDs > HC
de Zwaan et al.	1995	DSM-IV	Males and females, outpatient, obese + BED (83), obese + no BED (99)	TAS	TAS Total: no group differences
Deborde et al.	2008	MINI	Females, AN-R (10), AN-B/P (7), BN (30), HC (253)	TAS-20	Alexithymic: EDs (53.2%), HC (13.83%)
Eizaguirre et al.	2004	DSM-IV	Females, AN-R (25), AN-BP (44), BN (82), HC (43)	TAS-20	Alexithymic: AN-R (56%), AN-B/P (68.2%), BN (47%), HC (2.3%), TAS-20 Total, DIF, DDF, EOT: EDs > HC, DIF: AN-B/P > BN, AN-R, EOT: BN > AN-B/P, group differences disappeared when controlling for depression and anxiety
Gilboa-Schechtman et al.	2006	DSM-IV	Females, outpatient, AN (20), BN (20), HC (20)	TAS-20	TAS-20 DIF, DDF: EDs > HC, DDF scores: AN > BN, group differences disappeared when controlling for distress
Guttman et al.	2002	DSM-III-R	Females, outpatient, AN-R (34), HC (33)	TAS-20	TAS-20 Total, DIF, DDF: AN-R > HC
Jimerson et al.	1994	DSM-III-R	Females, outpatient, BN (20), HC (20)	TAS	Alexithymic: BN (40%), HC (0%); TAS Total, DIF, DDF: BN > HC, group differences disappeared for DDF when controlling for anxiety and depression
Lawson et al.	2008	DSM-IV	Females, outpatient, AN (11), BN (21), EDNOS (38)	TAS-20	TAS-20 Total, DIF, DDF: no group differences
Montebarocci et al.	2006	DSM-IV	Females, outpatient, AN-R (18), BN (16), HC (18)	TAS-20	Alexithymic: AN-R (50%), BN (56%), HC (22%); TAS-20 Total: AN-R, BN > HC, DIF: BN, AN-R > HC, EOT: AN-R > BN, HC, group differences disappeared when controlling for anxiety and depression
Nandrino et al.	2006	DSM-IV	Females, inpatient, AN-R (25), HC (25)	TAS-20	TAS-20 Total: AN-R > HC
Parling et al.	2010	DSM-IV	Females, outpatient, AN (35), HC (34)	TAS-20	TAS-20 DIF, DDF: AN > HC, group differences disappeared when controlling for anxiety and depression

Table 1 Studies investigating alexithymia in clinical samples of patients with anorexia nervosa, bulimia nervosa, and binge eating disorder *(Continued)*

Pascual et al.	2011	Self-report questionnaires	Females, BN-P (17), BN-NP (17), nonspecific AN (22), nonspecific BN (42)	TAS-20	DDF: nonspecific AN > nonspecific BN, BN-NP
Pinaquy et al.	2003	DSM-IV	Females, obese + BED (40), obese + no BED (129)	TAS-20	TAS-20 Total, DIF, DDF: obese + BED > obese + no BED
Rastam et al.	1997	DSM-III-R	Males and females, AN-R (48), HC (51)	TAS-20	Alexithymic: AN-R (23%), HC (6%)
Schmidt et al.	1993	DSM-III-R	Females, outpatient, BN (93), AN-R (55), AN-B/P (25), HC (48 females and 47 males)	TAS	Alexithymic: AN-R (56%), AN-B/P (48%), BN (50%), HC (17.8%); TAS Total: All EDs > HC, AN-R > BN
Sexton et al.	1998	DSM-IV	Females, inpatients, AN-R (15), AN-B/P (16), BN (22), HC (14)	TAS	TAS Total: AN-R, AN-B/P > HC; DIF, DDF: AN-B/P, BN > HC; DDF: AN-R > BN; after controlling for depression: TAS Total: AN-R > HC; DDF: AN-R > BN, HC
Sureda et al.	1999	DSM-III-R	Females, outpatient, BN (35), HC hospital staff (35)	TAS-20	Alexithymic: BN (51.4%), HC (6.3%); TAS-20 Total, DIF, DDF: BN > HC
Speranza et al.	2005	DSM-IV	Females, outpatient, AN-R (105), AN-B/P (49), BN (89), HC (279)	TAS-20	TAS-20 DIF, DDF: all EDs > HC, when controlling for depression; DIF: BN > HC; DDF: AN-R > HC
Taylor et al.	1996	DSM-III-R	Females, outpatient, AN (48), HC hospital staff (30), HC undergraduates (234)	TAS-20	Alexithymic: AN (68.8%), HC hospital staff (3.3%), HC undergraduates (13.7%); TAS-20 Total, DIF, DDF: AN > all HC groups
Torres et al.	2011		Females, outpatient, AN-R (52), AN-B/P (28), HC (80)	TAS-20	TAS-20 DIF, DDF, EOT: AN > HC
Troop et al.	1995	DSM-III-R	Females, outpatient, AN-R (29), AN-B/P (15), BN (83), HC (79)	TAS	TAS Total, DIF: EDs > HC; lack of fantasy: AN-R > BN, HC
Zeeck et al.	2011	DSM-IV	Females, outpatient, BED (20), obese (23), HC (20)	TAS-20	TAS-20 Total: BED > obese, HC
Zonnevijlle-Bender et al.	2002	DSM-IV	Females, outpatient, AN (16), BN (8), EDNOS (6), HC (33)	TAS-20	Alexithymic: AN (60%), BN (50%), EDNOS (14%), HC (10%), TAS-20 Total: EDs > HC
Zonnevijlle-Bender et al.	2004	DSM-IV	Females, AN-R (48), psychiatric control (anxiety and depression; 21), HC (48)	TAS-20	Alexithymic: AN (60%), psychiatric control (52%), HC (27%); TAS-20 Total, DIF, DDF: AN > HC

EDI = Eating Disorder Inventory [44]; MINI = The Mini-International Neuropsychiatric Interview [45]; DSM-III-R = Diagnostic Statistical Manual of Mental Disorders 3rd Edition Revised [46]; DSM-IV = Diagnostic Statistical Manual of Mental Disorders 4th Edition [47]; AN-R = Anorexia Nervosa – Restricting Type; AN-B/P = Anorexia Nervosa – Bingeing/Purging Type; BN = Bulimia Nervosa; BED = Binge Eating Disorder; HC = healthy control; TAS = Toronto Alexithyma Scale 26-item Version [13]; TAS-20 = Toronto Alexithymia Scale 20-item Version [16]; TAS Total = Toronto Alexithymia Scale Total Score; DIF = Toronto Alexithymia Scale Difficulties Identifying Feelings factor; DDF = Toronto Alexithymia Scale Difficulties Describing Feelings factor, EOT = Toronto Alexithymia Scale Externally Orienting Thinking factor.

alexithymia levels even when controlling for general distress [5,24,27,40,56]. For instance, controlling for depression levels, Bourke and colleagues [24] found significantly higher total alexithymia scores, as measured by the TAS, in a sample of 48 female outpatients who met DSM-III-R diagnostic criteria for AN compared to 30 female controls. Similarly, in a sample of 20 female outpatients who met DSM-III-R criteria for BN and 20 matched female controls, patients with BN had significantly higher scores on the TAS difficulties identifying and describing feelings factors as well as the TAS total score compared to matched female controls. When anxiety and depression were controlled, group differences remained for the total alexithymia score and the difficulties identifying feelings factor [5]. A recent study by Rozenstein and colleagues [56] found that depression explained group differences for the TAS-20 total score and the difficulties identifying feelings and difficulties describing feelings factor scores for patients with AN-R but not for patients with BN and AN-B/P. Rozenstein and colleagues [56] suggested that different mechanisms might underlie difficulties with identifying and communicating emotions for patients who restrict versus patients who engage in bingeing and purging behaviors. Specifically, while depression may directly contribute to difficulties with identifying and expressing emotions in patients who restrict, it may be the increased impulsivity and affective instability that underlies the affective difficulties of patients with bingeing and purging behaviors.

Our review of the literature on the role of depression in explaining group differences on alexithymia levels partially supports Rozenstein and colleagues' [56] proposal. Two of the studies that found that depression did not explain group differences in alexithymia levels focused solely on patients with BN [5,27]. Furthermore, although Eizaquirre and colleagues [4] found that group differences on alexithymia levels disappeared when controlling for both depression *and* anxiety, when only depression was controlled for, group differences between the control group and the AN-B/P and BN groups for the difficulties identifying feelings factor remained. It should be noted, however, that both Bydlowski and colleagues [25] and Gilboa-Schechtman and colleagues [36] failed to find any differences between patients who restricted and those who engaged in bingeing and purging behaviors after controlling for anxiety and depression levels. Further, using a sample of 53 female inpatients, Sexton and colleagues [40] found that after controlling for depression levels, only the AN-R group had significantly higher scores on the TAS total score and the difficulties communicating feelings factor compared to the control group.

As illustrated above, the findings for the role of anxiety and depression in accounting for group differences in alexithymia are mixed. There is a need for further research to clarify this pattern of findings. One of the limitations to date is that many of the studies in this area fail to distinguish between patients with AN-R and patients with AN-B/P. This differentiation is important in order to further test Rozenstein and colleagues' [56] suggestions regarding the differential influence of depression on alexithymia in patients who restrict versus patients who engage in bingeing and purging behaviors. Furthermore, with the exception of a few studies [5,32,36,41], most studies do not report comorbid diagnoses for participants, thus failing to differentiate between subclinical depressive and anxiety symptoms and comorbid major depressive disorder and anxiety disorders. Given the potential identified role of depression and anxiety in alexithymia symptoms, this important information should be included in future studies in order to better understand the role of anxiety and depression in alexithymia.

Do levels of alexithymia differ amongst the eating disorder diagnoses?

While some studies have not reported significant differences in alexithymia levels across the eating disorders [2,25,43,57,58], others have suggested that individuals with a diagnosis of AN experience higher levels of alexithymia [4,26,31,36,59]. In one of the first studies to investigate differences between eating disorders, Schmidt and colleagues [31] found that patients in the AN-R group reported significantly higher total alexithymia scores compared to patients in the AN-B/P and BN groups. Following these findings, a number of studies have examined group differences among eating disorders, further delineating alexithymia into its separate factors.

Three studies have found that individuals with AN report higher scores on the difficulties describing feelings factor compared to individuals with BN [36,40,59]. For instance, Pascual and colleagues [59] investigated group differences on the TAS-20 factors using a sample of 98 females divided into 4 groups: BN-purging type (n = 17), BN-non purging type (n = 17), nonspecific BN (met the majority of criteria for BN; n = 42), and nonspecific AN (met the majority of criteria for AN; n = 22). Participants in the nonspecific AN group reported significantly higher scores on the difficulties describing feelings factor compared to participants in the nonspecific BN group as well as the BN-non purging group. Participants in the BN-purging group had an intermediate profile such that their scores on difficulties describing feelings were lower than the nonspecific AN group but higher than the nonspecific BN group and the BN-non purging group. Similarly, Gilboa-Schechtman and colleagues [36] found that patients who met the DSM-IV criteria for AN reported significantly greater difficulties describing feelings compared to patients who met the criteria for BN. Based on the research to date, it appears that individuals with AN have elevated alexithymia levels, specific to difficulties expressing emotions, compared to individuals with BN.

Is alexithymia elevated in binge eating disorder?

Studies focusing on BED samples have generally found an association between alexithymia and BED symptom severity [60-63], but see [64] for an exception. For instance, Carano and colleagues [60] found that difficulties identifying and describing feelings, as measured by the TAS-20, predicted the severity of BED in 101 patients who met DSM-IV diagnostic criteria for BED. Similarly, female obese patients who met DSM-IV criteria for BED had significantly higher total scores as well as higher scores on difficulties identifying and describing emotions compared to female obese patients who did not meet DSM-IV criteria for BED [61]. Consistent with the pattern of findings in AN and BN, individuals with BED have higher levels of alexithymia, specifically with regards to identifying and communicating emotions.

What role does alexithymia play in the development of eating disorders?

To date, a paucity of research has specifically examined the potential etiological role of alexithymia in eating disorders, and the few studies that have been conducted have focused on childhood maltreatment and personality. Across studies using non-clinical undergraduate samples, childhood maltreatment has been indirectly associated with eating disorder symptoms through its relations with alexithymia and depression [65-69]. For instance, using a sample of 406 female undergraduates, Mazzeo and Espelage [67] found that high family conflict and low family cohesion were significantly associated with childhood physical and emotional abuse and neglect, and that the association between childhood maltreatment and disordered eating symptomatology was fully mediated by alexithymia and depression. This model was cross-validated and replicated using a second sample of 406 female undergraduate students [67]. Thus, in females, childhood physical and emotional abuse and neglect all increase the risk for depression and alexithymia, which in turn increase the risk for disordered eating symptoms. However, this pattern of results appears to vary with sex and ethnicity. For instance, in males, the relation between childhood maltreatment and bulimic symptoms appears to be mediated only by depression [69]. Furthermore, there appear to be differences between ethnic groups. Mazzeo and colleagues [68] found that the association of childhood maltreatment with eating disorder symptoms was mediated by self-reported anxiety, depression, and alexithymia in both African American and European American undergraduate female students. However, only the European American female sample had a positive relation between depression and alexithymia.

To date, only one study has investigated the relationship between personality factors and alexithymia in the development of eating disorders. Using a clinical sample of 49 patients with eating disorders, Ruggiero and colleagues [70] found that perfectionism mediated the relation between alexithymia and eating disorders, such that alexithymia increased the risk of perfectionism, which in turn increased the risk of developing an eating disorder.

In summary, the research to date suggests that low family cohesion and high levels of family conflict are associated with an increased risk for childhood physical and emotional abuse and neglect. In turn, childhood maltreatment increases the risk for depression and alexithymia, which both increase the risk for eating disorder behaviors. As noted above, sex and ethnic background might moderate these relationships, highlighting the importance of further examining sex and cultural differences in the eating disorder literature. In addition to familial factors, preliminary research also suggests a potential role of perfectionism in mediating the relation between alexithymia and eating disorders.

Do alexithymia levels change following treatment?

To date, six studies, three of which have been uncontrolled, have examined the effects of treatment on alexithymia levels in patients with eating disorders. These studies have shown that alexithymia scores decrease significantly post-treatment in patients with AN, BN, and BED [27,71-75]. For instance, Becker-Stoll and Gerlinghoff [71] examined the effects of a 4-month day hospital treatment on alexithymia levels in a sample of 47 patients (AN = 18, BN = 25, and EDNOS = 4). The treatment program was multi-modal, including psychoeducation, cognitive behavior therapy, and interpersonal therapy. As well, during group therapy an emphasis was placed on encouraging patients to experience and communicate their emotions. Across diagnostic groups, patients who completed the treatment reported significant reductions in eating disorder symptomatology as well as significant reductions in TAS-20 total scores. When the TAS-20 subscales were examined, across diagnostic groups, only the difficulties identifying feelings factor showed a statistically significant reduction from pre- to post-treatment. Similarly, Storch and colleagues [75] found that following inpatient treatment for eating disorders (i.e., AN-R, AN-B/N, and BN) patients evidenced a significant increase in their ability to identify emotions.

Clyne and Blampied [73] found that an 11-week group treatment for BED with a strong focus on identifying, communicating and managing emotions lead to significant reductions in alexithymia and depression scores from pre-treatment to post-treatment, as well as from post-treatment to follow-up, in a sample of 11 females who met criteria for BED according to self-report questionnaires. Similarly, Ciano and colleagues [72] compared the effects of group-analytic therapy (n = 6) and group psychoeducation (n = 5) on alexithymia levels in patients with BED. The group-analytic therapy focused on identifying and accepting intrapsychic conflicts that underlie disordered eating behaviors while the psychoeducation focused on communication and assertiveness skills training, nutrition education, and problem solving. While patients in both treatments evidenced significant symptom improvement at post-treatment and at the 6- and 12-month follow-up assessments, only patients in the psychoeducation group also showed a significant improvement in their ability to describe their feelings.

In sum, evidence suggests that psychological treatment leads to a significant improvement in alexithymia scores from pre- to post-treatment. However, the question remains about the clinical significance of the decrease in alexithymia scores. That is, after patients receive treatment, are their alexithymia scores still elevated compared to controls? To date, only one controlled study has investigated this question. de Groot and colleagues [27] examined the effectiveness of a group day hospital treatment program in 31 female patients with a diagnosis of BN. Patients completed the TAS pre- and post-treatment, and a group of 20 nurses who served as the control group, completed the TAS at one time-point. de Groot and colleagues [27] found that, despite a statistically significant reduction in the alexithymia total score and the difficulties identifying and describing feelings factor scores, the patients still had significantly higher alexithymia scores at post-treatment compared to the controls. Furthermore, although there was a significant decrease in the percentage of patients who were categorized as alexithymic from pre- to post-treatment, the percentage of patients who were alexithymic at post-treatment was still significantly higher compared to the percentage of controls who were alexithymic. This is the only controlled treatment study to date that has investigated alexithymia levels pre and post-treatment, and unfortunately the implications of its results are limited by the biased control group (i.e., nurses working in the hospital). An examination of alexithymia scores across studies, however, shows that across non-treatment studies, the control group scores on the TAS and TAS-20 range from 53.0 [5] to 63.7 [43] and 43.10 [28] to 47.0 [41], respectively. An examination of the alexithymia scores in the treatment studies reviewed shows that, with the exception of the study by Becker-Stoll and Gerlinghoff [71], the post-treatment alexithymia scores are still higher compared to the control scores reported in the literature. Thus, the decrease in alexithymia scores from pre to post-treatment, although statistically significant, may not lower alexithymia levels to the values reported by controls.

Given the clear association between alexithymia and depression, a critical question is whether the changes in alexithymia scores from pre-treatment to post-treatment can be explained by changes in depression scores. Surprisingly, only two studies to date have examined this question. Sexton and colleagues [40] found that scores for difficulties identifying and difficulties describing feelings decreased following inpatient psychological treatment in a sample of 53 female inpatients with eating disorders (AN-R, AN-BP, and BN). However, this change was accounted for by a decrease in depressive symptoms. The authors did not describe the treatment protocol used, thus making it difficult to determine whether special emphasis was placed on helping patients to identify and communicate their feelings. In another study, de Groot and colleagues [27] found that in a sample of 31 females with a diagnosis of BN who completed a group day hospital treatment program, both alexithymia, as measured by the TAS, and depression decreased significantly from pre-treatment to post-treatment. Although there was a statistically significant relation between alexithymia and depression scores both at pre-treatment and at post-treatment, it was found that both patients who were depressed at pre-treatment but not at post-treatment, as well as patients who were not depressed at either time-point, had statistically significant decreases in alexithymia scores from pre-treatment to post-treatment. Thus, although alexithymia and depression may be significantly related, there is evidence that alexithymia is not simply a by-product of depression because there was improvement in alexithymia scores even when depression scores were stable.

Based on the research reviewed, it appears that psychological treatments for eating disorders lead to statistically significant decreases in alexithymia scores from pre-treatment to post-treatment, although in the majority of cases, the alexithymia scores are still elevated at post-treatment compared to controls. There is a need for more controlled treatment studies to better understand changes in alexithymia from pre- to post-treatment and the potential mediators of this change.

Review

In summary, there is a robust body of literature illustrating that alexithymia levels, both from a continuous and a categorical perspective, are elevated in individuals with eating disorders compared to healthy controls. Furthermore, individuals with eating disorders have specific deficits in identifying and communicating emotions. One question that arises is whether alexithymia is a state or trait variable. There is strong evidence that alexithymia is not simply a by-product of eating disorder symptomatology. However, the evidence is mixed regarding whether alexithymia is independent of general distress. Although some studies have found that individuals with eating disorders no longer display elevated alexithymia scores once depression levels are controlled for [4,26,36,39], other studies have shown that individuals with eating disorders continue to have elevated alexithymia scores, even when depression levels are controlled for [5,24,27,40]. Furthermore, research evidence from treatment studies suggests that alexithymia levels decrease even when depression levels remain stable [27] and pharmacotherapy with antidepressants decreases depression levels but not alexithymia levels in individuals with high levels of both alexithymia and depression [31]. Lastly, genetic studies have shown that alexithymia has its own heritability component that cannot be fully explained by depression or a genetic susceptibility to general distress and psychopathology [76]. Consequently, although the evidence is mixed, it does suggest that alexithymia, although significantly related to depression, is an independent construct that needs to be considered separately from depression.

From a developmental perspective, structural equation modeling has suggested that childhood maltreatment has an indirect influence on eating disorder symptomatology such that the association between childhood maltreatment and eating symptomatology is mediated by alexithymia and depression, although there are some sex and cultural differences in these relations [65-69]. The identification of children with a history of childhood maltreatment and early intervention focused on depressive symptoms and the identification and communication of emotions may act as a protective factor and decrease the risk for the development of later disordered eating.

With respect to treatment, alexithymia levels decrease significantly in response to psychological treatments that place an emphasis on identifying and describing emotions in addition to symptom reduction [27,71-75]. However, despite these significant decreases in alexithymia scores from pre- to post-treatment, alexithymia scores still remain elevated compared to control scores at post-treatment, suggesting that more intensive treatment focused on emotion regulation may be needed.

Critical appraisal of the research

The research that has been conducted to date has a number of strengths, including the use of large clinical and non-clinical samples to cover the entire spectrum of eating disorder behaviors, and the use of psychometrically valid measures for the assessment of eating disorder behaviors and alexithymia. However, there are a number of limitations that should be taken into consideration when conducting future research on the role of alexithymia in eating disorders.

First, almost all of the studies to date have been cross-sectional in nature, thus making it difficult to determine the direction of causality. The treatment studies conducted to date, although more longitudinal in nature, are also limited by the fact that alexithymia was measured only at pre-treatment and at post-treatment, again raising questions about causality. For instance, do alexithymia scores decrease before eating disorder symptomatology? Does eating disorder symptomatology decrease before alexithymia? What is the relation between changes in depression scores and changes in eating disorder symptomatology and alexithymia scores? Are there specific aspects of the treatment protocol that facilitate the decrease of alexithymia scores? These important empirical questions remain unanswered.

The assessment of alexithymia, eating disorder symptomatology, and depression at multiple time-points during treatment would be helpful in understanding the sequence of change during treatment, as well as the factors that may contribute to the decrease in alexithymia scores during treatment. Furthermore, with regards to treatment, longer follow-up periods are required to examine the maintenance of changes in alexithymia scores over time. As mentioned previously, although alexithymia scores decrease significantly from pre to post-treatment, the post-treatment alexithymia scores are still elevated compared to controls. However, it is possible that alexithymia scores continue to decrease following the completion of treatment as patients generalize the skills learned in treatment. Thus, a study that included multiple follow-up assessments (i.e., 1-month, 3-months, 6-months, 12-months post-treatment) would elucidate the long-term effects of treatment on alexithymia scores.

Longitudinal family-based studies may also enhance our understanding of the role of alexithymia in eating disorders. Given that eating disorders have a genetic basis [77], offspring of parents with a history of eating disorders are at an increased risk for developing disordered eating. Thus, assessing alexithymia levels and eating patterns in children of patients with eating disorders over time may help to better define the role of alexithymia in the development of eating disorders.

In addition to the cross-sectional nature of the studies, another limitation of the research to date is the reliance on self-report measures of alexithymia. Across studies, alexithymia has been assessed through a self-report measure that requires participants to reflect on their ability to identify and describe emotions as well as their cognitive style. However, individuals who struggle with these skills may experience difficulties reflecting on their abilities and may not report accurately on their skills. In response to this challenge, a few studies have begun to use observer-rated and skills-based measures of alexithymia. For instance, Berthoz and colleagues [57] found significant relations between self-reported TAS-20 scores and scores on the Observer Alexithymia Scale completed by a selected family member in a sample of 75 females with a diagnosis of an eating disorder. Using a skills-based approach, Zonnevijlle-Bender and colleagues [34] found that females between the ages of 12 and 18 years who met DSM-IV diagnostic criteria for AN self-reported significantly higher scores on the TAS-20 compared to controls, and also performed significantly worse on an emotion recognition task that required them to label pictures of emotional facial expressions. In a later study, Zonnevijlle-Bender and colleagues [78] identified a similar pattern of results in adult females with AN.

As described above, some studies using skill-based assessments have found consistency across self-report and skills-based assessments of alexithymia. Others, however, have produced inconsistent findings. For example, despite significant group differences on the TAS-20, female patients with AN and controls did not differ on the Levels of Emotional Processing Scale (LEAS) [79,80], a task which requires participants to rate how they would feel in 20 different scenarios [39,81]. There is some suggestion that the LEAS may measure a different aspect of alexithymia than the TAS-20 because the LEAS is not significantly correlated with the TAS-20 difficulties identifying and describing emotions factors, but is significantly correlated with the externally-oriented thinking factor [81]. Thus, the lack of group differences on the LEAS may be accounted for by the fact that identifying and describing emotions appear to be the main emotional processing deficits in eating disorders. The discrepant findings between the LEAS and the TAS-20 highlight the need to more precisely define the specific constructs that are being assessed by the various measures of alexithymia, and to identify overlapping and unique features.

Research on alexithymia and eating disorders has primarily been conducted using female Caucasian samples. Thus, there is a paucity of research that considers sex differences, especially with regards to AN and BN, as well as variability due to ethnicity. The few studies that have considered sex and ethnicity, however, suggest that they may be important moderating variables that warrant further investigation [68,69].

From a theoretical perspective, it is important to consider whether the application of the term alexithymia to the emotion deficits observed in patients with eating disorders is accurate. As described in the introduction, the original conceptualization of alexithymia consisted of 4 characteristics: 1) difficulties identifying feelings and differentiating between feelings and bodily sensations; 2) difficulties describing feelings; 3) lack of fantasy; and 4) an externally-oriented thinking style. Based on the studies to date, individuals with eating disorders only endorse two out of four of the characteristics of alexithymia, although the lack of fantasy life factor has not been adequately assessed. It is important to consider whether applying the term alexithymic to patients with eating disorders is accurate based on the research to date, or whether it would be more accurate to highlight specific deficits in identifying and describing emotions.

Moreover, questions have been raised regarding the similarities and differences between alexithymia and interoceptive awareness. Interoceptive awareness has been defined as the ability to "recognize and accurately respond to emotional states" [82], p. 6, and it is typically assessed using the Interoceptive Awareness subscale of the Eating Disorder Inventory (EDI) [43]. The EDI defines low interoceptive awareness as "confusion and apprehension in recognizing and accurately responding to emotional states" [82], p. 6. Research has demonstrated that individuals with eating disorders have low levels of interoceptive awareness [83]. During the development of the TAS, Bagby and colleagues [13] incorporated 4 items from the Interoceptive Awareness Scale of the EDI [44] for the difficulties identifying feelings factor. Across studies, it has been shown that alexithymia and interoceptive awareness are significantly positively correlated, even when controlling for the overlapping questions [28,51]. The main factors that differentiate between alexithymia and interoceptive awareness are that alexithymia also focuses on cognitive factors, such as an externally-oriented cognitive style. However, as seen through the present review, individuals with eating disorders only have elevated scores on the difficulties identifying and communicating emotions factors. Therefore, based on the research to date, it appears that alexithymia and interoceptive awareness both refer to the same concept. Thus, consolidating the two lines of research may help in creating a more parsimonious explanation for emotional processing deficits in eating disorders.

Strengths and limitations of this review paper

The current paper provides a thorough, comprehensive review of the literature on alexithymia and eating disorders. It is important, however, to note some of the methodological limitations of the current review paper. First, although limiting the review paper to studies that used the TAS to assess alexithymia enhanced our ability to compare results across studies, it is also a limitation, as the paper does not include studies using other self-report and behavioral measures of alexithymia. Second, only one database (i.e., PsycInfo) was used to identify relevant articles and the database search was limited to English language papers. Third, only one author extracted the articles from the database and appraised them. Thus, we do not have reliability data for the extraction and appraisal process. Despite these limitations, to the best of our knowledge, this is the first comprehensive review paper focused on alexithymia and eating disorders, and the findings of the paper have theoretical and clinical implications for our understanding of eating disorders.

Clinical implications

Cognitive behavior therapy and interpersonal therapy are the most widely used and studied psychological treatments for eating disorders. Cognitive behavior therapy focuses on teaching behavioral strategies to help patients restore normal eating, identifying and understanding triggers for their eating disorder behaviors, and examining and modifying their cognitions related to food, shape, and weight [84,85]. Interpersonal therapy views interpersonal problems as underlying eating disorder symptoms and focuses on helping patients learn more effective strategies for dealing with interpersonal challenges, such as improving communication skills, modifying expectations in relationships, and identifying and modifying problematic interaction styles [86]. According to the National Institute for Health and Clinical Excellence guidelines [87], CBT is the first line treatment for BN and BED while IPT is a second line treatment for BN. To date, no one treatment has been identified as clearly superior for AN (see [88] for a review).

It is important to note, however, that even with CBT, fewer than 50% of patients with BN experience a full recovery and the outcomes are even worse for patients with AN [88]. Thus, a significant proportion of individuals with eating disorders are not being helped considerably by our current treatment approaches. Given the significant role of emotion dysregulation in eating disorders and the finding that alexithymia is a negative predictor of treatment outcome [89], a treatment approach that emphasizes identifying and coping with emotions, in combination with traditional CBT strategies for normalizing eating, may assist in improving treatment efficacy. One treatment approach that has emotion dysregulation as a key pillar to its theoretical orientation is dialectical behavior therapy (DBT) [90,91]. Dialectical behavior therapy combines CBT approaches with acceptance-based approaches [92] and suggests that maladaptive behaviors, such as self-harm, function to regulate negative emotions in individuals who lack emotion regulation skills [90]. Thus, from a DBT perspective, the behaviors that are considered maladaptive in eating disorders, such as bingeing, purging, restricting food intake, exercising excessively, and using laxatives/diuretics, are negatively reinforced, as they function to regulate emotions and decrease feelings of distress [93,94]. Consequently, helping patients develop more adaptive strategies to cope with their emotions should help patients improve their eating disorder behaviors.

Dialectical behavior therapy includes learning a number of strategies, often in group format, that are directly focused on increasing patients' skills to adaptively cope with strong urges and emotions. These strategies include: mindfulness, emotion regulation, distress tolerance, and interpersonal effectiveness [91].

The empirical evidence on DBT for BED and BN is currently in its infancy. To date, two case studies [95-97], an uncontrolled group treatment study [98], two wait-list studies and one active control treatment study [93,98,99] have been conducted. Across these studies, there is evidence that DBT leads to significant reductions in binge eating and purging behaviors from pre-treatment to post-treatment in patients with BN and BED, and that these reductions are maintained at 6-month follow-up [93,95,98]. There is also evidence of significant reductions in the tendency to eat when feeling anxious, depressed, or angry in patients with BN [95], but not in patients with BED [93,98].

To date, no studies have examined DBT for AN. However, there is some very preliminary evidence for the effectiveness of various emotion-based treatments for AN, including emotion-focused therapy [100], cognitive remediation and emotion skills training [101], and emotion acceptance behavior therapy [102]. Below, we provide a brief overview of these newer treatment approaches, highlighting key findings with regards to changes in emotion regulation skills. A detailed review of these newer treatment approaches is beyond the scope of the current paper.

Dolhanty and Greenberg [100] describe a single case study involving a 24-year old female with severe AN-R who experienced significant reductions in alexithymia scores following emotion-focused therapy. Emotion-focused therapy views emotions as being essential in helping individuals to understand the world and to respond effectively to various demands, challenges, and situations [103]. However, when individuals are raised in an environment that models emotions as being unacceptable (e.g., children being told that they should not cry) or overwhelming (e.g., mothers becoming overwhelmed by their children's anxiety) then people are at an increased risk for developing emotional difficulties due to an inability to identify and/or regulate their emotions. Thus, the goal of emotion-focused therapy is to help patients increase their awareness and expression of their emotions while learning to react to their emotions in a more adaptive and healthy way that will aid their personal growth and development [104,105].

There is also some evidence regarding the effectiveness of skills-based treatments for AN. Money and colleagues [101] developed a skills-based adjunct to inpatient treatment for AN focused on modifying cognitive rigidity and developing skills in identifying and regulating emotions. In a case study of an adult female patient with AN, Money and colleagues [101] showed that the treatment was acceptable to the patient and lead to a small reduction in alexithymia scores, especially with regards to difficulties with identifying feelings [101]. Another recently developed treatment for AN is emotion acceptance behavior therapy [102]. This therapeutic approach combines the standard components of treatment for AN (i.e., weight restoration, normalizing eating behaviors) with "psychotherapeutic techniques designed to increase emotional awareness, decrease emotional avoidance, and encourage resumption of valued activities and relationships outside the eating disorder" ([102], p. 422). A series of case studies has shown that this treatment is effective in reducing AN symptoms, increasing awareness and tolerance of emotions, and is also rated as acceptable by patients [102].

In conclusion, a number of different emotion-focused treatment protocols have been developed for eating disorders. The research on the majority of these protocols is still in its infancy and there is a need for more studies with larger sample sizes and controlled study designs to provide more insights as to the effectiveness of emotion-focused therapy for eating disorders, especially AN.

Conclusion

In summary, there is a robust body of literature showing that individuals with eating disorders experience difficulties identifying and describing emotions. Given these affect-related difficulties, it is important that eating disorder treatment protocols also incorporate a focus on emotions and emotion regulation. Future research should aim to address some of the methodological limitations in the research to date, including sole reliance on self-report measures of alexithymia, lack of experimental studies, lack of consideration of sex and ethnic differences, and an exclusive focus on negative emotions. An improved understanding of the role of emotions in eating disorders will help to enhance treatment protocols and better understand the etiological and maintenance factors involved in eating disorders.

Competing interests

The authors do not have any competing interests to report.

Authors' contributions

MN conceived the topic, conducted the literature review and drafted the manuscript. TM and SC helped with developing the topic, and drafting and editing the manuscript. All authors read and approved the final manuscript.

Acknowledgements

The preparation of this paper was supported by an Ontario Mental Health Foundation Research Studentship awarded to the first author.

Author details

[1]Department of Psychology, Ryerson University, 350 Victoria Street, Toronto, Ontario M5B 2K3, Canada. [2]Eating Disorder Program, The Toronto General Hospital, 200 Elizabeth Street, Toronto, Ontario M5G 2C4, Canada.

References

1. Sifneos PE: **The prevalence of 'alexithymic' characteristics in psychosomatic patients.** *Psychother Psychosom* 1973, **22**:255–262.
2. Cochrane CE, Brewerton TD, Wilson DB, Hodges EL: **Alexithymia in the eating disorders.** *Int J Eat Disorder* 1993, **14**:219–222.
3. De Berardis D, Carano A, Gambi F, Campanella D, Giannetti P, Ceci A, Mancini E, La Rovere R, Cicconetti A, Penna L, Di Matteo D, Scorrano B, Cotellessa C, Salerno RM, Serroni N, Ferro FM: **Alexithymia and its relationships with body checking and body image in a non-clinical female sample.** *Eat Behav* 2007, **8**:296–304.
4. Eizaguirre AE, de Cabezon AOS, de Alda IO, Olariaga LJ, Juaniz M: **Alexithymia and its relationships with anxiety and depression in eating disorders.** *Pers Indiv Differ* 2004, **36**:321–331.
5. Jimerson DC, Wolfe BE, Franko DL, Covino NA, Sifneos PE: **Alexithymia ratings in bulimia nervosa: clinical correlates.** *Psychosom Med* 1994, **56**:90–93.
6. Karukivi M, Hautala L, Korpelainen J, Haapasalo-Pesu KM, Liuksila PR, Joukamaa M, Saarijarvi S: **Alexithymia and eating disorder symptoms in adolescents.** *Eat Disord* 2010, **18**:226–238.
7. Kiyotaki Y, Yokoyama K: **Relationships of eating disturbances to alexithymia, need for social approval, and gender identity among Japanese female undergraduate students.** *Pers Indiv Differ* 2006, **41**:609–618.
8. Rastam M, Gillberg C, Gillberg IC, Johansson M: **Alexithymia in anorexia nervosa: a controlled study using the 20-item Toronto Alexithymia Scale.** *Acta Psychiat Scand* 1997, **95**:385–388.
9. Cooper MJ: **Cognitive theory in anorexia nervosa and bulimia nervosa: progress, development and future directions.** *Clin Psychol Rev* 2005, **25**:511–531.
10. Cooper MJ, Wells A, Todd G: **A cognitive theory of bulimia nervosa.** *Brit J Clin Psychol* 2004, **43**:1–16.
11. Fairburn CG, Cooper Z, Shafran R: **Cognitive behaviour therapy for eating disorders: a 'transdiagnostic' theory and treatment.** *Behav Res Ther* 2003, **41**:509–528.
12. Corstorphine E: **Cognitive-emotive-behavioural therapy for the eating disorders: working with beliefs about emotions.** *Eur Eat Disord Rev* 2006, **14**:448–461.
13. Bagby RM, Taylor GJ, Parker JDA: **Construct validity of the Toronto Alexithymia Scale.** *Psychother Psychosom* 1988, **50**:29–34.
14. Tylka TL, Subich LM: **Exploring the construct validity of the eating disorder continuum.** *J Couns Psychol* 1999, **46**:268–276.
15. Taylor GJ, Bagby RM, Parker JDA: **The Revised Toronto Alexithymia Scale: some reliability, validity, and normative data.** *Psychother Psychosom* 1992, **57**:34–41.
16. Bagby RM, Parker JDA, Taylor GJ: **The twenty-item Toronto Alexithymia Scale: I. item selection and cross-validation of the factor structure.** *J Psychosom Res* 1994, **38**:23–32.
17. Bressi C, Taylor G, Parker J, Bressi S, Brambilla V, Aguglia E, Allegranti I, Bongiorno A, Giberti F, Bucca M, Todarello O, Callegari C, Vender S, Gala C, Invernizzi G: **Cross validation of the factor structure of the 20-item Toronto Alexithymia Scale: an Italian multicenter study.** *J Psychosom Res* 1996, **41**:551–559.
18. Loas G, Corcos M, Stephan PH, Pellet J, Bizouard P, Venisse JL, Perez-Diaz F, Guelfi JD, Flament M, Jeammet P: **Factorial structure of the 20-item Toronto Alexithymia Scale: confirmatory factorial analyses in nonclinical and clinical samples.** *J Psychosom Res* 2001, **50**:255–261.
19. Pandey R, Mandal MK, Taylor GJ, Parker JD: **Cross-cultural alexithymia: development and validation of a Hindi translation of the 20-Item Toronto Alexithymia Scale.** *J Clin Psychol* 1996, **52**:173–176.

20. Parker JDA, Bagby RM, Taylor GJ, Endler NS, Schmitz P: **Factorial validity of the 20-item Toronto Alexithymia Scale.** *Eur J Personality* 1993, **7:**221–232.
21. Erni T, Lotscher K, Modestin J: **Two-factor solution of the 20-item Toronto Alexithymia Scale confirmed.** *Psychopathology* 1997, **30:**335–340.
22. Haviland MG: **Structure of the twenty-item Toronto Alexithymia Scale.** *J Pers Assess* 1996, **66:**116–125.
23. Beales DL, Dolton R: **Eating disordered patients: personality, alexithymia, and implications for primary care.** *Brit J Gen Pract* 2000, **50:**21–26.
24. Bourke MP, Taylor GJ, Parker JD, Bagby RM: **Alexithymia in women with anorexia nervosa: a preliminary investigation.** *Brit J Psychiat* 1992, **161:**240–243.
25. Bydlowski S, Corcos M, Jeammet P, Paterniti S, Berthoz S, Laurier C, Chambry J, Consoli SM: **Emotion-processing deficits in eating disorders.** *Int J Eat Disord* 2005, **37:**321–329.
26. Corcos M, Guilbaud O, Speranza M, Paterniti S, Loas G, Stephan P, Jeammet P: **Alexithymia and depression in eating disorders.** *Psychiatry Res* 2000, **93:**263–266.
27. de Groot JM, Rodin G, Olmsted MP: **Alexithymia, depression, and treatment outcome in bulimia nervosa.** *Compr Psychiat* 1995, **36:**53–60.
28. De Panfilis C, Rabbaglio P, Rossi C, Zita G, Maggini C: **Body image disturbance, parental bonding and alexithymia in patients with eating disorders.** *Psychopathology* 2003, **36:**239–246.
29. Deborde AS, Berthoz S, Wallier JM, Fermanian J, Falissard B, Jeammet P, Corcos M: **The Bermond-Vorst Alexithymia Questionnaire cutoff scores: a study in eating-disordered and control subjects.** *Psychopathology* 2008, **41:**43–49.
30. Montebarocci O, Codispoti M, Surcinelli P, Franzoni E, Baldaro B, Rossi N: **Alexithymia in female patients with eating disorders.** *Eat Weight Disord-St* 2006, **11:**14–21.
31. Schmidt U, Jiwany A, Treasure J: **A controlled study of alexithymia in eating disorders.** *Compr Psychiat* 1993, **34:**54–58.
32. Sureda B, Valdes M, Jodar I, de Pablo J: **Alexithymia, type A behaviour and bulimia nervosa.** *Eur Eat Disord Rev* 1999, **7:**286–292.
33. Taylor G, Parker JDA, Bagby MR, Bourke MP: **Relationships between alexithymia and psychological characteristics associated with eating disorders.** *J Psychosom Res* 1996, **41:**561–568.
34. Zonnevijlle-Bender MJS, van Goozen SHM, Cohen-Kettenis PT, van Elburg A, van Engeland H: **Do adolescent anorexia nervosa patients have deficits in emotional functioning?** *Eur Child Adoles Psy* 2002, **11:**38–42.
35. Zonnevylle-Bender MJS, van Goozen SHM, Cohen-Kettenis PT, van Elburg A, van Engeland H: **Emotional functioning in adolescent anorexia nervosa patients: a controlled study.** *Eur Child Adoles Psy* 2004, **13:**28–34.
36. Gilboa-Schechtman E, Avnon L, Zubery E, Jeczmien P: **Emotional processing in eating disorders: specific impairment or general distress related deficiency?** *Depress Anxiety* 2006, **23:**331–339.
37. Guttman H, Laporte L: **Alexithymia, empathy, and psychological symptoms in a family context.** *Comp Psychiatr* 2002, **43:**448–455.
38. Nandrino JL, Doba K, Lesne A, Christophe V, Pezard L: **Autobiographical memory deficit in anorexia nervosa: Emotion regulation and effect of duration of illness.** *J Psychosom Res* 2006, **61:**537–543.
39. Parling T, Mortazavi M, Ghaderi A: **Alexithymia and emotional awareness in anorexia nervosa: time for a shift in the measurement of the concept?** *Eat Behav* 2010, **11:**205–210.
40. Sexton MC, Sunday SR, Hurt S, Halmi KA: **The relationship between alexithymia, depression, and Axis II psychopathology in eating disorder inpatients.** *Int J Eat Disorder* 1998, **23:**277–286.
41. Speranza M, Corcos M, Loas G, Stephan P, Guilbaud O, Perez-Diaz F, Venisse JL, Bizouard P, Halfon O, Flament M, Jeammet P: **Depressive personality dimensions and alexithymia in eating disorders.** *Psychiat Res* 2005, **135:**153–163.
42. Torres S, Guerra MP, Lencastre L, Roma-Torres A, Brandao I, Queiros C, Vieira F: **Cognitive processing of emotions in anorexia nervosa.** *Eur Eat Disorders Rev* 2011, **19:**100–111.
43. Troop NA, Schmidt UH, Treasure JL: **Feelings and fantasy in eating disorders: a factor analysis of the Toronto Alexithymia Scale.** *Int J Eat Disorder* 1995, **18:**151–157.
44. Garner DM, Olmsted MP: *The Eating Disorder Inventory Manual.* Florida: Psychological Assessment Resources; 1984.
45. Lecrubier Y, Sheehan DV, Weiller E, Amorin P, Bonora I, Harnet Sheehan K, Janavs J, Dunbar GC: **The MINI International Neuropsychiatric Interview (MINI) a short diagnostic structured interview: reliability and validity according to the CIDI.** *Eur Psychiat* 1999, **12:**224–231.
46. American Psychiatric Association: *Diagnostic statistical manual of mental disorders, Third Edition.* District of Columbia: Author; 1987.
47. American Psychiatric Association: *Diagnostic statistical manual of mental disorders, Fourth Edition.* 4th edition. District of Columbia: Author; 1994.
48. De Berardis D, Serroni N, Campanella D, Carano A, Gambi F, Valchera A, Conti C, Sepeda G, Caltabiano M, Pizzorno AM, Cotollessa C, Salerno RM, Ferro FM: **Alexithymia and its relationships with dissociative experiences, body dissatisfaction and eating disturbances in a non-clinical female sample.** *Cognitive Ther Res* 2009, **33:**471–479.
49. Fukunishi I: **Eating attitudes in female college students with self-reported alexithymic characteristics.** *Psychol Rep* 1998, **82:**35–41.
50. Hayaki J: **Negative reinforcement eating expectancies, emotion dysregulation, and symptoms of bulimia nervosa.** *Int J Eat Disorder* 2009, **42:**552–556.
51. Laquatra TA, Clopton JR: **Characteristics of alexithymia and eating disorders in college women.** *Addict Behav* 1994, **19:**373–380.
52. Markey M, Vander Wal JS: **The role of emotional intelligence and negative affect in bulimic symptomatology.** *Compr Psychiat* 2007, **48:**458–464.
53. Quinton S, Wagner HL: **Alexithymia, ambivalence over emotional expression, and eating attitudes.** *Personal Indiv Differ* 2005, **38:**1163–1173.
54. Ridout N, Thom C, Wallis DJ: **Emotion recognition and alexithymia in females with non-clinical disordered eating.** *Eat Behav* 2010, **11:**1–5.
55. Sasai K, Tanaka K, Hishimoto A: **Alexithymia and its relationships with eating behavior, self esteem, and body esteem in college women.** *Kobe J Med Sci* 2010, **56:**E231–E238.
56. Rozenstein MH, Latzer Y, Stein D, Eviatar Z: **Perception of emotion and bilateral advantage in women with eating disorders, their healthy sisters, and nonrelated healthy controls.** *J Affect Disorders* 2011, **134:**386–395.
57. Berthoz S, Perdereau F, Godart N, Corcos M, Haviland MG: **Observer- and self-rated alexithymia in eating disorder patients: levels and correspondence among three measures.** *J Psychosom Res* 2007, **62:**341–347.
58. Lawson R, Waller G, Sines J, Meyer C: **Emotional awareness among eating-disordered patients: the role of narcissistic traits.** *Eur Eat Disord Rev* 2008, **16:**44–48.
59. Pascual A, Etxebarria I, Cruz MS: **Emotional differences between women with different types of eating disorders.** *Int J Psychol Psychol Therapy* 2011, **11:**1–11.
60. Carano A, De Berardis D, Gambi F, Di Paolo C, Campanella D, Pelusi L, Sepede G, Mancini E, La Rovere R, Salini G, Cotellessa C, Salerno RM, Ferro FM: **Alexithymia and body image in adult outpatients with binge eating disorder.** *Int J Eat Disorder* 2006, **39:**332–340.
61. Pinaquy S, Chabrol H, Simon C, Louvet J, Barbe P: **Emotional eating, alexithymia, and binge-eating disorders in obese women.** *Obes Res* 2003, **11:**195–201.
62. Wheeler K, Greiner P, Boulton M: **Exploring alexithymia, depression, and binge eating in self-reported eating disorders in women.** *Perspect Psychiatr C* 2005, **41:**114–123.
63. Zeeck A, Stelzer N, Linster HW, Joos A, Hartmann A: **Emotion and eating in binge eating disorder and obesity.** *Eur Eat Disorders Rev* 2011, **19:**426–437.
64. de Zwaan M, Bach M, Mitchell JE, Ackard D, Specker SM, Pyle RL, Pakesch G: **Alexithymia, obesity, and binge eating disorder.** *Int J Eat Disorder* 1995, **17:**135–140.
65. Hund AR, Espelage DL: **Childhood sexual abuse, disordered eating, alexithymia, and general distress: a mediation model.** *J Couns Psychol* 2005, **52:**559–573.
66. Hund AR, Espelage DL: **Childhood emotional abuse and disordered eating among undergraduate females: mediating influence of alexithymia and distress.** *Child Abuse Negl* 2006, **30:**393–407.
67. Mazzeo SE, Espelage DL: **Association between childhood physical and emotional abuse and disordered eating behaviors in female undergraduates: an investigation of the mediating role of alexithymia and depression.** *J Consult Psychol* 2002, **49:**86–100.
68. Mazzeo SE, Mitchell KS, Williams LJ: **Anxiety, alexithymia, and depression as mediators of the association between childhood abuse and eating disordered behavior in African American and European American women.** *Psychol Women Quart* 2008, **32:**267–280.
69. Mitchell KS, Mazzeo SE: **Mediators of the association between abuse and disordered eating in undergraduate men.** *Eat Behav* 2005, **6:**318–327.

70. Ruggiero GM, Scarone S, Marseno S, Bertelli S, Sassaroli S: **The relationship between alexithymia and maladaptive perfectionism in eating disorders: a mediation moderation analysis methodology.** *Weight Disorders* 2011, **16**:e182–e187.
71. Becker-Stoll F, Gerlinghoff M: **The impact of a four-month day treatment programme on alexithymia in eating disorders.** *Eur Eat Disord Rev* 2004, **12**:159–163.
72. Ciano R, Rocco PL, Angarano A, Biasin E, Balestrieri M: **Group-analytic and psychoeducational therapies for binge-eating disorder: an exploratory study on efficacy and persistence of effects.** *Psychother Res* 2002, **12**:231–239.
73. Clyne C, Blampied NM: **Training in emotion regulation as a treatment for binge eating: a preliminary study.** *Behav Change* 2004, **21**:269–281.
74. Shiina A, Nakazato M, Mitsumori M, Koizumi H, Shimizu E, Fujisaki M, Iyo M: **An open trial of outpatient group therapy for bulimic disorders: combination program of cognitive behavioral therapy with assertive training and self-esteem enhancement.** *Psychiat Clin Neuros* 2005, **59**:690–696.
75. Storch M, Keller F, Weber J, Spindler A, Milos G: **Psychoeducation in affect regulation for patients with eating disorders: a randomized controlled feasibility study.** *Am J Psychother* 2011, **65**:81–93.
76. Picardi A, Fagnani C, Gigantesco A, Toccaceli V, Lega I, Stazi MA: **Genetic influences on alexithymia and their relationship with depressive symptoms.** *J Psychosom Res* 2011, **71**:256–263.
77. Klump KL, Suisman JL, Burt AS, McGue M, Iacono WG: **Genetic and environmental influences on disordered eating: an adoption study.** *J Abnorm Psychol* 2009, **118**:797–805.
78. Zonnevylle-Bender MJS, van Goozen SHM, Cohen-Kettenis PT, van Elburg A, de Wildt M, Stevelmans E, van Engeland H: **Emotional functioning in anorexia nervosa patients: Adolescents compared to adults.** *Depress Anxiety* 2004, **18**:35–42.
79. Lane RD: *LEAS scoring manual and glossary.* Arizona: Department of Psychiatry, University of Arizona Health Sciences Center; 1991.
80. Lane RD, Quinlan DM, Schwartz GE, Walker PA, Zeitlin SB: **The Levels of Emotional Awareness Scale: a cognitive-developmental measure of emotion.** *J Pers Assess* 1990, **55**:124–134.
81. Subic-Wrana C, Bruder S, Thomas W, Lane RD, Kohle K: **Emotional awareness deficits in inpatients of a psychosomatic ward: a comparison of two different measures of alexithymia.** *Psychosom Med* 2005, **67**:483–489.
82. Garner DM: *Eating Disorder Inventory-2: professional manual.* Florida: Psychological Assessment Resources; 1991.
83. Fassino S, Piero A, Garmaglia C, Abbate-Daga G: **Interoceptive awareness in anorexia nervosa, bulimia nervosa, and obesity.** *Psychopathology* 2004, **37**:168–174.
84. Brownell KD, Fairburn CG: *Eating disorders and obesity: a comprehensive handbook.* 2nd edition. New York: Guilford Press; 2002.
85. Fairburn CG, Marcus MD, Wilson GT: **Cognitive behaviour therapy for binge eating and BN: a comprehensive treatment manual.** In *In Binge eating: nature, assessment, and treatment.* Edited by Fairburn CG, Wilson GT. New York: Guilford Pre; 1993:361–404.
86. Garner DM, Garfinkel PE: *Handbook of treatment for eating disorders.* New York: Guilford Press; 1997.
87. National Institute for Clinical Excellence: *Eating disorders - Core interventions in the treatment and management of anorexia nervosa, bulimia nervosa and related eating disorders.*; 2004. www.nice.org.uk/guidance/CG9.
88. Wilson GT, Grilo CM, Vitousek KM: **Psychological treatment of eating disorders.** *Am Psychol* 2007, **62**:199–216.
89. Speranza M, Loas G, Wallier J, Corcos M: **Predictive value of alexithymia in patients with eating disorder: a 3-year prospective study.** *J Psychosom Res* 2007, **63**:365–371.
90. Linehan MM: *Cognitive-behavioral treatment of borderline personality disorder.* New York: Guilford Press; 1993.
91. Linehan MM: *Skills training manual for treating borderline personality disorder.* New York: Guilford Press; 1993.
92. Linehan MM: **Commentary on innovations in dialectical behavior therapy.** *Cogn Behav Pract* 2001, **7**:478–481.
93. Telch CF, Agras WS, Linehan MM: **Dialectical behavior therapy for binge eating disorder.** *J Consult Clin Psych* 2001, **69**:1061–1065.
94. Waller G: **The psychological factors in a functional analysis of binge eating.** In *Eating disorders and obesity: A comprehensive handbook.* 2nd edition. Edited by Fairburn CG, Brownell KD. New York: Guilford Press; 2003.
95. Safer DL, Telch CF, Agras SW: **Dialectical behavior therapy adapted for bulimia: a case report.** *Int J Eat Disorder* 2001, **30**:101–106.
96. Telch CF: **Skills training treatment for adaptive affect regulation in a woman with binge-eating disorder.** *Int J Eat Disorder* 1997, **22**:77–81.
97. Telch CF, Agras WS, Linehan MM: **Group dialectical behavior therapy for binge-eating disorder: a preliminary uncontrolled trial.** *Behav Ther* 2000, **31**:569–582.
98. Safer DL, Robinson AH, Jo B: **Outcome for a randomized controlled trial of group therapy for binge eating disorder: comparing dialectical behavior therapy adapted for binge eating to an active comparison group.** *Behav Ther* 2010, **41**:106–120.
99. Safer DL, Telch CF, Agras SW: **Dialectical behavior therapy for bulimia nervosa.** *Am J Psychiat* 2001, **158**:632–634.
100. Dolhanty J, Greenberg L: **Emotion-focused therapy in a case of anorexia nervosa.** *Clin Psychol Psychot* 2009, **16**:366–382.
101. Money C, Davies H, Tchanturia K: **A case-study introducing cognitive remediation and emotion skills training for anorexia nervosa inpatient care.** *Clinical Case Studies* 2011, **10**:110–121.
102. Wildes JE, Marcus MD: **Development of emotion acceptance behavior therapy for anorexia nervosa: a case series.** *Int J Eat Disord* 2011, **44**:421–427.
103. Greenberg L: **Emotion-focused therapy: a clinical synthesis.** *J Lifelong Learn Psychiatry* 2010, **VIII**:32–42.
104. Greenberg L: *Emotion-focused therapy: coaching clients to work through feelings.* District of Columbia: American Psychological Association; 2002.
105. Greenberg L, Watson J: *Emotion-focused therapy of depression.* District of Columbia: American Psychological Association; 2006.

Maternal and family factors and child eating pathology: risk and protective relationships

Karina L Allen[1,2*], Lisa Y Gibson[1], Neil J McLean[2], Elizabeth A Davis[1,3] and Susan M Byrne[2]

Abstract

Background: Previous studies have found associations between maternal and family factors and child eating disorder symptoms. However, it is not clear whether family factors predict eating disorder symptoms specifically, or relate to more general child psychopathology, of which eating disorder symptoms may be one component. This study aimed to identify maternal and family factors that may predict increases or decreases in child eating disorder symptoms over time, accounting for children's body mass index z-scores and levels of general psychological distress.

Methods: Participants were 221 mother-child dyads from the Childhood Growth and Development Study, a prospective cohort study in Western Australia. Participants were assessed at baseline, 1-year follow-up and 2-year follow-up using interview and self-report measures. Children had a mean age of 10 years at baseline and 46% were male. Linear mixed models and generalised estimating equations were used to identify predictors of children's eating disorder symptoms, with outcome variables including a global index of eating disorder psychopathology, levels of dietary restraint, levels of emotional eating, and the presence of loss of control ('binge') eating.

Results: Children of mothers with a current or past eating disorder reported significantly higher levels of global eating disorder symptoms and emotional eating than other children, and mothers with a current or past eating disorder reported significantly more concern about their children's weight than other mothers. Maternal concern about child weight, rather than maternal eating disorder symptoms, was significant in predicting child eating disorder symptoms over time. Family exposure to stress and low maternal education were additional risk factors for eating disorder symptoms, whilst child-reported family satisfaction was a protective factor.

Conclusions: After adjusting for relevant confounding variables, maternal concern about child weight, children's level of family satisfaction, family exposure to stress, and maternal education are unique predictors of child eating disorder symptoms.

Keywords: Eating disorders, Children, Loss of control eating, Family, Risk factors, Protective factors, Running head, Family factors and eating pathology

Background

It is recognised that families do not cause eating disorders [1] and there is robust evidence to support a strong genetic component to these conditions [2]. Nonetheless, certain family characteristics may increase risk for eating disorders and/or problematic eating behaviours in childhood and adolescence (e.g., [3-5]). This study sought to extend previous research by elucidating risk and protective factors in the relationships between family variables and eating disorder symptoms in children, with attention to the specificity of any identified effects.

Previous research has focused on two main categories of family characteristics, including maternal eating disorder history, maternal eating disorder symptoms and a family emphasis on eating, weight and shape; and general family functioning and parenting practices, which incorporate family conflict, family support and the frequency and nature of parent–child interactions. Moreover, studies have considered two main categories of child eating behaviour, including feeding patterns and difficulties in

* Correspondence: karina@ichr.uwa.edu.au
[1]Telethon Institute for Child Health Research, Centre for Child Health Research, The University of Western Australia, PO Box 855, West Perth, WA, Australia
[2]School of Psychology, The University of Western Australia, Crawley, WA, Australia
Full list of author information is available at the end of the article

infancy and early childhood; and eating, weight and shape concerns, dieting, binge eating and purging in later childhood and adolescence. The following sections review key findings across these areas.

Maternal and family emphasis on eating, weight and shape

Available data suggest that mothers with an eating disorder history are more likely to have infants with feeding difficulties, to restrict their child's eating in early and middle childhood, and to use food for non-nutritive purposes (e.g., reward, distraction) when compared to mothers without an eating disorder history [6-11]. Mothers with an eating disorder history may also be more likely to experience concern about their child's eating and weight, and to have children who themselves report elevated concerns about eating, weight and shape [6,12]. There is some evidence that these effects are gender-specific, with female children of mothers with an eating disorder history being affected to a greater degree than male children [6]. There is little evidence for associations between maternal eating disorder history and children's body mass index (BMI), self-esteem, or parent-reported emotional and behavioural problems [12].

Maternal and/or familial emphasis on eating, weight and shape (e.g., parental dieting, comments about weight and shape in the home environment) may also predict weight loss attempts, weight and shape concerns, binge eating and purging in children and adolescents. Data suggest that these links apply cross-sectionally [13,14] and longitudinally [15-20], but may only occur when other predisposing factors (such as neuroticism or a general vulnerability to psychological difficulties) are present in children [21] or mothers [22]. Again, there appear to be gender differences in the strength of associations between variables, with girls, in particular, more likely to experience (or perceive) family-based pressures regarding eating or weight than boys [23-25].

Results in this area are consistent with sociocultural theories of eating disorders, which view internalisation of the 'thin ideal' and/or perceived pressure to be thin as key contributors to body dissatisfaction and eating pathology [26]. In childhood and adolescence, the family environment is an important source of information about cultural values and ideals. Mothers with an eating disorder history, or current eating disorder symptoms, may also find it difficult to know when and how to feed their children, or doubt their judgement in this area [10]. As noted by others [10,27,28], it is likely that these family environmental factors work in conjunction with genetic vulnerability to increase eating disorder risk.

Family functioning and relationships

The second category of research has focused on associations between family functioning and parenting style (e.g., frequency of family interactions, family conflict) and child and adolescent eating disorder symptoms. Several groups have found prospective associations between low family affection or high family conflict and later onset of eating disorder symptoms [5,29-31] or increasing weight and shape concerns [32] in male and female adolescents. It is generally accepted that child eating disorder symptoms are likely to impact deleteriously on family interactions, meaning that cross-sectional links between family conflict and eating pathology are difficult to interpret [1]. However, parent-adolescent connectedness (i.e., the presence of parents at home, parental knowledge of their adolescent's behaviour) and frequent family communication have been identified as significant, cross-sectional protective factors for adolescent dieting and eating disorder symptoms [33]. Greater parent-adolescent connectedness and greater family meal frequency have also been identified as significant prospective protective factors for dieting, binge eating and purging in adolescent girls [31,34].

These findings suggest that a positive family environment may help to reduce vulnerability to eating disorder symptoms in adolescence. This is consistent with the broader literature on links between family support and adolescent resilience and coping [35], and the potential for positive environmental factors to help negate risks associated with negative environmental exposures and/or underlying genetic vulnerabilities [36].

The specificity of identified risk effects

Overall, there is evidence for associations between certain family characteristics and both feeding behaviour in early childhood, and eating disorder symptoms in later childhood and adolescence. Less is known about the specificity of these associations. In the case of maternal eating disorder symptoms, it is important to distinguish between the effects of maternal eating pathology and those of more general psychiatric morbidity. Research from the Avon Longitudinal Study of Parents and Children (ALSPAC) [11] helps to address this issue. In the ALSPAC sample (n = 12,050), women with a self-reported history of anorexia nervosa (AN; n = 247) or bulimia nervosa (BN; n = 194) reported more feeding difficulties in the first 12 months post-partum than general control participants [12]. In most cases, however, these feeding difficulties were comparable to those reported by ASLPAC women with a non-eating related psychiatric disorder ('psychiatric control participants') (n = 1,148). This suggests that feeding difficulties in infancy may be associated with general maternal psychiatric distress, rather than eating disorders specifically. This possibility was supported by follow-up analyses in the ALSPAC cohort, which showed that associations between maternal eating disorder history and infant feeding difficulties were mediated by maternal anxiety and depressive symptoms [28]. A recent publication extends these infant findings to child emotional and behaviour problems at 3 to 4 years of age [37]. The ALSPAC mothers with an eating disorder history in pregnancy reported greater emotional and behavioural difficulties in their children at 3.5 years, compared to control mothers, but these associations were largely accounted for by anxiety and depressive symptoms during pregnancy. The direct effect of a maternal eating disorder history on child functioning was small [37].

These results highlight that maternal eating disorder history may be a proxy for other relevant maternal or family factors, rather than a strong specific predictor of child eating pathology. Comparing children of mothers with an eating disorder history to children of mothers with a history of another, non-eating related psychiatric disorder is important if the effects of maternal eating pathology are to be fully understood. Further, any effects of eating pathology should be evaluated in the context of general maternal psychological distress (e.g., depressive and anxiety symptoms).

It is also important to determine if family characteristics predict child eating disorder symptoms specifically, or are associated with general psychological distress, of which eating disorder symptoms may be one component. This is particularly true for studies on family functioning, which is likely to have a diverse influence on offspring development [35]. To address this, studies need to consider if family functioning predicts offspring eating disorder symptoms after children's general psychological functioning has been accounted for.

The current study

This study sought to extend previous research by examining risk and protective relationships between family characteristics (including maternal eating disorder history, maternal eating disorder symptoms, family emphasis on eating, weight and shape, and indices of family functioning) and child eating behaviours (early feeding practices and later eating disorder symptoms), with attention to the specificity of any identified effects. Children were followed from pre to early adolescence, a high risk period for the emergence of eating disorder symptoms, and early feeding practices were assessed retrospectively.

Specific aims were as follows:

Aim 1. To compare children of mothers with a current or past eating disorder ('eating disorder group'), children of mothers with a non-eating related current or past psychiatric disorder ('psychiatric control group'), and children of mothers with no psychiatric history ('general control group') on early feeding practices, child eating disorder symptoms, and child psychological well-being.

Aim 2. To identify family characteristics that can predict increases or decreases in child eating disorder symptoms over time, taking into account child body mass and general psychological distress.

The following hypotheses were tested:

Hyp. 1. Children in the maternal eating disorder group would score significantly higher on measures of early feeding difficulties (shorter breastfeeding duration, early commencement of solids) and eating disorder symptoms (overall eating, weight and shape concern, dieting, emotional eating, binge eating) than children in the general and psychiatric control groups (Aim 1).

Hyp. 2. Maternal anxiety and depressive symptoms would be stronger predictors of increases in child eating disorder symptoms over time than maternal eating disorder history or maternal eating disorder symptoms (Aim 2).

Hyp. 3. Positive family interactions (assessed through parent and child report) would protect against increases in child eating disorder symptoms over time (Aim 2).

Methods

Design

This research involved data from the Childhood Growth and Development (GAD) Study. The GAD Study is a prospective cohort study based in Perth, Western Australia, which has a central focus on weight and eating behaviour in childhood. Children were recruited from Perth primary schools and interviewed at baseline (Time 1), 1-year follow-up (Time 2), and 2-year follow-up (Time 3). Additional details of the GAD Study methodology, including detailed recruitment information, have been reported previously [38-40].

Participants

Participants were community-recruited mother-child dyads where the child was aged between 8 and 13 years at baseline and where baseline, 1-year follow-up and 2-year follow-up assessments were completed between January 2004 and January 2009. This equated to 221 children (46% male) and, due to 55 sibling pairs or triplets, 166 mothers. Family clustering was accounted for in analyses. There were 15 father-child dyads who were excluded from analyses, due to the small number of participating fathers and the focus on maternal characteristics in analyses.

Participant attrition over the 2-year period was 32% (baseline N = 325 children). Differences between families included in this study and those lost to follow-up are discussed under Preliminary Analyses, below.

At the baseline assessment, children had a mean age of 10.78 years (SD 1.72, range = 8-13 years) and mothers had a mean age of 40.98 years (SD 5.17, range = 30-54 years). As the mean age of the sample exceeded 12 years at Time 3, pubertal stage was considered as a possible confounder of the results. This was assessed via self-report Tanner stages [41], which have been found to converge well with physical examination in pre-adolescent samples [42,43]. All boys were pre-pubertal at baseline and 93% (n = 95/102) remained pre-pubertal at 2-year follow-up. There were no significant differences between pre- and post-pubertal boys at 2-year follow-up, for any of the assessed variables. Most girls (94%; n = 112/119) were pre-pubertal at baseline and 72% (n = 86/119) were pre-pubertal at 2-year follow-up. Girls who were post-pubertal were significantly older than girls who were not at both time points, but pubertal status did not relate significantly to the family variables of interest or children's eating disorder symptoms. Thus, pubertal status was not included as a covariate in analyses.

Procedure

Children and mothers were assessed separately by trained GAD Study researchers, at baseline, 1-year follow-up, and 2-year follow-up. Assessments were conducted in the family's own home, at the Telethon Institute for Child Health Research or at Princess Margaret Hospital for Children, according to family preference. With the exception of the GAD Study interview questions and the Eating Disorder Examination (EDE; [44]), all maternal measures were completed as self-report questionnaires. In contrast, all child measures were administered verbally. The same measures were administered at all assessment points.

All GAD Study researchers received comprehensive training prior to conducting assessments, and had Honours level qualifications or above in psychology, medicine or exercise physiology. Training for the EDE and ChEDE was conducted by the first and last authors, who have extensive experience with the administration of these interviews. The first author also checked all EDE/ChEDE scores prior to data entry, to ensure adherence to scoring protocols.

Ethics approval was provided by the Ethics Committee of Princess Margaret Hospital for Children. Mothers provided written informed consent for participation.

Outcome variables: child feeding problems and eating disorder symptoms

Child feeding problems (maternal report)

Questions about early feeding practices were included in the GAD Study parent interview. Specifically, two questions were used to determine the age at which mothers stopped breastfeeding their child(ren) (to the nearest week; 0 weeks if they did not breastfeed at all) and the age at which they started their child(ren) on solid food (to the nearest month).

Child eating disorder symptoms (child report)

Child eating disorder symptoms were assessed using the Child Eating Disorder Examination (ChEDE) [45] and Children's Affect Regulation Scale (CARES) [46].

The ChEDE is a semi-structured interview adapted from the adult Eating Disorder Examination (EDE) [44]. Like the adult version, it generates four subscale scores (Restraint, Eating Concern, Weight Concern, Shape Concern) and a Global score (the mean of the four subscale scores). A Brief Global score appears to be a more reliable index of eating pathology than the original four subscales, which are not supported by factor analysis [47,48]. The brief scale consists of eight items from the original Weight Concern and Shape Concern scales, and the resulting index correlates very highly with the original Global score and moderately to highly with each of the original four subscales [47,48]. This study used the Brief Global score as an index of overall child eating disorder psychopathology ($\alpha = .88$ at baseline). To allow a specific focus on dietary restraint, we also made use of the ChEDE Restraint scale, which consists of 5 items regarding actual and intended dieting behaviour (α at baseline = .69).

The ChEDE also allows children to be categorised according to whether or not they experienced loss of control or 'binge' eating. Loss of control eating encompasses objective binge eating (feeling out of control of one's eating and consuming an objectively large amount of food) and subjective binge eating (feeling out of control of one's eating but not consuming a large amount of food). It is established that loss of control, regardless of the amount of food eaten, is the key component of binge eating behaviour in childhood [49] and objective and subjective binge eating were both considered for this research.

The CARES was used to assess emotional eating. The measure includes 10 items that assess the tendency to eat as a means of affect regulation. Scores can range from 0 (no emotional eating) to 4 (very frequent emotional eating). The alpha coefficient was .82 at baseline.

Predictor variables: family characteristics

Maternal eating disorder and psychiatric disorder history (maternal report)

Five questions in the GAD Study parent interview were used to determine if mothers (i) had ever had an eating disorder or been suspected of having one and, if yes, (ii) the nature of the disorder, (iii) when it occurred, (iv) if it was diagnosed, and (v) if it was treated.

Five additional questions in the GAD Study parent interview were used to determine if mothers (i) had ever experienced an emotional or psychological problem not related to eating and, if yes, (ii) the nature of the problem/s, (iii) when they occurred, (iv) if they were diagnosed, and (v) if they were treated.

Responses to these items were used to categorise mothers according to whether they had a past eating disorder history, a non-eating related current or past psychiatric disorder, or no history of a psychiatric disorder.

Current maternal eating disorder symptoms (maternal report)

The adult EDE version 12 was used to assess current maternal eating disorder symptoms. As per the ChEDE, this semi-structured interview generates four subscale scores (Restraint, Eating Concern, Weight Concern, Shape Concern) and a Global score (the mean of the four subscale scores), and includes diagnostic items for determining eating disorder diagnoses. The measure is established as reliable and valid [50-53]. Again, there is greater support for the Brief Global scale than the original subscales [47]. This study used the Brief Global score as an index of overall maternal eating disorder psychopathology ($\alpha = .85$ at baseline). Diagnostic items were used to determine current *DSM-5* eating disorder diagnoses in mothers.

Maternal concern about child weight (maternal report)

One question in the GAD Study parent interview was used to assess mother's level of concern about their child(ren)'s weight, with the available response options being "not at all", "a little", "moderately" or "very" concerned. If the mother had multiple children participating in the study, separate ratings were made for each. As very few mothers reported being "very" concerned, responses in the two highest categories were collapsed to give a moderate-high concern group.

An additional question was used to assess mother's level of concern about their child(ren)'s overall health. Mothers rated their child(ren)'s current physical health on a 5-point scale ranging from "poor" (1) to "excellent" (5).

Family relationships (maternal and child report)

Family relationships were assessed in two ways. First, mothers completed the self-report General Functioning Scale (GFS) of the McMaster Family Functioning Device [54]. The GFS includes 12 items regarding family relationships, arguments and interactions, and has been established as reliable and valid with a variety of clinical and non-clinical groups [54-57]. Higher scores indicate greater family conflict and disharmony. The alpha coefficient in this sample was .90 at baseline.

Second, the Family Satisfaction subscale of the Students' Life Satisfaction Scale (SLSS; [58]) was verbally administered to children. This subscale is designed to assess children's level of satisfaction with their family, parents, and the nature of family interactions. It contains seven items, and subscale scores can range from 0 to 5; higher scores indicate greater family satisfaction. The measure has been established as reliable and valid [58-60], and the alpha coefficient in this sample was .78 at baseline.

Parenting style (maternal report)

The Parenting Scale [61] was used to assess for unhelpful parenting practices. The scale includes 30 items regarding overly permissive discipline ("Laxness"), inappropriate displays of anger, meanness or irritability ("Overreactivity"), and the use of lengthy verbal responses or instructions even when ineffective ("Verbosity"). It can be used to generate subscale scores for each of these categories of items, as well as an overall global score. In each instance, scores can range from one to seven, with higher scores indicating less positive parenting. The measure has acceptable psychometric properties, although the factor structure of the three subscales has been debated [62,63]. Global scores were used in this study and the 30 items were internally consistent ($\alpha = .78$).

Family exposure to stressful life events (maternal report)

The List of Threatening Experiences [64], otherwise known as the Life Events Scale, was used to assess family exposure to stressful life events. The scale asks respondents to indicate if they have experienced each of 12 negative life events (e.g., unemployment, significant illness) over the past 6 months, with scores calculated by summing the number of "yes" responses. It has been established as a valid index of life stress [65-67].

Maternal depressive, anxiety and stress symptoms (maternal report)

The 21-item self-report Depression Anxiety Stress Scale (DASS) [68] was used to assess maternal depressive, anxiety and stress symptoms experienced over the previous week. The DASS generates three subscale scores (Depression, Anxiety and Stress) that can range from 0 to 42. It has been established as reliable and valid [68-72]. Scores on the Depression subscale correlate highly with scores on other measures of depression, and scores on the Anxiety subscale correlate highly with those on other measures of anxiety [68,69,71]. Alpha coefficients were satisfactory in this sample (=.77 - .86).

Maternal self-esteem (maternal report)

The Rosenberg Self-Esteem Scale (RSES) [73] was used to assess overall maternal self-esteem. The scale includes 10 items and scores can range from 10 to 40, with higher scores indicating greater self-esteem. It has well-established psychometric properties [73-75]. The alpha coefficient at baseline was .88.

Covariates and additional descriptive variables

Child psychosocial functioning (child report)

Indices of child psychosocial functioning were considered as potential confounders of associations between family characteristics and child eating disorder symptoms.

The short form of the Child Depression Inventory (CDI) [76] was used to assess depressive symptoms. The CDI is a modification of the Beck Depression Inventory, and is the most commonly used instrument for assessing depressive symptoms in children. The short-form CDI contains 10 items that assess negative mood, anhedonia, ineffectiveness, and negative self-esteem, and it has been established as internally consistent and successfully used to screen children for depression [76]. It was internally consistent in this sample ($\alpha = .73$ at baseline).

The Global Self-Worth subscale of the Self-Perception Profile for Children (SPPC) [77] was used to assess children's overall or global level of self-esteem. The SPPC is a multi-dimensional measure of self-esteem and has been validated for use with participants aged eight years and older [77,78]. The alpha coefficient for the Global Self-Worth scale at baseline was .71.

The Multidimensional Media Influences Scale (MMIS) [79] was used to assess children's awareness and internalisation of the thin-ideal, and their perceived level of media pressure to achieve the thin ideal. It has acceptable psychometric properties [79] and the total score was used in this study ($\alpha = .75$).

Family sociodemographic information (maternal report)

Questions in the GAD Study parent interview were used to assess total family income, mother's marital status, mother's highest level of education and mother's general health, for consideration as covariates in analyses.

For family income, a dichotomous variable was created to reflect whether or not the family could be considered to have a low income relative to Australian standards. "Low income" was defined as an annual pre-tax income in the lowest population quartile, which equated to approximately $35,000 per annum. For marital status, a dichotomous variable was created to reflect whether or not the mother was married or in an equivalent long-term de facto relationship. For education, a dichotomous variable was created to reflect whether or not the mother had completed high school. For maternal health, mothers rated their current physical health on a 5-point scale ranging from "poor" (1) to "excellent" (5).

Maternal and child Body Mass Index (BMI)

Height and weight were measured during the GAD Study interview. For mothers, BMI was calculated using the standard formula (weight [kg]/height [m]^2). For children, age- and sex-specific BMI z-scores were calculated using the CDC 2000 reference data [80].

Statistical analyses

Responses to the EDE and GAD Study interview questions were used to categorise mothers into one of three groups: an *eating disorder group,* if they met criteria for a current eating disorder on the EDE or had a previous eating disorder as diagnosed by a health professional; a *psychiatric control group,* if they had a current or previous non-eating related psychiatric disorder as diagnosed by a health professional; or a *general control group,* if there was no evidence of a current or past eating or psychiatric disorder. Groups were compared on maternal and family factors.

To address Aim 1, linear mixed models were constructed to examine the effects of maternal group (eating disorder vs. psychiatric control vs. general control) on early child feeding practices (breastfeeding duration, age of introduction of solids), child eating disorder symptoms, child psychological functioning, general child health, and level of maternal concern about child weight. Mixed linear models allow grouping variables (i.e., family status) to be controlled for, meaning that any effects of clustering of children within families could be accounted for in the analyses. These models considered the effects of maternal group on early child feeding practices as reported at a single time point (retrospectively assessed at baseline) and childhood variables as assessed annually from baseline to 2-year follow-up. Support for Hypothesis 1 would come from children of mothers with a past or current eating disorder showing greater eating disorder symptoms, on average, over the 2-year study period than children of mothers in the psychiatric and general control groups.

To address Aim 2, linear mixed models and generalised estimating equations were used to identify significant predictors of changes in child eating disorder symptoms over time. Continuous outcome variables (for use in linear mixed models) included ChEDE Brief Global scores and Restraint scores, and CARES emotional eating scores. The categorical outcome variable (for use in generalised estimating equations) was loss of control eating. Time invariant and time-varying family factors were considered as predictor variables and child BMI z-score was included as a covariate in all multivariate models.

Time invariant predictors were those variables assessed at baseline only, or which showed considerable stability over the 2 year assessment period and so were used at baseline only. These included maternal group (eating disorder vs. psychiatric control vs. general control) and level of maternal concern about child weight (no concern vs. slight concern vs. moderate-high concern) as family predictor variables, and family income (low vs. medium-high), mother's marital status (married/de facto vs. no long-term relationship) and maternal education (high school vs. less than high school) as potential covariates. For these variables, associations were between the predictor variable at baseline and average levels of the outcome variable over the 2 year study period. A significant interaction between a time invariant predictor and time would show that the predictor variable at baseline predicted changes in the outcome variable over the subsequent 2 years.

Time-varying predictors were those variables that were assessed annually from baseline to 2-year follow-up, and which showed variation over the assessment period. These included scores for the EDE Brief Global scale, DASS, RSES, Life Event Scale, Parenting Scale, McMaster Family Functioning scale and SLSS, as family predictor variables, as well as maternal BMI as a potential covariate. For these variables, associations were between changes in the predictor variable over the 2 year study period and changes in the outcome variable over the same time frame.

Predictors were initially examined in univariate models, and those that were significant at $p < .05$ were later entered in multivariate analyses. As note, all multivariate models included child BMI z-score. In addition, a more complex model was specified that included child BMI z-score as well as child depressive symptoms and global self-esteem. If family factors predicted child eating disorder symptoms after depressive symptoms and self-esteem were accounted for, evidence would be provided for a specific association between family factors and child eating disorder symptoms.

Models were constructed for boys and girls together, with gender interaction terms used to explore possible gender differences in the degree or nature of associations between variables. Consistent with recommendations, analyses were initially conducted using non-interaction variables only and subsequently conducted using non-interaction and interaction terms [81]. Interaction terms were only retained if they contributed to a model significantly.

Support for Hypothesis 2 would come from mother's DASS scores being significant longitudinal predictors of increasing child eating disorder symptoms. Support for Hypothesis 3 would come from mother's McMaster Family Functioning scores and/or children's SLSS family satisfaction scores being significant longitudinal predictors of decreasing eating disorder symptoms.

Results

Preliminary analyses

Consistent with other longitudinal studies, GAD Study families lost to follow-up tended to be more socially disadvantaged at baseline than families who remained in the study. Specifically, mothers lost to follow-up (n = 100) were less likely to have completed high school ($p = .002$), more likely to be single or divorced ($p = .041$), and more likely to report family exposure to stressful live events ($p = .010$) at baseline than mothers included in analyses (n = 166). However, there were no significant baseline differences between children lost to follow-up (n = 104) and those included in this study (n = 221) on any of the child variables assessed, including eating disorder symptoms.

Of the 166 mothers included in analyses, eight met criteria for a current *DSM-5* eating disorder. Of these, five women met criteria for binge eating disorder (BED), two met criteria for bulimia nervosa (BN) and one met criteria for anorexia nervosa (AN). A further 10 women were determined to have a history of an eating disorder, and had previously been diagnosed with AN (n = 5) or an AN-like disorder (n = 2), BN (n = 2), or AN and BN at different time points (n = 1). These 10 participants and the eight current eating disorder cases were included in the maternal eating disorder group (n = 18; 11% of the maternal sample).

Of the women who did not meet criteria for a current or past eating disorder, 36 (22%) reported experiencing a current or past emotional problem that had warranted diagnosis and/or treatment. In most cases, the problem was depression (with or without anxiety; n = 28) and was treated with medication (n = 25). Other reported problems included generalised anxiety (without depression; n = 2), post-traumatic stress disorder (n = 2), substance abuse/dependence (n = 1), and agoraphobia (n = 1). These 36 participants were included in the maternal psychiatric disorder group. A further 10 women reported experiencing a current or past emotional problem that had not been diagnosed or treated. Due to difficulties in validating the nature and severity of these problems, these participants were not included in the psychiatric disorder group, and were instead excluded from analyses.

The 102 mothers (61%) who did not report a current or past eating disorder or psychiatric disorder were included in the general (non-psychiatric) control group.

Baseline demographic details and mean scores on maternal and family-based measures are shown in Table 1 by maternal group. Significant between-group differences are also shown, as identified using a one-way ANOVA (for continuous variables) and chi square tests (for categorical variables).

Aim 1: Effects of maternal eating disorder history on child eating behaviour and general psychological functioning

Linear mixed model analyses identified significant main effects of maternal group (eating disorder vs. psychiatric control vs. general control) on the age at which solids were introduced, $F(2, 512) = 5.65$, $p = .004$, degree of maternal concern about child weight, $F(2, 507) = 7.79$, $p < .001$, ChEDE Brief Global scores, $F(2, 558) = 3.30$, $p = .038$, and child emotional eating $F(2, 562) = 3.27$, $p = .039$, after controlling for the clustering of children within families. Children born to mothers with an eating disorder history were given solids significantly earlier,

Table 1 Maternal characteristics (mean [SD] unless otherwise indicated) at baseline, by maternal psychiatric group (Ns refer to number of mothers)

	General control (n = 102)	Psychiatric control (n = 36)	Eating disorder (n = 18)
Age	41.38 (5.52)	41.50 (5.39)	38.90 (6.17)
% married or de facto	73.5% (75/102)	58.3% (21/36)	66.7% (12/18)
% low family income	5.9% (6/102)$_a$	22.2% (8/36)$_b$	0% (0/0)$_a$
% completed high school	61.8% (63/102)$_a$	66.7% (24/36)$_a$	27.8% (5/18)$_b$
BMI	25.83 (5.33)	24.97 (4.37)	28.11 (6.47)
Maternal health	3.59 (0.92)$_a$	3.54 (1.01)	3.07 (1.03)$_b$
EDE brief global	0.82 (0.83)$_a$	0.92 (1.35)$_a$	2.05 (1.57)$_b$
DASS depression	1.22 (1.48)$_a$	2.65 (3.95)	6.57 (5.53)$_b$
DASS anxiety	1.01 (1.35)$_a$	2.00 (2.58)	4.80 (4.61)$_b$
DASS stress	3.87 (3.01)	5.56 (3.87)	5.80 (6.34)
Rosenberg self-esteem scale	32.96 (3.82)$_a$	30.50 (4.70)$_b$	28.33 (5.85)$_b$
Family stress – life events scale	1.38 (1.53)	1.45 (1.78)	2.20 (2.70)
Parenting scale	3.03 (0.53)	3.11 (0.58)	3.12 (0.60)
McMaster family functioning scale	1.68 (0.41)	1.59 (0.44)	1.91 (0.26)

Note. Columns with different subscripts are significantly different at $p < .05$ as identified through analysis of variance (continuous variables) or Chi square (categorical variables) comparisons.
BMI = Body Mass Index; EDE = Eating Disorder Examination; DASS = Depression Anxiety Stress Scale.

had significantly higher levels of eating disorder psychopathology (on average from baseline to 2-year follow-up), and were significantly more likely to report emotional eating (on average from baseline to 2-year follow-up) than children born to mothers in the psychiatric disorder and general control groups (see Table 2). In addition, there was a significant main effect of maternal group on the likelihood of mothers reporting slight concern, Wald χ^2 (2) = 6.94, $p = .031$, or moderate-high concern, Wald χ^2 (2) = 14.91, $p = .001$, about their child's weight. Follow-up analyses revealed that mothers in the eating disorder group were more concerned about their child's weight than mothers in the general control group, but did not differ significantly from mothers in the psychiatric control group (see Table 2).

There were no significant effects of maternal group on the age at which breastfeeding stopped, ChEDE Restraint scores, loss of control eating, CDI scores, or SLSS scores (*ps* = .081 - .645). There were trend level, though non-significant, effects of maternal group on child BMI z-score ($p = .051$), SPPC Global self-esteem scores ($p = .052$) and MMIS scores ($p = .057$).

Table 2 summarises baseline information for each of the dependent variables and the identified between-group effects.

Aim 2: Maternal and family predictors of child eating disorder symptoms

ChEDE Brief Global score

Parenting Scale scores, family exposure to stressful life events, maternal depressive, anxiety and stress symptoms, and children's SLSS family satisfaction scores were identified as significant time-varying predictors of ChEDE Brief Global scores in univariate analyses. Baseline maternal concern about child weight and maternal education were identified as significant time invariant predictors. There were no significant interaction effects between time and concern about child weight or between time and maternal education.

When the above variables were entered in a multivariate model with child BMI z-score as a covariate, DASS depression scores, SLSS family satisfaction scores, maternal education, and maternal concern about child weight contributed to the model significantly (see Table 3, Model 1). When the multivariate model was re-run with child depressive symptom and self-esteem scores as additional covariates (Table 3, Model 2), maternal education and maternal concern about child weight continued to predict eating disorder symptoms, but maternal depression and children's family satisfaction did not. Model coefficients showed that ChEDE Brief Global scores were 0.18 points lower, on average over the 2-year period, when mothers had completed high school relative to when they had not. Brief Global scores were 0.64 points higher, on average over the 2-year period, when maternal concern about child weight was moderate-high at baseline relative to minimal (no concern) at baseline. There were no significant interaction effects with child sex (see Table 3).

ChEDE Restraint score

Parenting Scale scores were the only significant time-varying predictor of ChEDE Restraint scores in univariate

Table 2 Child characteristics (mean [SE] unless indicated) at baseline, by maternal psychiatric group (Ns refer to number of children)

	No eating disorder/psychiatric history (n = 154)	Psychiatric history (n = 49)	Eating disorder history (n = 18)
Child BMI z-score	0.67 (0.08)	0.74 (0.14)	1.18 (0.28)
Child gender – % male	47.4% (73/ 154)	44.9% (22/ 49)	54.5% (10/ 18)
	Maternal report variables		
Age started solids (weeks)	21.86 (0.49)$_a$	20.40 (0.88)$_a$	15.96 (1.79)$_b$
Age stopped breastfeeding (weeks)	39.75 (1.66)	36.70 (2.97)	36.09 (6.25)
Child health	4.04 (0.07)	3.95 (0.13)	3.91 (0.25)
Concern for child weight			
% no concern	77.9% (120/154)$_a$	59.2% (29/49)	27.8% (5/18)$_b$
% slight concern	14.9% (23/154)$_a$	26.5% (13/49)	44.4% (8/18)$_b$
% moderate-high concern	7.1% (11/154)$_a$	14.3% (7/49)	27.8% (5/18)$_b$
	Child report variables		
ChEDE brief global	0.52 (0.07)$_a$	0.42 (0.13)$_a$	1.02 (0.27)$_b$
ChEDE restraint	0.24 (0.53)	0.26 (0.65)	0.40 (0.78)
Loss of control eating – %	7.8% (12/ 154)	6.1% (3/ 49)	11.1% (2/ 18)
CARES	0.46 (0.04)$_a$	0.51 (0.08)$_a$	0.78 (0.15)$_b$
CDI	1.77 (0.22)	1.73 (0.41)	2.45 (0.82)
SPPC global	3.32 (0.05)	3.41 (0.09)	3.08 (0.17)
MMIS	1.57 (0.42)	1.51 (0.39)	1.77 (0.46)
SLSS	4.17 (0.06)	4.21 (0.10)	3.96 (0.20)

Note. Columns with different subscripts are significantly different at $p < .05$ as identified through linear mixed models (continuous variables) or generalised estimating equations (categorical variables). Effects apply at baseline and when considering average scores over the full 2-year study period.
BMI = Body Mass Index, ChEDE = Child Eating Disorder Examination, CARES = Children's Affect Regulation Scale, CDI = Child Depression Inventory, SPPC = Self-Perception Profile for Children, MMIS = Multidimensional Media Influences Scale, SLSS = Student's Life Satisfaction Scale.

analyses, and baseline maternal concern about child weight was the only significant time invariant predictor. The interaction between time and concern about child weight was not significant.

When Parenting Scale scores and maternal concern about child weight were entered in a multivariate model with child BMI z-score as a covariate, both remained significant in predicting ChEDE Restraint scores (see Table 3, Model 1). When the multivariate model was re-run with child depressive symptoms and self-esteem scores as additional covariates (Table 3, Model 2), maternal concern about child weight remained significant in predicting ChEDE Restraint but Parenting Scale scores did not. Model coefficients showed that ChEDE Restraint scores were 0.25 points higher, on average over the 2-year period, when maternal concern about child weight was moderate-high at baseline relative to minimal (no concern) at baseline. There were no significant interaction effects with child sex (see Table 3).

Emotional eating

Family exposure to stressful life events and maternal depressive symptoms were identified as significant time-varying predictors of emotional eating in univariate analyses. There were no significant time invariant predictors of emotional eating.

When family stress and maternal depressive symptoms were entered in a multivariate model with child BMI z-score as a covariate, family stress was significant in predicting emotional eating scores in children (Table 3, Model 1). This relationship remained significant when child depressive symptoms and self-esteem scores were added as covariates (Table 3, Model 2). Model coefficients showed that for every stressful event experienced over the 2-year study period, CARES emotional eating scores may be expected to increase by 0.04 over the same time frame. There were no significant interaction effects with child sex (see Table 3).

Loss of control eating

Maternal anxiety symptoms and children's SLSS family satisfaction scores were identified as significant time-varying predictors of loss of control eating in univariate analyses. There were no significant time invariant predictors of loss of control eating.

When maternal anxiety symptoms and children's family satisfaction scores were entered in a multivariate model with child BMI z-score as a covariate, family satisfaction

Table 3 Multivariate models for the longitudinal relationship between maternal and family variables and child eating disorder symptoms

	Model 1		Model 2	
ChEDE brief global	Coefficient (95% CI)	*p*	Coefficient (95% CI)	*p*
Parenting scale	0.01 (−0.12, 0.14)	.875	−0.03 (−0.16, 0.10)	.636
Life events scale	0.01 (−0.04, 0.07)	.562	0.02 (−0.03, 0.07)	.402
DASS depression	0.02 (0.01, 0.04)	.033*	0.02 (−0.01, 0.04)	.094
DASS anxiety	−0.01 (−0.03, 0.01)	.431	−0.02 (−0.04, 0.01)	.121
DASS stress	−0.01 (−0.02, 0.02)	.833	0.01 (−0.01, 0.02)	.645
SLSS family satisfaction	−0.27 (−0.38, −0.16)	<.001**	−0.05 (−0.17, 0.07)	.408
Maternal education (ref: completed high school)				
< High school	0.19 (0.03, 0.35)	.021*	0.18 (0.02, 0.33)	.023*
Concern about child weight (ref: no concern)				
Slight concern	0.01 (−0.19, 0.21)	.931	-.01 (−0.20, 0.18)	.908
Moderate-high concern	0.67 (0.40, 0.93)	<.001**	0.64 (0.39, 0.88)	<.001**
ChEDE restraint scale	Coefficient (95% CI)	*p*	Coefficient (95% CI)	*p*
Parenting scale	0.10 (0.02, 0.18)	.021*	0.07 (−0.01, 0.16)	.100
Concern about child weight (ref: no concern)				
Slight concern	−0.01 (−0.13, 0.13)	.968	−0.02 (−0.16, 0.11)	.745
Moderate-high concern	0.27 (0.11, 0.44)	.001**	0.25 (0.08, 0.41)	.003**
CARES emotional eating	Coefficient (95% CI)	*p*	Coefficient (95% CI)	*p*
Life events scale	0.05 (0.02, 0.08)	.001**	0.04 (0.01, 0.07)	.017*
DASS depression	0.01 (−0.01, 0.02)	.056	0.01 (−0.01, 0.02)	.292
Loss of control eating	Odds ratio (95% CI)	*p*	Odds ratio (95% CI)	*p*
DASS anxiety	1.06 (1.02, 1.14)	.150	1.03 (0.95, 1.12)	.470
SLSS family satisfaction	0.44 (0.29, 0.72)	<.001**	0.56 (0.35, 0.90)	.026*

Note. Models include variables that predicted the outcome significantly in univariate analyses. Model 1 is adjusted for child body mass index (BMI) z-score only. Model 2 is adjusted for child BMI z-score and child depressive symptom and global self-esteem scores. Coefficients show the predicted change in the dependent variable per unit change in the predictor variable, as identified through linear mixed models. Generalised estimating equations were used to determine odds ratios for the categorical outcome of loss of control eating.
$^{*}p < .05$ $^{**}p < .001$.

was significant in predicting loss of control eating (Table 3, Model 1). This relationship remained significant when child depressive symptoms and self-esteem scores were added as covariates (Table 3, Model 2). A 1 point increase in family satisfaction scores over time (equivalent to moving from mildly to moderately satisfied) was associated with a 44% reduction in risk for loss of control eating, although there was some uncertainty around this estimate with 95% confidence intervals suggesting a 10% to 65% reduction in risk (see Table 3). Again, there were no significant interaction effects with child sex.

Discussion

This study aimed to determine whether eating disorder symptoms and psychological well-being would differ significantly across children of mothers with an eating disorder history, children of mothers with a history of another psychiatric disorder, and children of mothers with no past or present eating or psychiatric disorder. In addition, it aimed to identify family factors that could predict increases or decreases in child eating disorder symptoms over time, with attention to the specificity of any identified effects. In final multivariate models, maternal education and maternal concern about child weight were significant in predicting general eating disorder psychopathology; maternal concern about child weight was significant in predicting dietary restraint; family exposure to stressful life events was significant in predicting emotional eating; and children's family satisfaction scores were significant in predicting loss of control eating. Results did not differ significantly across boys and girls.

Partial support was provided for Hypothesis 1. Children in the maternal eating disorder group did score significantly higher on the Brief Global index of eating disorder psychopathology and the CARES index of emotional eating than children in the general and psychiatric control groups. Mothers with a past or present eating disorder also introduced solids significantly earlier than other mothers, and were more concerned about their children's weight. These results are consistent with previous findings (e.g., [6,12]), and were specific to children of mothers with an eating disorder history: children of mothers with another psychiatric disorder were not affected. We found no significant between-group differences for dietary restraint or rates of loss of control eating in children. This may reflect a genuine lack of association between maternal disorders and these offspring behaviours, or stem from the relatively small number of mothers with a past or present eating disorder, combined with relatively low rates of dieting and loss of control eating amongst children. Stein et al. [12] did find higher rates of dieting, as well as heightened weight and shape concerns, in their sample of 10-year-old children born to mothers with an eating disorder. Thus, further research may be required to determine whether dieting is consistently inflated amongst children of mothers past or present eating disorders.

The second phase of analyses provides insight into the mechanisms through which maternal eating disorder history may influence child eating behaviour. Contrary to Hypothesis Two, maternal depressive and anxiety symptoms did not predict child eating disorder symptoms. Maternal eating disorder history and maternal eating disorder symptoms also failed to predict child eating pathology. Instead, the most robust predictor in multivariate models was maternal concern about child weight. In almost all cases (>90%), this concern was in relation to perceived child overweight rather than underweight. Parent-perceived child overweight also emerged as a significant risk factor for adolescent eating disorders in a separate Australian study [82], lending support to the generalizability of these findings. In this study, it deserves note that maternal concern about child weight was relatively stable across the study period, and baseline levels did not predict subsequent *changes* in child eating disorder symptoms. Instead, baseline maternal concern was significant in predicting children's eating disorder symptoms on average over the next 2 years. Children of mothers who were concerned about their weight at baseline had consistently high levels of weight and shape concern and dietary restraint over the next 2 years.

Maternal education was an additional baseline predictor of Brief Global ChEDE scores, such that children of mothers who had not completed high school had higher levels of eating disorder psychopathology across the 2-year study period than children of mothers who had completed high school. Maternal education may be a marker of general socio-demographic status, whereby children from more disadvantaged or 'resource poor' families are more vulnerable to heightened weight and shape concerns. Alternatively, mothers who do not complete high school may differ from other mothers in their capacity to model healthy eating and body image messages, and/or in the emphasis they place on weight and shape. Further research is needed to address these possibilities, and to elucidate the mechanisms through which maternal education may influence child eating disorder psychopathology. It is interesting to note that, in this sample, media influences regarding the thin-ideal were not significant in predicting children's eating disorder symptoms. This suggests that family factors may be more important than media influences in accounting for eating disorder features in this age group. With adolescent samples, some studies have found family, peer and personality factors to be more important than media influences in predicting eating disorder symptoms [83,84], whilst other data suggest that family and media influences are more important than peer factors [16]. Regardless of age, it seems important that studies on media influences and eating pathology also attend to family predictors.

Two variables predicted changes in child eating disorder symptoms over time. Consistent with Hypothesis 3, child-reported family satisfaction was a significant protective factor for loss of control eating, with increases in SLSS scores over time predicting decreases in vulnerability to loss of control eating. This relationship applied even after child BMI z-score and general psychological distress were accounted for. Increases in SLSS scores over time were also significant in predicting decreases in children's Brief Global ChEDE scores over the same time period, but this relationship ceased to reach statistical significance after adjusting for child psychological distress. These results highlight the potential benefits of family support in protecting against child and adolescent eating disorder symptoms, particularly loss of control eating. Research with adolescents has also linked positive family relationships to lower rates of adolescent dieting [31,34], a finding not observed here. This difference may stem from cross-study variation in the age of participants (late childhood / early adolescence for the current sample, versus later adolescence in prior reports) and/or in the assessment approach used. In this research, the ChEDE was used to assess a mix of dietary restriction (actual restriction of eating) and restraint (intent to restrict eating) over the past month. Previous studies have tended to rely on single item assessing self-reported dieting frequency in the past year [31,34], which may capture a different type of behaviour. Ongoing attention to the potential protective benefits of positive family relationships, and their impact on different eating disorder symptoms over adolescence, seems warranted.

Family stress was also a significant longitudinal predictor of emotional eating. The magnitude of this effect was small, with 25 stressful events in 2 years being required to predict an increase in emotional eating from "sometimes" to "often" on the CARES scale. Nonetheless, emotional eating may be understood as a coping mechanism for children who are exposed to repeated or pronounced stressful events over time. Exposure to stressful life events has also been linked to the development of binge eating disorder [85], and found to precipitate and maintain emotional eating in adolescent [86] and adult [87] samples. To our knowledge, this is the first study to identify a prospective association between family exposure to stress and increases in emotional eating in childhood.

There are four main implications arising from these results. First, maternal concern about child weight appears to be a strong predictor of child eating disorder symptoms, even after objective body weight and general child psychological distress are adjusted for. Thus, interventions designed to prevent or reduce child eating pathology may benefit from targeting mother's concerns about, and attitudes towards, their children's weight. This may need to occur early in childhood as, in the current study, mothers' levels of concern about their child(ren)'s weight were already stable, tracking from middle childhood onwards.

Second, family satisfaction may be a protective factor for loss of control eating. The transition to adolescence is a high risk time for eating disorder onset and a period of changing family dynamics, with children starting to individuate and develop an identity autonomous from their family. Working to enhance family support and relationships during this period may be beneficial for eating disorder prevention.

Third, family stress and low maternal education may increase risk for emotional eating and weight and shape concerns, respectively. Accordingly, children who experience repeated exposure to family stress and children of mothers who did not complete high school education may benefit from additional support during their adolescent years. As noted, there is also a need for more research to identify the mechanisms through which low maternal education may influence child eating disorder symptoms.

Fourth, maternal eating disorder symptoms and general maternal psychological distress do not predict child eating disorder symptoms when other family and child variables are accounted for. This is important, because these features have traditionally been viewed as risk factors for child eating pathology and may distract from family variables that genuinely do serve as a marker of risk.

This study has a number of strengths. The use of interview-based measures to assess eating disorder symptoms provides support for the validity of the data, and the longitudinal design allows issues of causality to be considered. Additional advantages include the use of general and psychiatric control participants; the use of mother and child report data; and consideration of gender differences in the effects of maternal and family factors. The study also has limitations, including the reliance on self-report data for determining maternal psychiatric disorders and past maternal eating disorders, the small number of mothers in the eating disorder group, participant attrition over time, and the use of single-item measures for some constructs. Although all mothers stated that they had been diagnosed or treated for a psychiatric condition or eating disorder, information on the validity of those diagnoses was not available. Moreover, women who did not wish to disclose a psychiatric history, and those who did not seek diagnosis or treatment for psychiatric difficulties, would not have been identified in this study. If larger group sizes were available, it would be beneficial for past and current maternal eating disorders to be distinguished, along with different eating disorder diagnoses. Finally, families with lower maternal education and greater exposure to stress at baseline were more likely to be lost to follow-up. As maternal education and family stress predicted eating disorder symptoms in children, efforts should be made to try and retain families with these characteristics in future studies of this nature. For the current research, effect estimates for these predictor variables may be conservative in nature.

Conclusions

This study has provided insight into associations between maternal and family factors and child eating disorder symptoms, with attention to the relative importance of different maternal and family predictors and the specificity of identified effects. Consistent with previous findings, children of mothers with a current or past eating disorder reported significantly higher levels of some eating disorder symptoms than other children, and mothers with a current or past eating disorder reported significantly more concern about their children's weight than other mothers. Maternal concern about child weight, rather than maternal eating disorder symptoms, was significant in predicting child eating disorder symptoms. Other family variables of importance included children's level of family satisfaction, family exposure to stress, and maternal education.

Abbreviations

ALSPAC: Avon longitudinal study of parents and children; BMI: Body mass index; CARES: Children's affect regulation scale; ChEDE: Child eating disorder examination; CDI: Child depression inventory; DASS: Depression anxiety stress scale; EDE: Eating disorder examination; GAD Study: Childhood growth and development study; MoBa: Norwegian Mother and Child Cohort Study; MMIS: Multidimensional media influences scale; RSES: Rosenberg self-esteem scale; SLSS: Students' life satisfaction scale; SPPC: Self-perception profile for children.

Competing interests
The authors declare that they have no competing interests.

Authors' contributions
ED and SB contributed to the design of the Childhood Growth and Development Study. KA, LG, ED and SB collected data for the Childhood Growth and Development Study. KA, NM and SB designed the current research study. KA performed the statistical analyses and drafted the manuscript. All authors read and approved the final manuscript.

Acknowledgments
We are extremely grateful to the schools, children and parents who gave their time to participate in the Childhood Growth and Development Study, and to all staff who contributed to the running of the study. We would like to acknowledge Felicity Watt, Dr Katie Suriano and Dr Deborah Blumberg for their contributions to data collection.
The Childhood Growth and Development Study was funded by Healthway and the Raine Medical Foundation. The first author is supported by an early career research fellowship from the National Health and Medical Research Council (NHMRC) of Australia.

Author details
[1]Telethon Institute for Child Health Research, Centre for Child Health Research, The University of Western Australia, PO Box 855, West Perth, WA, Australia. [2]School of Psychology, The University of Western Australia, Crawley, WA, Australia. [3]Department of Endocrinology and Diabetes, Princess Margaret Hospital for Children, Subiaco, Australia.

References

1. Le Grange D, Lock J, Loeb KL, Nicholls D: **Academy for eating disorders position paper: the role of the family in eating disorders.** *Int J Eat Disord* 2010, **43:**1–5.
2. Campbell IC, Mill J, Uher R, Schmidt U: **Eating disorders, gene-environment interactions and epigenetics.** *Neurosci Biobehav Rev* 2011, **35:**784–793.
3. Patel P, Wheatcroft R, Park RJ, Stein A: **The children of mothers with eating disorders.** *Clin Child Fam Psychol Rev* 2002, **5:**1–19.
4. Schmidt U, Humfress H, Treasure J: **The role of general family environment and sexual and physical abuse in the origins of eating disorders.** *Eur Eat Disord Rev* 1997, **5:**184–207.
5. Johnson JG, Cohen P, Kasen S, Brook JS: **Childhood adversities associated with risk for eating disorders or weight problems during adolescence or early adulthood.** *Am J Psychiatry* 2002, **159:**394–400.
6. Agras WS, Hammer LD, McNicholas F: **A prospective study of the influence of eating-disordered mothers on their children.** *Int J Eat Disord* 1999, **25:**253–262.
7. Stice E, Agras SW, Hammer LD: **Risk factors for the emergence of childhood eating disturbances: a five-year prospective study.** *Int J Eat Disord* 1999, **25:**375–387.
8. Koubaa S, Hällstrom T, Hirschberg AL: **Early maternal adjustment in women with eating disorders.** *Int J Eat Disord* 2008, **41:**405–410.
9. Waugh E, Bulik CM: **Offspring of women with eating disorders.** *Int J Eat Disord* 1999, **25:**123–133.
10. Reba-Harreleson L, Von Holle A, Hamer RM, Torgersen L, Reichborn-Kjennerud T, Bulik CM: **Patterns of maternal feeding and child eating associated with eating disorders in the Norwegian mother and child cohort study (MoBa).** *Eat Behav* 2010, **11:**54–61.
11. Micali N, Simonoff E, Treasure J: **Infant feeding and weight in the first year of life in babies of women with eating disorders.** *J Pediatr* 2009, **154:**55–60.
12. Stein A, Woolley H, Cooper S, Winterbottom J, Fairburn CG, Cortina-Borja M: **Eating habits and attitudes among 10-year-old children of mothers with eating disorders: longitudinal study.** *Br J Psychiatry* 2006, **189:**324–329.
13. Hill AJ, Weaver C, Blundell JE: **Dieting concerns of 10-year-old girls and their mothers.** *Br J Clin Psychol* 1990, **29:**346–348.
14. Edmunds H, Hill AJ: **Dieting and the family context of eating in young adolescent children.** *Int J Eat Disord* 1999, **25:**435–440.
15. Linville D, Stice E, Gau J, O'Neil M: **Predictive effects of mother and peer influences on increases in adolescent eating disorder risk factors and symptoms: a 3-year longitudinal study.** *Int J Eat Disord* 2011, **44:**745–751.
16. Field AE, Camargo CAJ, Taylor CB, Berkey CS, Roberts SB, Colditz GA: **Peer, parent and media influences on the development of weight concerns and frequent dieting among preadolescent and adolescent girls and boys.** *Pediatrics* 2001, **107:**54–60.
17. McCabe MP, Ricciardelli LA: **A prospective study of pressures from parents, peers, and the media on extreme weight change behaviors among adolescent boys and girls.** *Behav Res Ther* 2005, **43:**653–668.
18. Field AE, Javaras KM, Aneja P, Kitos N, Camargo CA, Taylor CB, Laird NM: **Family, peer, and media predictors of becoming eating disordered.** *Arch Pediatr Adolesc Med* 2008, **162:**574–579.
19. Helfert S, Warschburger P: **A prospective study on the impact of peer and parental pressure on body dissatisfaction in adolescent girls and boys.** *Body Image* 2011, **8:**101–109.
20. Neumark-Sztainer D, Bauer KW, Friend S, Hannan PJ, Story M, Berge JM: **Family weight talk and dieting: how much do they matter for body dissatisfaction and disordered eating behaviors in adolescent girls?** *J Adolesc Health* 2010, **47:**270–276.
21. Davis C, Shuster B, Blackmore E, Fox J: **Looking good- family focus on appearance and the risk for eating disorders.** *Int J Eat Disord* 2004, **35:**136–144.
22. Farrow CV, Blissett J: **Do obsessive compulsive symptoms mediate the relationship between maternal eating psychopathology and restrictive feeding practices?** *Int J Eat Disord* 2009, **42:**76–80.
23. Smolak L, Levine MP, Schermer F: **Parental input and weight concerns among elementary school children.** *Int J Eat Disord* 1999, **25:**263–271.
24. Peterson KA, Paulson SE, Williams KK: **Relations of eating disorder symptomology with perceptions of pressures from mother, peers, and media in adolescent girls and boys.** *Sex Roles* 2007, **56:**629–639.
25. Phares V, Steinberg AR, Thompson JK: **Gender differences in peer and parental Influences: body image disturbance, self-worth, and psychological functioning in preadolescent children.** *J Youth Adolesc* 2004, **33:**421–429.
26. Stice E: **Risk and maintenance factors for eating pathology: a meta-analytic review.** *Psychol Bull* 2002, **128:**825–848.
27. Reichborn-Kjennerud T, Bulik CM, Tambs K, Harris JR: **Genetic and environmental influences on binge eating in the absence of compensatory behaviors: a population-based twin study.** *Int J Eat Disord* 2004, **36:**307–314.
28. Micali N, Simonoff E, Stahl D, Treasure J: **Maternal eating disorders and infant feeding difficulties: maternal and child mediators in a longitudinal general population study.** *J Child Psychol Psychiatry* 2011, **52:**800–807.
29. Beato-Fernandez L, Rodriguez-Cano T, Belmonte-Llario A, Martinez-Delgado C: **Risk factors for eating disorders in adolescents: a Spanish community-based longitudinal study.** *Eur Child Adolesc Psychiatry* 2004, **13:**287–294.
30. Moorhead DJ, Stashwick CK, Reinherz HZ, Giaconia RM, Streigel-Moore RM, Paradis AD: **Child and adolescent predictors for eating disorders in a community population of young adult women.** *Int J Eat Disord* 2003, **33:**1–9.
31. Berge JM, Wall M, Larson N, Eisenberg ME, Loth KA, Neumark-Sztainer D: **The unique and additive associations of family functioning and parenting practices with disordered eating behaviors in diverse adolescents.** *J Behav Med* 2014, **37:**205–217.
32. May AL, Kim JY, McHale SM, Crouter AC: **Parent-adolescent relationships and the development of weight concerns from early to late adolescence.** *Int J Eat Disord* 2006, **39:**729–740.
33. Fonseca H, Ireland M, Resnick MD: **Familial correlates of extreme weight control behaviors among adolescents.** *Int J Eat Disord* 2002, **32:**441–448.
34. Haines J, Kleinman KP, Rifas-Shiman SL, Field AE, Austin B: **Examination of shared risk and protective factors for overweight and disordered eating among adolescents.** *Arch Pediatr Adolesc Med* 2010, **164:**336–343.
35. Viner RM, Ozer EM, Denny S, Marmot M, Resnick M, Fatusi A, Currie C: **Adolescence and the social determinants of health.** *Lancet* 2012, **379:**1641–1652.
36. Belsky J, Pluess M: **Beyond diathesis stress: differential susceptibility to environmetal influences.** *Psychol Bull* 2009, **135:**885–908.
37. Micali N, Stahl D, Treasure J, Simonoff E: **Childhood psychopathology in children of women with eating disorders: understanding risk mechanisms.** *J Child Psychol Psychiatry* 2013, **2013:** In press.

38. Allen KL, Byrne SM, Blair EM, Davis EA: **Why do some overweight children experience psychological problems? The role of weight and shape concern.** *Int J Pediatr Obes* 2006, **1**:239–247.
39. Allen KL, Byrne SM, McLean NJ, Davis EA: **Overconcern with weight and shape is not the same as body dissatisfaction: evidence from a prospective study of pre-adolescent boys and girls.** *Body Image* 2008, **5**:261–270.
40. Gibson LY, Byrne SM, Jacoby P, Davis E: **The role of family and maternal factors in childhood obesity.** *Med J Aust* 2007, **186**:591–595.
41. Tanner JM: *Growth at adolescence.* Springfield: Charles C Thomas; 1962.
42. Brooks-Gunn J, Warren MP, Rosso J, Gargiulo J: **Validity of self-report measures of girls' pubertal status.** *Child Dev* 1987, **58**:829–841.
43. Duke PM, Lit IF, Gross RT: **Adolescents' self-assessment of sexual maturation.** *Pediatrics* 1980, **66**:918–920.
44. Fairburn CG, Cooper Z: **The Eating Disorder Examination.** In *Binge eating: Nature, assessment and treatment.* 12th edition. Edited by Fairburn CG, Wilson GT. New York: Guilford Press; 1993:317–360.
45. Bryant-Waugh RJ, Cooper PJ, Taylor CL, Lask BD: **The use of the eating disorder examination with children: a pilot study.** *Int J Eat Disord* 1996, **19**:391–397.
46. Allen KL, Byrne SM, McLean NJ: **The dual-pathway and cognitive-behavioural models of binge eating: prospective evaluation and comparison.** *Eur Child Adolesc Psychiatry* 2012, **21**:51–62.
47. Byrne SM, Allen KL, Lampard AM, Dove ER, Fursland A: **The factor structure of the eating disorder examination in clinical and community samples.** *Int J Eat Disord* 2010, **43**:260–265.
48. Jongenelis MI, Byrne SM, Pettigrew S, Allen KL, Watts F: **A psychometric examination of a modified 8-item version of the children's eating disorder examination.** *Psychol Assess* 2014, In press.
49. Tanofsky-Kraff M, Marcus MD, Yanovski SZ, Yanovski JA: **Loss of control eating disorder in children age 12 years and younger: proposed research criteria.** *Eat Behav* 2008, **9**:257–380.
50. Luce KH, Crowther JH: **The reliability of the eating disorder examination-self-report questionnaire version (EDE-Q).** *Int J Eat Disord* 1999, **25**:349–351.
51. Grilo CM, Masheb RM, Lozano-Blanco C, Barry DT: **Reliability of the eating disorder examination in patients with binge eating disorder.** *Int J Eat Disord* 2004, **35**:80–85.
52. Guest T: **Using the eating disorder examination in the assessment of bulimia and anorexia: issues of reliability and validity.** *Soc Work Health Care* 2000, **31**:71–83.
53. Rizvi SL, Peterson CB, Crow SJ, Agras SW: **Test-retest reliability of the eating disorder examination.** *Int J Eat Disord* 2000, **28**:311–316.
54. Epstein NB, Baldwin LM, Bishop DS: **The McMaster family assessment device.** *J Marital Fam Ther* 1983, **9**:171–180.
55. Georgiades K, Boyle MH, Jenkins JM, Sanford M, Lipman E: **A multilevel analysis of whole family functioning using the McMaster family assessment device.** *J Fam Psychol* 2008, **22**:344–354.
56. Byles J, Byrne C, Boyle MH, Offord DR: **Ontario child health study: reliability and validity of the general functioning subscale of the McMaster family assessment device.** *Fam Process* 1988, **27**:97–104.
57. McDermott BM, Batik M, Roberts L, Gibbon P: **Parent and child report of family functioning in a clinical child and adolescent eating disorders sample.** *Aust N Z J Psychiatry* 2002, **36**:509–514.
58. Heubner ES: **Preliminary development and validation of a multidimensional life satisfaction scale for children.** *Psychol Assess* 1994, **6**:149–158.
59. Huebner E, Laughlin JE, Ash C, Gilman R: **Further validation of the multidimensional students' life satisfaction scale.** *J Psychoeduc Assess* 1998, **16**:118–134.
60. Greenspoon PJ, Saklofske DH: **Validity and reliability of the multidimensional students' life satisfaction scale with Canadian children.** *J Psychoeduc Assess* 1997, **15**:138–155.
61. Arnold DS, O'Leary SG, Wolff LS, Acker MM: **The parenting scale: a measure of dysfunctional parenting in discipline situations.** *Psychol Assess* 1993, **5**:137–144.
62. Arney F, Rogers H, Baghurst P, Sawyer M, Prior M: **The reliability and validity of the parenting scale for Australian mothers of preschool-aged children.** *Aust J Psychol* 2008, **60**:44–52.
63. Rhoades KA, O'Leary SG: **Factor structure and validity of the parenting scale.** *J Clin Child Adolesc Psychol* 2007, **36**:137–146.
64. Brugha T, Bebbington P, Tennant C, Hurry J: **The list of threatening experiences: a subset of 12 life event categories with considerable long-term contextual threat.** *Psychol Med* 1985, **15**:189–194.
65. Wagner C, Abela JR, Brozina K: **A comparison of stress measures in children and adolescents: a self-report checklist versus an objectively rated interview.** *J Psychopathol Behav Assess* 2006, **28**:251–261.
66. Brugha T, Cragg D: **The list of threatening experiences: the reliability and validity of a brief life events questionnaire.** *Acta Psychiatr Scand* 1990, **82**:77–81.
67. McQuaid JR, Monroe SM, Roberts JE, Johnson SL, Garamoni DJ, Kupfer DJ, Frank E: **Toward the standardization of life stress assessment: definitional discrepancies and inconsistencies in methods.** *Stress Med* 1992, **8**:47–56.
68. Lovibond SH, Lovibond PF: *Manual for the Depression Anxiety Stress Scales.* 2nd edition. Sydney: Psychology Foundation; 1995.
69. Antony MM, Bieling PJ, Cox BJ, Enns MW, Swinson RP: **Psychometric properties of the 42-item and 21-item versions of the depression anxiety stress scales in clinical groups and a community sample.** *Psychol Assess* 1998, **10**:176–181.
70. Gloster AT, Rhoades HM, Novy D, Klotsche J, Senior A, Kunik M, Wilson N, Stanley MA: **Psychometric properties of the depression anxiety and stress scale-21 in older primary care patients.** *J Affect Disord* 2008, **110**:248–259.
71. Henry JD, Crawford JR: **The short-form versions of the depression anxiety stress scales (DASS-21): construct validity and normative data in a large non-clinical sample.** *Br J Clin Psychol* 2005, **44**:227–239.
72. Norton PJ: **Depression anxiety and stress scales (DASS-21): psychometric analysis across four racial groups.** *Anxiety Stress Coping* 2007, **20**:253–265.
73. Rosenberg M: *Society and the adolescent self-image (revised).* Princeton, CT: Princeton University Press; 1989.
74. Robins RW, Hendin HM, Trzesniewski KH: **Measuring global self-esteem: construct validation of a single-item measure and the rosenberg self-esteem scale.** *Pers Soc Psychol Bull* 2001, **27**:151–161.
75. Shevlin ME, Bunting BP, Lewis CA: **Confirmatory factor analysis of the Rosenberg self-esteem scale.** *Psychol Rep* 1995, **76**:707–710.
76. Kovacs M: *The Child Depression Inventory (CDI) manual.* Toronto, Canada: Multi Health Systems; 1992.
77. Harter S: *Manual for the Self-Perception Profile for Children.* Denver, CO: University of Denver; 1985.
78. Muris P, Meesters C, Fijen P: **The self-perception profile for children: further evidence for its factor structure, reliability, and validity.** *Pers Individ Dif* 2003, **35**:1791–1802.
79. Cusumano DL, Thompson JK: **Media influence and body image in 8–11-year-old boys and girls: a preliminary report on the multidimensional media influence scale.** *Int J Eat Disord* 2001, **29**:37–44.
80. Ogden CL, Kuczmarski RJ, Flegal KM, Mei Z, Guo S, Wei R, Grummer-Strawn LM, Curtin LR, Roche AF, Johnson CL: **Centers for disease control and prevention 2000 growth charts for the United States: improvements to the 1977 National Center for Health Statistics version.** *Pediatrics* 2002, **109**:45–60.
81. Aiken LS, West SG: *Multiple regression: Testing and interpreting interactions.* Newbury Park, CA: Sage; 1991.
82. Allen KL, Byrne SM, Forbes D, Oddy WH: **Risk factors for full- and partial-syndrome early adolescent eating disorders: a population-based pregnancy cohort study.** *J Am Acad Child Adolesc Psychiatry* 2009, **48**:800–809.
83. Ferguson CJ, Munoz ME, Winegard B, Winegard B: **The influence of heritability, neuroticism, maternal warmth and media use on disordered eating behaviors: a prospective analysis of twins.** *Psychiatr Q* 2012, **83**:353–360.
84. Ferguson CJ, Munoz ME, Garza A, Galindo M: **Concurrent and prospective analyses of peer, television and social media influences on body dissatisfaction, eating disorder symptoms and life satisfaction in adolescent girls.** *J Youth Adolesc* 2013, In press.
85. Striegel-Moore RH, Dohm FA, Kraemer HC, Schreiber GB, Taylor CB, Daniels SR: **Risk factors for binge-eating disorders: an exploratory study.** *Int J Eat Disord* 2007, **40**:481–487.
86. Nguyen-Rodriguez ST, Chou C-P, Unger JB, Spruijt-Metz D: **BMI as a moderator of perceived stress and emotional eating in adolescents.** *Eat Behav* 2008, **9**:238–246.
87. Adam TC, Epel ES: **Stress, eating and the reward system.** *Physiol Behav* 2007, **91**:449–458.

Factors impacting treatment and recovery in Anorexia Nervosa: qualitative findings from an online questionnaire

Sarah Fogarty[1,2*] and Lucie M. Ramjan[3,4]

Abstract

Background: Anorexia nervosa (AN) is characterised by restriction of energy intake, fear of gaining weight and severe disturbances in weight or shape. Recovery from AN is a complicated and often multifaceted experience that can take many years to achieve. Qualitative research has found that support, being understood, hope, desire for recovery, positive experiences in treatment, self-efficacy, motivation and relationships are important in recovery from AN. The experience of treatment for patients with an eating disorder is an important aspect of recovery with the potential to enhance recovery or hinder it. The aim of the questionnaire was to better understand factors impacting the care experiences during treatment and or recovery from self-reported Anorexia Nervosa (AN).

Method: An online questionnaire was developed and administered to past or current sufferers of Anorexia Nervosa, ≥18 years of age. Participants were recruited through eating disorder organisations both in Australia and the United Kingdom. The questionnaire was a mixture of quantitative and qualitative questions. The quantitative data was analysed using descriptive statistics and the qualitative data was analysed using conventional content analysis (CCA).

Results: Of those who responded, most currently experienced self-reported AN. The quantitative results identified that most participants had trust and confidence in their health care provider and felt listened to and supported yet on the subject of the suitability of treatment this had varied opinions. Being understood, hope (life after AN) and self-acceptance were considered the top three important factors in the treatment and recovery from Anorexia Nervosa. The qualitative results revealed the factors hindering or benefiting treatment and recovery, and individuals' needs during the four phases of recovery.

Conclusion: Factors were identified that could either hinder or benefit treatment and recovery and these included whether treatment supported the individual to cope with change, whether the individual found the treatment to be appropriate for their personal needs and whether treatment addressed underlying factors. Individuals' needs differed during the four phases of recovery. The findings of the study may help treatment providers address key factors involved in recovery at the right stage of treatment however by the nature of the qualitative methodology conclusions are putative and further definitive research is indicated.

Keywords: Anorexia nervosa, Treatment, Recovery

* Correspondence: s.fogarty@westernsydney.edu.au
[1]School of Medicine, Western Sydney University, Richmond, Australia
[2]National Institute of Complementary Medicine, Western Sydney University, PO Box 2002, Homebush West, NSW 2140, Australia
Full list of author information is available at the end of the article

Background

Anorexia nervosa (AN) is a mental illness which is characterised by restriction of energy intake, fear of gaining weight and severe disturbances in weight or shape [1]. Recovery from AN is a complicated and often multifaceted experience that can take many years to achieve [2]. Research into recovery has commonly employed a qualitative methodology however a small number of researchers have used quantitative methods to explore recovery from AN. Support, being understood, hope, desire for recovery, positive experiences in treatment, self-efficacy, motivation and relationships are the quantitative themes that have been identified as important in recovery from AN [3–8].

The experience of treatment for patients with an eating disorder is an important aspect of recovery with the potential to enhance recovery [3] or hinder it [9]. Patients diagnosed with AN entering a treatment program may encounter difficulties including facing the challenges of changing unhealthy eating behaviors [10, 11]. The challenges of changing unhealthy eating behaviors is often complicated by patients displaying an ambivalence to making changes related to eating behaviors [10, 11]. Long-term exposure to eating disorder pathology and repeated failed attempts at reducing eating disorder symptoms may lead to an increase in ambivalence and a sense of hopelessness (from the patient as well as the clinician/therapist perspective), creating even more barriers to attaining healthy eating behaviors. Recent research has identified and categorised four phases involved in the recovery process; Unable and/or unready to change, Tipping point of change, Active pursuit of recovery and, Reflection and rehabilitation [4]. Given the influence of the treatment experience in recovery, understanding what is considered reliable and efficient treatment, is particularly important. Understanding the needs of AN sufferers during the different phases of recovery is an emerging area of research and a more in-depth understanding of AN patients' experience of care in each of these phases is needed. Using an explorative qualitative methodology the paper aimed to better understand the care experience during treatment for AN in individuals with self-reported AN or recovery from AN".

Method

The treatment experiences questionnaire specifically examined the therapeutic relationship and care experience during treatment for AN. Ethical approval was obtained from the University of Western Sydney's Human Research and Ethics Committee (HREC), H10825.

Questionnaire development

The authors developed an anonymous questionnaire, which consisted of 30-items and, included 14 closed questions and 16 open-ended questions. The open-ended items encouraged written responses on individuals' personal experience of care during the treatment of AN. Questions were included to elicit responses to the therapeutic relationships encountered and the care received during treatment for AN. Recent research revealed there are four phases in the recovery process: Unable and/or unready to change, Tipping point of change, Active pursuit of recovery and, Reflection and Rehabilitation [4]. There were a number of questions in the questionnaire that elicited a response about care encountered during these four stages.

The questionnaire used a purposive sampling technique which aims to recruit those who have particular expertise in the relevant topic of interest [12]. The sample in this case was recovered or recovering individuals with AN.

Patient sample and procedure

The survey was completed online. A number of eating disorder associations including The Butterfly Foundation, BEAT UK (Beat Eating Disorders) and the Centre of Excellence for Eating Disorders advertised the study and provided a link to the online questionnaire. Sites advertised the study for a period of nine months. The questionnaire was anonymous. Inclusion criteria included being 18 years of age or over and having self-reported AN or having recovered from self-reported AN. Exclusion criteria included not being able to read and write in English. One hundred and sixty-eight individuals with self-reported AN consented to participate in the online questionnaire. Of the 168, seven agreed to participate but did not complete any questions thus 161 participants completed a combination of some to all of

Table 1 Demographics of participants

Demographic Questions	Completed	% Answered
Completed	68 ($n = 142$)	47.89
Age		
Mean	25.11	
SD	6.44	
eOccupation		
Full time student	20	41.18
Employed	27	44.11
Other [a]	5	7.35
Place of Birth	$n = 67$	
Australia	29	
United Kingdom	26	
Other [b]	12	

[a] part time student/employed, homemaker, unemployed
[b] Scotland, Wales, Northern Ireland, United States of America, Canada, New Zealand, Italy, Africa, Germany, Portugal

the questions. The 46.6 % of participants that answered the gender and age questions, were all women, average age 25.8 years ± 7.0 and the majority were students. One responder mentioned they were male but did not answer the gender question. No responder identified as an Aboriginal or Torres Straight Islander. See Table 1 for demographic details.

Accessing participants in both the UK and Australia was chosen to increase study participant numbers, taking into consideration ethics and similarities in treatments. The 'standard' treatment offered for Anorexia Nervosa is similar with both the UK and Australia utilising a multidimensional treatment approach, addressing the physical, psychological, psychosocial and family needs of the individual. Treatment can include psychiatrists, psychologists, primary care physicians, social workers, nurses and dieticians [13, 14]. In general both countries have similar treatment aims; to restore the individual's weight within a normal range for their height and age, to reduce abnormal eating behaviours, and weight and shape cognitions, and manage co-morbidities (both mental and physical) [13, 14]. In both the UK and Australia we were able to provide contact details for support services should any study participants experience distress.

Data analysis

Descriptive statistics were used to analyse demographic data such as overall sample size, demographic characteristics (location, age) and the responses to the closed questions. Data were analysed using Microsoft Excel for Mac, version 14.4.7.

The responses to the open-ended questions was analysed using a *Conventional Content Analysis* (CCA) technique [15]. The CCA approach allows the analysis (categories and names for the categories) to be derived directly from the text data, rather than being preconceived [15]. The purpose of CCA is to identify patterns in textual material. CCA is a dynamic form of textual analysis which summarises the informational content of data [16].

The first author read all the survey responses multiple times to achieve immersion [15]. Responses were then read in depth and frequently repeated words (e.g. understanding) denoting main views on treatment and recovery were manually circled on hard copy data extracts. First impressions of data were noted and formed the basis of development of 'Sub Categories' for grouping into main 'Categories' [15]. A quasi-statistical analysis style was used to determine a hierarchical summary of the 'important features of recovery and treatment' based on the frequency of views expressed [16]. Associations and relationships within sub categories and categories were identified and where relevant they were combined into a smaller number of sub categories and categories which reflected the perceptions of the individuals with AN [15]. The first author coded and analysed all questionnaire data. Results were checked by the second author to determine if categories and subcategories were mutual. Any differences were discussed until consensus was reached.

Results

Sixty-eight (42.5 %) of the responders currently had self-reported AN and over 97 % received some form of treatment (either inpatient or outpatient care or a combination of both inpatient and outpatient care or another version of care) (See Table 2). The majority or responders felt they were treated well ($n = 64$), able to trust and had confidence in their treatment providers ($n = 93$) and felt that their treatment providers listened and understood their issues ($n = 100$). The appropriateness of the treatment program was mixed with some responders feeling that treatment was suitable ($n = 55$) and others feeling it did not suit them ($n = 63$). The majority of responders felt they were unready and or unable to change when they sought treatment ($n = 62$). Being understood, hope (possibility of life after AN), and self-acceptance were all viewed as important factors in the treatment of AN.

Results of the open-ended questions

The open-ended questions addressed two main areas: factors hindering or benefiting treatment and recovery and identifying what was needed during the four phases of recovery.

> The three themes that were seen to both hinder and contribute to recovery were: *1) supporting a person to cope with change* (*subthemes of hope, being listened to and understood, and empowerment/disempowerment*), 2) *treatment suitability and*, 3) *treat underlying factors.*

Supporting a person to cope with change

The treatment experience impacted on the individuals' perception of support with treatment either providing support for the patient to change and benefiting recovery or not providing support for change and disempowering the individual and hindering recovery. The elements of treatment that contributed to participants experiencing support included hopefulness, being listened to and understood, having input into recovery, increased self-worth and learning new skills and coping mechanisms. These elements contributed to make the individuals with AN feel stronger and more confident, especially in controlling their AN and facing the challenges that 'recovery' entails.

Table 2 Quantitative Results

Question 1. How long ago did you have Anorexia Nervosa (AN)? (*n* = 154, 100.00 %)		%
Have it now	63	40.91
Less than 12 months ago	20	12.99
12 months to less than 2 years ago	11	7.14
2 years to less than 5 years ago	23	14.94
5 years to less than 10 years ago	20	12.99
Greater than 10 years ago	15	9.74
Other	2	1.30
Question 2. What type of treatment did you receive for your AN? (*n* = 153, 99.35 %)		%
Combination of both (in and out patient)	77	50.33
In-patient	14	9.15
Outpatient	53	34.64
Other	9	5.88
Question 3a. How well were you treated when you first sought treatment? (*n* = 133, 86.36 %)		%
I was treated well	64	48.12
I was not treated so well	57	42.86
No opinion	12	9.02
Question 3b. How suitable is/was the treatment program for you? (*n* = 133, 86.36 %)		
It has suited me	55	41.35
It did not suit me	63	47.37
No opinion	15	11.28
Question 3c. Do you think your treatment providers have been able to listen and understand the things you have brought up during treatment? (*n* = 133, 86.36 %)		
Yes, to a great extent	33	25.00
Yes to some extent	67	50.76
No	32	24.24
Question 3d. Did/Do you feel trust and confidence in the treatment providers? (*n* = 133, 86.36 %)		
Yes, to a great extent	33	24.81
Yes to some extent	60	45.11
No, not sufficiently	40	30.08
Question 3e. Are/Were you and the treatment providers in agreement about the goals of your treatment? (*n* = 132, 85.71 %)		
Yes, to a great extent	30	22.72
Yes to some extent	72	54.55
No	30	22.72
Question 4. Please indicate which phase you believed you were in when you sought treatment (multiple answers allowed) (*n* = 93, 60.39 %)		
Unready and or unable to change	62	67.39
The Tipping point of change	37	43.53
Active pursuit of recovery	26	30.59
Reflection and rehabilitation	5	5.88

Table 2 Quantitative Results *(Continued)*

Question 7. Research has identified key themes of recovery factors in AN. Please indicate which factors you feel are important in the treatment of AN (multiple answers allowed) (*n* = 93, 60.39 %)		
Being Understood	71	76.34
Self-discovery	44	47.31
Hope (possibility of change)	63	67.74
Hope (possibility of life after AN)	68	73.12
Self-acceptance	64	68.82
Improved self-esteem	55	59.14
Engagement with therapist or treatment provider	62	66.67
None	1	1.08

The elements of treatment that contributed to participants feeling unsupported included not being heard, or understood, control taken away, being infantised, threats and punishments. These elements largely attributed to the individuals with AN feeling unsafe, incapable and undeserving of being able to face the challenges that 'recovery' entails.

Subtheme: Hope

Imbuing hope through treatment helped individuals feel supported, normal and believed in and provided them with the motivation when confronted with challenges. A participant described positive experiences with her therapist: "[*she*] *invested her time and hope into me which made me feel worthy and deserving of life* (*112*)". Hope that recovery was possible was either inherent and experienced by individuals with AN, as illustrated in the following quote: "*hope, the possibility of life after AN. We all want to know that we can beat this and that there is a life that doesn't involve AN* (*63*)". Alternatively it was nurtured through others such as a treatment provider: "*others having hope when I had lost all of mine* (*76*)".

Subtheme: Feeling listened to and understood

Feeling listened to and understood helped individuals to feel safe, validated and worthy and supported to open up and make changes. This is conveyed by the following participant quotes: *I trusted her 100 % (a therapist) and she understood me so well, she made recovery feel more safe and achievable* (*60*)" and "*I feel understood, not alone in this horrible battle which makes me comfortable to be honest and open up about things I would find hard to discus with others due to embarrassment and fear of judgment* (*40*)"..

Not being heard and not being understood created an environment that was not conducive to coping with change: "*if you are misunderstood it's hard to get to the cause of a problem and to find solutions or skills that a person is capable of implementing to overcome distress (84)*". It also eroded trust in providers and lead to feelings of not being safe and unsupported during times of stress and change. For instance a participant explained that she did not feel understood, which "*made me feel I couldn't be as honest about my ED behaviours (40)*" while another participant felt her treatment providers "*didn't listen to how I really felt, didn't care. Never once did I feel supported or cared for or safe* (68)". Not being heard enforced feelings of not being 'normal' and feelings that "*the opinions about myself were wrong and stupid which left me feeling alienated* (94)".

Subtheme: Empowered/disempowered

The definition of empowerment is "to make (someone) stronger and more confident, especially in controlling their life and claiming their rights" [17]. Individuals with AN paradoxically display control regarding the structure and regime of their exercise and eating yet they feel out of control by that same routine and structure [18] and the inability to change it [19]. Participants who had input into their recovery or some control over their recovery/treatment felt empowered by the changes they were making and their capacity to confront aspects of their AN. This was demonstrated by a participant who commented: "(*my treatment provider*) *allowed me to set the pace, meaning I felt a great sense of self-satisfaction as I took charge of my own recovery* (75)". Consequently when individuals had more input into their own recovery their experience of treatment was positive: "*I have a great input into my own recovery which I believe has made it a better and more positive experience* (142)". A sense of empowerment was also experienced as participants regained some control through learning new coping strategies and skills to help combat the disorder such as increasing self-worth and respect. This has been captured in the following participant quotes: "*I had a very low sense of self worth and a huge sense of failure, and it was very important to me that my therapist respected me as a person and not just an illness. I needed to feel they could see my strengths* (88)", "*I was respected and taught the strategies for coping with emotions and difficult situations* (79)" and recovery was helped by "*improving self esteem*". *We want to be able to look at our bodies, and smile when we are in public or looking in the mirror, we want to be confident and proud* (63)". When control was felt to be taken away from participants they experienced powerlessness and this heightened their sense of being 'out of control' which is intrinsic in AN [18]. This was illustrated by the following participants: "*I was forced to do things I could not cope with, the pace things were moving at was uncomfortable and it made me even worse as things were so out of my control* (145)" and "*when suffering from anorexia, control is a big thing. And having that taken away from you by professionals making choices on your behalf is very demeaning* (68)".

A number of participants felt that they had been threatened and punished or treated like a child during their treatment for AN. Participants found this demoralising and damaging to their self-esteem. "*As patients it felt like we were treated like criminals.... We were punished regularly whenever we fell victim to our eating disorders and never encouraged for the times we were able to be strong and stand up to our distressing thoughts* (75)" One participant felt like she was "*constantly spoken to like a child or babied which actually fed my insecurities* (68)". In many cases it was fear that motivated change rather than a desire to be recovered: "*I gained weight and did what I was told out of fear of being punished rather than because I felt supported to get well* (41)".

Treatment suitability

Treatment suitability was an important aspect in treatment and recovery. This theme included multiple domains, including access to treatment, treatment itself and the treatment providers. When treatment was deemed suitable to the person with AN, it was viewed as "*systematic, compassionate and individualised* (46)" and available regardless of weight gain and cost. For one participant it was having "*no time limit on treatment and being able to remain as inpatient at a healthy maintenance weight was crucial* (96)" which was crucial to recovery. When treatment was suitable individuals also felt supported by practitioners, friends and or family: "*having the knowledge that they were loved through their replaces, that they were safe to break down* (19)". For some the non-clinical environment was "*warm and inviting... these things as well as the respectfulness of my treatment team made me feel safe and valued and my opinions respected* (79)". Individuals often experienced treatment and the treatment providers as conveying "*empathy, patience, humour and a genuine belief in my worth as a person* (82)".

When treatment was not suitable to the person with AN it was viewed as too rigid and not individualized such as having a "*one size fits all approach-if you don't improve on their regime, you must not be trying hard enough* (50)". Treatment was often, inaccessible, either due to cost or not being ill enough with participants experiencing *"being sent home until critical and in need of life saving (45)"* and trouble *"getting the GP to refer me to specialists as I was told my weight was not low enough (142)"*. Not being able to access treatment when needed and there is a genuine desire for help can lead to *"further distress"* and deterioration of health. One participant revealed that she struggled for three months to access treatment and *"by this point my BMI was so low I needed to be hospitalised. I believe, if I had support sooner, I would not have got that ill (104)"*. Treatment providers not having AN specific experience or skills negatively influenced recovery and the treatment experience with many participants experiencing treatment providers negatively: *"staff did not have a great knowledge or understanding about AN (28)"*. Treatment providers were often telling them to *"just eat"* which lead to participants feeling invalidated and helpless.

Treat underlying factors

"Eating disorders are not just about the weight on the scale (142)" and when treatment was perceived to address more than just weight gain it was viewed as beneficial. Treating underlying factors and separating the eating disorder from self enabled a treatment that allowed individuals to focus on *"what the eating disorder represents, explore personality traits, interests and life (113)"*, and *"deal with the dysfunction underlying the disorder (140)"*. Treatment that *"addressed psychological, dietetic, medical and practical (97)"* aspects of the eating disorder was viewed as holistic. Treating underlying causes was also viewed as facilitating the conditions to *"learn new healthy coping strategies (105, 140)"* and skills.

When treatment was perceived to address only weight then it was viewed as hindering recovery. Individuals felt strongly that there was a need to treat underlying factors, not just the signs/symptoms of AN. Individuals experienced a feeling of incomplete treatment, invalidation and lack of congruence about treatment and recovering. This occurred for individuals who were discharged at their 'target weight' and yet they still felt emotionally the same as explained by this participant: *"when in inpatient treatment the focus was on physical restoration so when I was discharged at the 'target weight', I was still the same emotionally as when I was admitted (141)"*. Some felt they had not learnt the skills they needed to cope during treatment: *"the goal was not to learn the coping skills necessary to overcome our illness, we were released as soon as we reached our 'goal weight' (75)'"*.

The stages of recovery

The stages of recovery involved different experiences of treatment and different needs (See Table 3). The first stage of recovery (unready or unwilling to change) saw individuals feeling alone as they were thrust into a situation they were not ready for or didn't understand. Support was important in stages 2-4 of recovery (tipping point of change, actively pursuing recovery and reflection and rehabilitation), but more important during the tipping point of change and in the reflection and rehabilitation stages. The right treatment and exceptional treatment providers were also important in stages 2-4 but more important in the active pursuit of recovery phase. Being understood was an important factor in the tipping point of change and self-directed recovery was important in the active pursuit of recovery phase.

Discussion

This paper investigated the care experience during treatment for AN in a self-selected volunteer sample of patients with or recovered from AN and three themes were identified; supporting a person to cope with change, treatment suitability and treat underlying factors. These themes were found to be important and either hindered and/or benefited recovery during treatment.

In this study, the theme of supporting a person to cope with change involved the following subthemes: hopefulness, being listened to and understood, control in recovery, increased self-worth, learning new skills and coping mechanisms. Not supporting a person to cope with change involved not being listened to, not being understood, a lack of control in recovery and punishments, and threats. Treatments that emphasise and limit these factors might, therefore, be helpful in promoting recovery from AN. Our study augments the current research on the impact of support to change on the treatment experiences of individuals with AN and may provide valuable identification of some of the key factors that should align with treatment for recovery to occur. Empowerment has been shown to lead to better experiences of the quality of care received, better patient-provider communication, increased motivation and higher patient involvement in decision making [20, 21]. Motivation and empowerment have been linked to a more favourable treatment response for patients with AN including completing the course of treatment [4, 5, 8, 22–25]. The study findings of not being supported to change, lack of control and disempowerment align with current research, which shows that feeling disempowered and that treatment was likened to being in prison, hinders the development of the therapeutic relationship and has the potential to exacerbate ambivalence to change for those with AN [9, 11, 24, 26]. The importance of hope in recovery has been emphasised in previous research findings [3, 4, 27, 28] and our study emphasises the importance of hope in supporting change,

Table 3 The phases of treatment and what impacted recovery

Four phases of AN treatment and what was experienced and or helped in each stage (ranked in order of importance)			
Unable or unready to change	*Tipping Point of Change*	*Actively pursuing recovery*	*Reflection and rehabilitation*
Forced into treatment	Supported (not alone)	Right treatment and great treatment providers	Support
Felt alone	Right treatment	Support	Right treatment & great treatment providers
Believed okay/didn't have AN	Felt understood	Recovery self-directed (responsible for self)	Self-acceptance/personal worth/self love/kindness to self
Wasn't ready to change	Involved in having a say in treatment	Set own goals	Encouraged
Wasn't ready so rebelled	Recognised illness severity	More than AN (life outside AN)/Hope)	Skills to cope/manage
Wasn't understood	Listened to		
Needed:	Trust		
More information (what to expect from treatment, how to manage AN)			
Treatment focusing on more than weight Support			
Time/space/therapy to recognise there was a problem			

recovery and the treatment experience. Although supporting patients is important and it might be one way of improving their perception and experience of care, which may have flow on effects for treatment efficacy and or compliance, it cannot wholly account or explain recovery. However focusing on the factors that promote individuals feeling supported might give treatment providers a piece of the puzzle. It may help in addressing the complex, multidimensional needs of individuals for recovery and keep patients engaged in treatment.

Treatment, which was viewed as suitable, involved individualised and accessible care with support during treatment however when treatment was deemed incompatible to the individual, it was too structured, not individualised and inaccessible. Difficulty accessing treatment for AN is not a new phenomenon with research identifying multiple causes including people not being 'thin' enough to access treatment [26]. Recovery has been shown to be influenced by intake BMI and age of first accessing treatment [26, 29], therefore it is imperative that individuals are able to access appropriate treatment without fear of denial or conditional prerequisites. The study findings draw attention to the importance of individualised treatment and are consistent with similar themes that characterise people with AN and their experience of treatment [24, 30–32]. These themes emphasise the struggle between the provision of effective AN treatment approaches and structure and the need for autonomy and a treatment structure that can meet the needs of the individuals. Consistent with earlier studies, treatment when experienced as incompatible to the individual, was felt to be too rigid and not tailored to the individuals' needs [26, 31, 32] with patients experiencing oppression, and of being in a prison and restricted [9, 24, 25, 32]. Dissatisfaction with treatment has been linked with treatment inefficiency, delays in accessing treatments, increased risk of relapse, and premature cessation of treatment [25, 33–36]. The studies findings add to the factors that can be improved in the treatment of AN to make a considerable difference in recovery. A positive finding of this study was the important impact treatment providers can and are making by providing treatment that suits the individual. Despite this some individuals are not experiencing treatment that is applicable and thus more research is needed on how to improve the treatment experience for more individuals with AN. Quantitative methodologies should be employed to test hypotheses generated from the present study's findings such as individualised treatment. For example for individualised treatment, a controlled trial employing programs that allow for individualised meal plans versus less flexible programs could be undertaken.

The importance of treating the underlying factors of AN, not just weight, is well established [26, 31, 37]. Our study findings reinforce the importance of treating underlying factors and provide an understanding of the factors that contribute to treatment being experienced as holistic. Treatment systems that have a strong emphasis on weight and food have been shown to have negative side effects including increased suicidal behaviour, restriction and reinforcing of AN behaviours [26, 38]. Being treated holistically has been identified as what is sought from AN treatments [26] but it is not clear what underlying factors require more emphasis and research. This study identifies treatment congruence with weight and life goals, the provision of coping and management skills, as important factors of a 'holistic' treatment and more research is needed on these factors such as a controlled trial program that employs a more 'holistic' treatment such as massage therapy or yoga versus more conventional treatments such as counseling.

Four phases or recovery have been identified and with that key factors associated with each phase [4]. The findings of this paper support initial research findings of not believing/understanding they had AN during the *unready* phase, feeling understood in the *tipping point of change* phase and self-acceptance in the *reflection* phase [3]. Our findings also support the theme of locus of control with the person moving from an external locus of control to an internal locus of control as recovery progresses. There were some original experiences found for each phase of recovery such as being forced into treatment and feeling alone during the *unready* phase, feeling supported and receiving the right treatment in the *tipping point of change*, the *active* and the *reflection* phases. Understanding how people with AN experience these phases might help treatment providers' address the key concerns and feelings at the right stage of the treatment phase and has the potential to improve treatment experiences and therefore treatment outcomes. Further research addressing key factors and experiences during the different phases of recovery is warranted such as a controlled trial program that identifies AN patients in the unready to change phase and allocates them to an adjunct program that focused on being understood and not feeling alone versus an additional psychological treatment.

The study has several limitations. The participants included both recovered and non-recovered individuals and as such some of the participants' experiences were retrospective. Participants were a self-selected volunteer sample with self-identified AN and as such were not representative of the diversity of people receiving treatment for AN. The study used qualitative exploratory methods and conclusions are thereby putative, not definitive. Future studies should investigate treatment experiences in representative samples such as clinical cohort studies with diagnostic and recovery status assessed by validated instruments. The time period of recover from AN for participants was not collected, in hindsight collection of this data should be have been collected. Another limitation was that participants were from two different geographic locations. However a strength of this study is the similarity of findings between both locations.

Conclusion

This paper investigated the care experience during treatment for AN in a self-selected volunteer sample of patients with or recovered from AN and three themes emerged that identified factors that either hindered and/or benefited recovery; the effect of treatment on empowerment/disempowerment, treatment suitability and treat underlying factors. The stages of recovery involved different experiences of treatment and identified different needs during each stage which with further research may help treatment providers address key concerns at the right stage or in the right treatment phase of AN. Similarly to other qualitative research undertaken on the treatment experiences of those with AN, our study reiterates that many important interrelated factors are important in recovery however the nature of the qualitative methodology conclusions are putative and further definitive research is indicated.

Competing interests

The authors declare that they have no competing interests.

Authors' contributions

SF and LR participated in the design of the study and the questionnaire. SF was responsible for the recruitment of participants. SF performed the statistical analysis. SF and LR performed the qualitative analysis. SF drafted the manuscript. All authors read and approved the final manuscript.

Acknowledgements

The authors would like to thank Professor Alan Bensoussan for sharing his knowledge and experience and providing guidance on the questionnaire design.

Author details

[1]School of Medicine, Western Sydney University, Richmond, Australia. [2]National Institute of Complementary Medicine, Western Sydney University, PO Box 2002, Homebush West, NSW 2140, Australia. [3]School of Nursing and Midwifery, Western Sydney University, Richmond, Australia. [4]Centre for Applied Nursing Research, Ingham Institute of Applied Medical Research, Richmond, Australia.

References

1. American Psychiatric Association. The Diagnostic and Statistical Manual of Mental Disorders, Fifth Edition (Feeding and Eating Disoders). The American Psychiatric Association (APA). 2013. www.dsm5.org/documents/eating disorders fact sheet.pdf. Accessed 6 September 2013.
2. Strober M, Johnson C. The need for complex ideas in Anorexia Nervosa: why biology, environment, and psyche all matter, why therapists make mistakes, and why clinical benchmarks are needed for managing weight correction. Int J Eat Disord. 2012;45:155–78.
3. Hay PJ, Cho K. A Qualitative Exploration of Influences on the Process of Recovery from Personal Written Accounts of People with Anorexia Nervosa. Women Health. 2013;53(7):730–40. doi:10.1080/03630242.2013.821694.
4. Dawson L, Rhodes P, Touyz S. "Doing the Impossible": The Process of Recovery From Chronic Anorexia Nervosa. Qual Health Res. 2014;24(4): 494–505. doi:10.1177/1049732314524029.
5. Federici A, Kaplan A. The patient's account of relapse and recovery in Anorexia Nervosa: a qualitative study. Eur Eat Disord Rev. 2008;16:1–10.
6. Darcy A, Katz S, Fitzpatrick K, Forsberg S, Utzinger L, Lock J. All Better? How Former Anorexia Nervosa Patients Define Recovery and Engaged in Treatment. Eur Eat Disor Rev. 2010;18(4):260–70.
7. Hsu L, Crisp A, Callender J. Recovery in anorexia nervosa: the patient perspective. Int J Eat Disord. 1992;11:341–50.
8. Tozzi F, Sullivan PF, Fear JL, McKenzie J, Bulik CM. Causes and Recovery in Anorexia Nervosa: The Patient's Perspective. Int J Eat Disord. 2003;33(2):143–54.
9. Ramjan LM, Gill BI. An inpatient program for adolescents with anorexia experienced as a metaphoric prison. Am J Nurs. 2012;112(8):24–33. doi:10.1097/01.NAJ.0000418094.31317.52.

10. Ramjan LM. Nurses and the theraputic relationship: caring for adolescents with anorexia nervosa. J Adv Nurs. 2004;45(5):495–503.
11. Wright KM. Theraputic relationship: Developing a new understanding for nurses and care workers within an eating disorder unil. J Psychiatr Ment Health Nurs. 2010;19:154–61.
12. Harrell BM. Data collection methods: semistructured interviews and focus groups. Arlington: VA: Rand Corporation; 2009.
13. National Collaborating Centre for Mental Health (UK). Eating Disorders: Core Interventions in the Treatment and Management of Anorexia Nervosa, Bulimia Nervosa and Related Eating Disorders. NICE Clinical Guidelines, No. 9, vol 6 Treatment and management of anorexia nervosa. Leicester (UK): British Psychological Society (UK); 2004.
14. Hay P, Chinn D, Forbes D, Madden S, Newton R, Sugenor L, et al. Royal Austalian and New Zealand College of Psychaitrists clinical practice guidelines for the treatment of eating disorders. Aust N Z J Psychiatry. 2014; 48(11):977–1008.
15. Hsieh H-F, Shannon SE. Three Approaches to Qualitative Content Analysis. Qual Health Res. 2005;15:1277–88. doi:10.1177/1049732305276687.
16. Sandelowski M. Focus on Reserach Methods. Whatever Happened to Qualitative Description? Res Nurs Health. 2000;223:334–40.
17. Collins. Collins Dictionary of the English Language. In: Wilkes GAE, editor. Collins Dictionary of the English Language. Sydney: Collins; 1979.
18. Lawrence M. Anorexia nervosa—The control paradox. Women's Studies International Quarterly. 1979;2 (1):93-101. doi:http://dx.doi.org/10.1016/S0148-0685(79)93118-X.
19. Kolnes L-J. 'Feelings stronger than reason': conflicting experiences of exercise in women with anorexia nervosa. J Eat Disord. 2016;4(1):1–15. doi:10.1186/s40337-016-0100-8.
20. Aardoom JJ, Dingemans AE, Boogaard LH, Van Furth EF. Internet and patient empowerment in individuals with symptoms of an eating disorder: A cross-sectional investigation of a pro-recovery focused e-community. Eat Behav. 2014;15 (3):350-6. doi:http://dx.doi.org/10.1016/j.eatbeh.2014.04.003.
21. Gabay G. Exploring perceived control and self-rated health in re-admissions among younger adults: A retrospective study. Patient Educ Couns. doi: http://dx.doi.org/10.1016/j.pec.2015.11.011.
22. Espel H, Goldstein S, Manasse S, Juarascio A. Experiential acceptance, motivation for recovery, and treatment outcome in eating disorders. Eat Weight Disord. 2015:1-6. doi:10.1007/s40519-015-0235-7.
23. Schlegl S, Diedrich A, Neumayr C, Fumi M, Naab S, Voderholzer U. Inpatient Treatment for Adolescents with Anorexia Nervosa: Clinical Significance and Predictors of Treatment Outcome. Eur Eat Disord Rev. 2015:n/a-n/a. doi:10.1002/erv.2416.
24. Smith V, Chouliara Z, Morris PG, Collin P, Power K, Yellowlees A, et al. The experience of specialist inpatient treatment for anorexia nervosa: A qualitative study from adult patients' perspectives. J Health Psychol. 2016; 21(1):16–27. doi:10.1177/1359105313520336.
25. Clinton D, Almlöf L, Lindström S, Manneberg M, Vestin L. Drop-in access to specialist services for eating disorders: a qualitative study of patient experiences. Eat Disord. 2014;22(4):279–91. doi:10.1080/10640266.2014.912553.
26. Rance N, Moller NP, Clarke V. 'Eating disorders are not about food, they're about life': Client perspectives on anorexia nervosa treatment. J Health Psychol. 2015:1-13. doi:10.1177/1359105315609088.
27. Dawson L, Rhodes P, Mullan B, Miskovic J, Touyz S. Recovery stories - helpful or unhelpful? A randomised controlled trial. J Eat Dis. 2014;2 ((Suppl 1):O50). doi:10.1186/2050-2974-2-S1-O50.
28. Lindgren B-M, Enmark A, Bohman A, Lundström M. A qualitative study of young women's experiences of recovery from Bulimia Nervosa. J Adv Nurs. 2015;71(4):860–9. doi:10.1111/jan.12554.
29. Errichiello L, Iodice D, Bruzzese D, Gherghi M, Senatore I. Prognostic factors and outcome in anorexia nervosa: a follow-up study. Eat Weight Disord. 2015:1-10. doi:10.1007/s40519-015-0211-2.
30. Micevski V, McCann TV. Developing interpersonal relationships with adolescents with anorexia nervosa. Contemp Nurse. 2005;20(1):102–16.
31. Offord A, Turner H, Cooper M. Adolescent inpatient treatment for Anorexia Nervosa: a qualitative study exploring young adults' retrospective views of treatment and discharge. Eur Eat Disord Rev. 2006;14:377–87.
32. Eli K. Between Difference and Belonging: Configuring Self and Others in Inpatient Treatment for Eating Disorders. PLoS One. 2014;9(9), e105452. doi:10.1371/journal.pone.0105452.
33. Lindstedt K, Neander K, Kjellin L, Gustafsson S. Being me and being us - adolescents' experiences of treatment for eating disorders. J Eat Disord. 2015;3(1):9.
34. Federici A, Kaplan A. The patient's account of relapse and recovery in anorexia nervosa: a qualitative study. Eur Eat Disor Rev. 2007;16:1.
35. Roots P, Rowland L, Gowers S. User satisfaction with services in a randomised controlled trial of adolescent Anorexia Nervosa. Eur Eat Disor Rev. 2009;17:331–7.
36. Paulson-Karlsson G, Nevonen L, Engstrom I. Anorexia Nervosa: treatment satisfaction. J Fam Ther. 2006;28:293–306.
37. Escobar-Koch T, Banker J, Crow S, Cullis J, Ringwood S, Smith G, et al. Service users' views of eating disorder services: an international comparison. Int J Eat Disord. 2010;43:249–60.
38. Gowers S, Weetman J, Shore A, Hossain F, Elvins R. Impact of hospitalisation on the outcome of adolescent anorexia nervosa. Br J Psychiatry. 2000;176(2):138–41.

19

The role of music therapy in reducing post meal related anxiety for patients with anorexia nervosa

Jennifer Bibb[1,2*], David Castle[3,4] and Richard Newton[1,3,4]

Abstract

Background: It is well known that mealtime is anxiety provoking for patients with Anorexia Nervosa. However, there is little research into effective interventions for reducing meal related anxiety in an inpatient setting.

Methods: This study compared the levels of distress and anxiety of patients with Anorexia Nervosa pre and post music therapy, in comparison to standard post meal support therapy. Data was collected using the Subjective Units of Distress (SUDS) scale which was administered pre and post each condition.

Results: A total of 89 intervention and 84 control sessions were recorded. Results from an unpaired t-test analysis indicated statistically significant differences between the music therapy and supported meal conditions.

Conclusions: Results indicated that participation in music therapy significantly decreases post meal related anxiety and distress in comparison to standard post meal support therapy. This research provides support for the use of music therapy in this setting as an effective clinical intervention in reducing meal related anxiety.

Keywords: Music therapy, Anorexia nervosa, Meal support therapy

Background

It is well documented that mealtimes are anxiety provoking for patients with Anorexia Nervosa (AN) [1]. Eating and weight gain is associated with feelings of fear and anxiety amongst AN patients [2, 3]. Psychological and physical discomfort are often experienced after meals when patients can become preoccupied with thoughts of purging or feelings of guilt [4]. Support from staff or family during meal times is acknowledged as an important therapeutic activity for decreasing meal-related distress [5–8]. Supported mealtimes are typically facilitated by inpatient staff but there is little research into effective interventions for reducing meal related anxiety in a ward setting [5].

Music therapy

Participation in music therapy can improve the quality of life, interpersonal relationships and social skills of people with mental illness [9–11]. Music therapy can help promote self-determination and collaboration with patients through focusing on strengths and resource-oriented practice [12]. Literature supports the relationship between music therapy practice in mental health recovery and emphasis on empowerment and patient led processes [12–14]. Use of music therapy to promote feelings of empowerment and equality are arguably expressly important in inpatient mental health settings that may otherwise provide little opportunity for self-determination [15, 16].

Music therapy and eating disorders

Music therapy may offer motivation for recovery from eating disorders, distraction from negative thoughts and feelings, a sense of autonomy and creative expression [17–19]. Case studies derived from patient experiences have described feelings of renewed self confidence and empowerment through participation

* Correspondence: bibb.jennifer@unimelb.edu.au
[1]Mental Health CSU, Austin Health, 145 Studley Road, Heidelberg 3084, Victoria, Australia
[2]National Music Therapy Research Unit, Melbourne Conservatorium of Music, University of Melbourne, 151 Barry Street, Parkville 3010, Victoria, Australia
Full list of author information is available at the end of the article

in music therapy [20]. In a qualitative study exploring the perceptions of group singing from eight people with eating disorders, participants reported several emotional and cognitive benefits including mental engagement and opportunity to distance themselves from life's problems [21]. Despite these reports of positive experiences during music therapy, there is no published research examining the role of music therapy during supported meal times. This study aimed to address this gap by evaluating post-meal music therapy amongst a group of inpatients with AN.

Method

Setting

The study was conducted in a specialist five bed inpatient eating disorders program situated within an acute psychiatric unit. The program primarily caters for adults with severe anorexia nervosa who have been unable to recover through outpatient treatment. The average age of patients admitted to the inpatient program is 22 years of age, predominately young women. A collaborative conceptualisation-based approach [22] is adopted which is patient-centred and focuses on individualised treatment. The therapy program includes a supported meal time (meal support therapy) that involves a period of post meal distress tolerance and support provided by a team member every lunchtime.

Design

The aim of this study was to evaluate post-meal music therapy amongst a group of inpatients with AN. The study aimed to both determine if participation in music therapy decreased subjective distress during post-meal support and to understand how participants described their experiences of music therapy during this time. The interest in both understanding and measuring post-meal music therapy suggested a mixed method approach, using different modes of self-reporting on the phenomenon [23]. An embedded mixed methods design was adopted where quantitative and qualitative data were collected within a quasi-experimental design [23]. The qualitative part of the study is not included in this article due to the authors' desire to conduct a deeper exploration of the participants' rich descriptions of their experience. The quantitative element which is presented in this article, was a non-randomised pre-post design comparing music therapy with treatment as usual following mealtime. This was considered a fitting design because the intention of the study was to evaluate an existing music therapy program and therefore acted as a pilot study, in an attempt to give indicators of the size of the effect of the clinical intervention and to check the feasibility for a possible larger scale study.

Quantitative data was collected using the Subjective Units of Distress (SUDS) scale which was administered pre and post each intervention and control condition. Participants attended the music therapy intervention twice per week for the duration of their admission. At all other times during the week participants continued with their usual ward program. This project was approved by Human Research Ethics Committee at Austin Health (HREC/14/Austin/75).

Participants

Adults admitted to the eating disorders program within the acute psychiatric unit, Mental Health Clinical Service Unit at Austin Health were invited to participate in the study. The primary researcher (Bibb) distributed the plain language statement and consent form to patients upon their admission to hospital. Informed consent to participate in the study was obtained from 18 of a total of 32 patients. During this time 89 intervention and 84 control sessions were recorded.

Inclusion criteria for the study were as follows:

- Current patient within the inpatient eating disorder program
- Between 18 and 65 years of age
- Able to read and write (in English) in order to complete data collection tool

Exclusion criteria were:

- Non-English speaking
- Severe cognitive impairment, language problems or hearing impairment

Materials

Participants were trained in the use of the Subjective Units of Distress Scale (SUDS) which is a self-report tool measuring the subjective intensity of distress or anxiety currently experienced by a participant [24]. Although originally used with a 0 to 100 rating scale, more recently scales of 0 to 10 have been adapted, with participants rating their anxiety on a scale ranging from '0 – totally relaxed' to '10 – highest distress/anxiety/fear/discomfort you have ever felt.' A visual analogue scale in the form of a 'feelings thermometer' aided in the visual representation of the SUDS ratings (see Fig. 1) [25].

Procedure

Music therapy

Two one-hour music therapy group sessions were held directly after lunch each week. The group was facilitated by a university trained Registered Music Therapist (first author; RMT) in a meeting room on the psychiatric unit. During music therapy sessions participants were

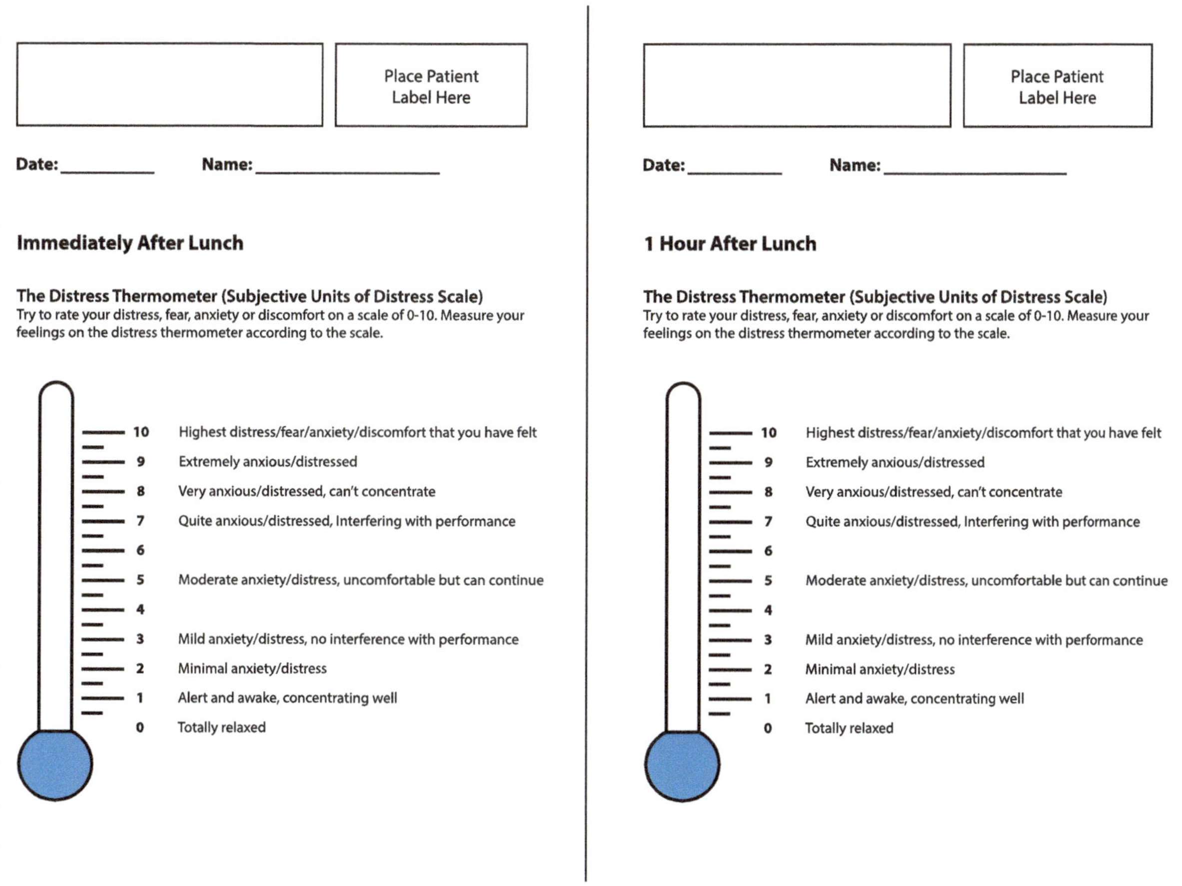

Fig. 1 Adapted subjective units of distress thermometers

encouraged to participate in singing and listening to songs, talking about and sharing music with others and writing songs together. The goal for the group was focused on offering participants a distraction and opportunity to practice coping skills through music. A humanistic approach [26] was adopted where participants were invited to collaborate together on the process of each session. The principles of humanism suggest that "all persons have innate capabilities for actualising their own unique potentials for health and wellbeing" (p.148). Thus, the music therapist maintained a perspective of unconditional positive regard instead of a more directive approach common to cognitive behavioural therapy groups in inpatient eating disorder programs. Group members were encouraged to listen to one another and engage in discussion about song lyrics and their preferred musical tastes. Other topics also emerged in discussions within the group which were often related to eating disorder recovery.

Post meal support therapy

Structured post meal support therapy acted as a control condition (treatment as usual) involving a one hour group session after mealtime and occurred on the remaining three days of the working week. These sessions included discussion of feelings, encouragement to focus on achieving the goals of admission and group activities such as playing games or art activities. Nursing and allied health staff facilitated post meal support therapy on a rotating roster.

Statistical analyses

The statistical software SPSS was used to analyse the data. Mean differences between pre and post scores and the standard deviation were calculated for both intervention and control group data. An unpaired t-test was then performed to explore statistical differences between the mean differences between the music therapy and control interventions.

Table 1 Raw data

Condition	n	Pre-test Mean	Pre-test Std error (m)	Post-test Mean	Post-test Std error (m)	Difference (m)	Std dev.
Intervention	89	8	0.23	5.6	0.26	2.4	1.9
Control	84	8.1	0.24	7.1	0.27	0.93	1.7

Results

A total of 18 patients participated in the study, including 17 females and one male. Participant's ages ranged between 20 and 58 years old. Length of admission ranged between 21 and 90 days. The 18 participants, attended 173 sessions in total for the music therapy ($n = 89$) and the control conditions ($n = 84$). Results can be seen in Table 1. The mean pre-test score for the intervention group was 8 and the mean post-test score was 5.6. The mean pre-test score for the control group was 8.1 and post-test was 7.1. Mean pre-post test difference for the intervention condition was 2.4 integers on the scale with a standard deviation of 1.9 integers. The mean pre-post test difference for the control condition was 0.93 integers on the scale with a standard deviation of 1.7 integers. The mean standard error for the intervention group was .23 pre-test and .26 post-test, while the mean standard error for the control group was .24 pre-test and .27 post-test. An ANOVA score of $f = 28.5$ and a highly statistically significant ($p = <0.0001$) difference between the control and intervention conditions was found. The combined mean pre-test score for both control and intervention conditions was higher (8.1) than the mean post-test score for both conditions (6.3), meaning that across all 173 occasions participants rated their anxiety higher prior to participation in either condition, than afterwards. Additionally, there was a statistically significant difference ($p = <0.0001$) between the pre-test scores and post-test scores of all combined 173 occasions.

Discussion

The aim of this study was to compare the levels of distress and anxiety of patients with AN pre and post group music therapy provided after meals, with standard post meal support therapy. The results are strongly positive and offer support for the use of music therapy in AN inpatient care. Participants in both conditions reported decreased anxiety post-session compared with straight after lunch (pre-session). This supports previous research suggesting that meal related distress and anxiety is a great concern for patients with AN [1]. Participants' levels of anxiety significantly decreased after both conditions which also aligns with previous research that suggests therapist facilitated support after meals is helpful for patients with AN [5–8].

Results from the current study also suggest that group music therapy is a more effective intervention for reducing meal related anxiety than standard post meal support therapy in an inpatient setting. The average age of eating disorder patients admitted to the inpatient program is 22 years of age. It is well known that music is an engaging activity for young people and is a motivating factor for participating in therapy [27]. It is likely that participants considered music therapy as a non-threatening and familiar activity in an often confronting medical setting [15, 16]. Participation in music therapy may have acted as a "cognitive divergence" (p. 111) for patients, allowing time for the body to digest food while the mind was attending to something else that was engaging for them [17].

AN is associated with emotion avoidance and dysphoria [28]. Patients report that AN helps them to avoid and control their emotions [29, 30]. Participation in music therapy after meal times is a way for distressing emotions to be experienced through the music. Using music therapy as a distress tolerance technique emphasises the therapy that occurs during the music rather than through discussion [27]. In this instance, the experience of musical process is the therapy [31]. As such, there are broader implications for the use of music therapy as an alternate coping technique for patients who are likely to avoid distressing emotions and often report feeling emotionally 'numb' [32].

Participants' anxiety decreased significantly pre-post the music therapy group compared with standard post meal support therapy. This is important knowledge for inpatient eating disorder programs. Previously it was known that support after mealtime was helpful but the kind of interventions that were effective in reducing anxiety during this time were not [5]. Incorporating music therapy into inpatient meal support programs can offer patients with AN an alternative distress tolerance technique, which they can translate into their external environments post discharge [33]. Previous music therapy research has focused on participants' experiences of music therapy sessions during their recovery from AN [17–19]. It is important to consider the heightened distress of patients with AN after meal times and the role music therapy can play in reducing anxiety during this time. The current study is the first to use music therapy post meal-time and offers support for further research into this area.

Limitations

The current study has positive implications for the use of music therapy in reducing meal related anxiety for patients with AN. However, the findings may be limited due to a number of factors. First, the research design was quasi-experimental and did not randomise participants to each condition. The same participants contributed to several occasions (both intervention and control conditions) during their admission which meant randomisation was impossible. Second, participants were recruited from one site which may effect the generalisabiltiy of the results. Third, the same music therapist facilitated the intervention group condition while a variety of therapists (allied health and nursing staff) facilitated the control group condition. The researchers attempted to reduce this potential bias by collecting a large number of occasions (173) over the 36 week period. A larger number of participants, randomisation to control and intervention conditions and recruitment from different hospital sites would benefit future research in this area.

Conclusions

Music therapy for the treatment of AN is under funded in adult mental health services in Australia. This study provides support for the future funding of inpatient music therapy programs and contributes to the evidence base for the use of music therapy with this population. Music therapy offers an important role in the management of meal related anxiety for patients with AN.

Competing interests

DC has received grant monies for research from Eli Lilly, Janssen Cilag, Roche, Allergen, Bristol-Myers Squibb, Pfizer, Lundbeck, Astra Zeneca, Hospira; Travel Support and Honoraria for Talks and Consultancy from Eli Lilly, Bristol-Myers Squibb, Astra Zeneca, Lundbeck, Janssen Cilag, Pfizer, Organon, Sanofi-Aventis, Wyeth, Hospira, Servier; and is a current Advisory Board Member for Lu AA21004: Lundbeck; Varenicline: Pfizer; Asenapine: Lundbeck; Bitopertin: Roche Aripiprazole LAI: Lundbeck; Lisdexamfetamine: Shire; Lurasidone: Servier. He has no stocks or shares in any pharmaceutical company.

Authors' contributions

All authors were involved in the design of the study. JB collected and analysed the data under the supervision of the other authors. All authors drafted and approved the final manuscript.

Acknowledgements

This research was financially supported by the Austin Medical Research Foundation (AMRF). The authors would like to thank the patients who generously participated in this study.

Author details

[1]Mental Health CSU, Austin Health, 145 Studley Road, Heidelberg 3084, Victoria, Australia. [2]National Music Therapy Research Unit, Melbourne Conservatorium of Music, University of Melbourne, 151 Barry Street, Parkville 3010, Victoria, Australia. [3]The Body Image & Eating Disorders Treatment & Recovery Service (BETRS), St Vincent's Hospital, 104 Studley Park Rd, Kew 3101Victoria, Australia. [4]Department of Psychiatry, University of Melbourne, Parkville 3010, Victoria, Australia.

References

1. Hage TW, Ro O, Moen A. "Time's up"- Staff's management of mealtimes on inpatient eating disorder units. J Eat Disord. 2015;3:13.
2. Breiner S. An evidence-based eating disorder program. J Pediatr Nurs. 2003;18:75–80.
3. Harvey T, Troop NA, Treasure JL, Murphy T. Fear, disgust, and abnormal eating attitudes: a preliminary study. Int J Eat Disord. 2002;32:213–8.
4. Leichner M, Standish K, Leichner P. Strategies for supporting youth with eating disorders when intensive treatment is needed. BCMJ. 2005;47(1):49–55.
5. Long S, Wallis D, Leung N, Meyer C. "All eyes are on you": Anorexia nervosa patient perspectives of in-patient mealtimes. J Health Psychol. 2012;17:419–28.
6. Clinton D, Bjorck C, Sohlberg S, Norring C. Patient satisfaction with treatment in eating disorders: Cause for complacency or concern? Eur Eat Disord Rev. 2004;12(4):240–6.
7. Federici A, Kaplan AS. The patient's account of relapse and recovery in anorexia nervosa: A qualitative study. Eur Eat Disord Rev. 2008;16(1):1–10.
8. Offord A, Turner H, Cooper M. Adolescent inpatient treatment for anorexia nervosa: A qualitative study exploring young adults' retrospective views of treatment and discharge. Eur Eat Disord Rev. 2006; 14(6):377–87.
9. Grocke D, Block S, Castle D. The effect of group music therapy on quality of life for participants living with a severe and enduring mental illness. J Music Ther. 2009;46:90–104.
10. Hayashi N, Tanabe Y, Nakagawa S, Noguchi M, Iwata C, Koubuchi Y, et al. Effects of group musical therapy on inpatients with chronic psychoses: A controlled study. Psychiatry Clin Neurosci. 2002;56:187–93.
11. Mossler K, Chen X, Heldal TO, Gold C. Music therapy for people with schizophrenia and schizophrenia-like disorders. Cochrane Database of Systematic Reviews. 2011; Issue 12. Art. No.: CD004025. doi:10.1002/14651858.CD004025.pub3.
12. Rolvsjord R. Resource-oriented music therapy in mental health care. Gilsum: Barcelona Publishers; 2010.
13. Baines S. A consumer-directed and partnered community mental health music therapy program. Voices: A World Forum for Music Therapy. 2003; 3. doi: http://dx.doi.org/10.15845/voices.v3i3.
14. Procter S. Empowering and enabling — Music therapy in non-medical mental health provision. In: Kenny C, Stige B, editors. Contemporary voices in music therapy. Oslo: Unipub Forlag; 2002.
15. Dalton JH, Elias MJ, Wandersman A. Community psychology, Linking individuals and communities. London: Wadsworth (Thomson Learning); 2001.
16. Fitzsimons S, Fuller R. Empowerment and its implications for clinical practice in mental health: A review. J Ment Health. 2002;11(5):481–99.
17. Hilliard RE. The use of cognitive-behavorial therapy in the treatment of women with eating disorders. Music Ther Perspect. 2001;19(2):109–13.
18. Robarts J, Sloboda A. Perspectives on music therapy with people suffering from anorexia nervosa. Br J Music Therapy. 1994;8(1):7–14.
19. McFerran K. Dangerous liaisons: Group work for adolescent girls who have anorexia nervosa. Voices: A World Forum for Music Therapy. 2005. doi: http://dx.doi.org/10.15845/voices.v5i1.
20. Lejonclou A, Trondalen G. "I've started to move into my own body": Music therapy with women suffering from eating disorders. Nord J Music Ther. 2009;18(1):79–92.
21. Pavlakou M. Benefits of group singing for people with eating disorders: Preliminary findings from a non-clinical study. Approaches Music Therapy Special Music Educ. 2009;1(1):30–48.
22. Newton R. Treating anorexia nervosa: a collaborative conceptualisation-based approach. In: Castle DJ, Hood S, Starcevic V, editors. Anxiety Disorders: Current Understandings, Novel Treatments. Melbourne: Australian Postgraduate Medicine; 2012. p. 153–64.
23. Creswell JW, Plano Clark VL. Designing and Conducting Mixed Methods Research. 2nd ed. Thousand Oaks: Sage Publications; 2011.
24. Wolpe J. The Practice of Behavior Therapy. New York: Pergamon Press; 1969.
25. Kendall P, Robin J, Hedtke K, Suveg C, Flannery-Schroeder E, Gosch E. Considering CBT with anxious youth? Think exposures. Cogn Behav Pract. 2005;12:136–50.
26. Abrams B. Humanistic approaches. In: Wheeler BL, editor. Music therapy handbook. New York, USA: The Guildford Press; 2015. p. 148–60.
27. McFerran K. Adolescents, Music and Music Therapy. London: Jessica Kingsley Publishers; 2010.

28. Wildes JE, Ringham RM, Marcus MD. Emotion Avoidance in Patients with Anorexia Nervosa: Initial Test of a Functional Model. Int J Eat Disord. 2010;43:398–404.
29. Gale C, Holliday J, Troop NA, Serpell L, Treasure J. The pros and cons of change in individuals with eating disorders: A broader perspective. Int J Eat Disord. 2006;39:394–403.
30. Corstorphine E, Mountford V, Tomlinson S, Waller G, Meyer C. Distress tolerance in the eating disorders. Eat Behav. 2007;8:91–7.
31. Aigen K. Music-Centred Music Therapy. Gilsum NH: Barcelona Publishers; 2005.
32. Schmidt U, Treasure J. Anorexia nervosa: Valued and visible. A cognitive-interpersonal maintenance model and its implications for research and practice. Br J Clin Psychol. 2006;45:343–66.
33. Gutierrez EOF, Camarena VAT. Music therapy in generalized anxiety disorder. Arts Psychotherapy. 2015;44:19–24.

Process evaluation of the MOSAIC trial: treatment experience of two psychological therapies for out-patient treatment of Anorexia Nervosa

Kelly Ann Zainal[1†], Beth Renwick[1†], Alexandra Keyes[1], Anna Lose[1], Martha Kenyon[1], Hannah DeJong[1], Hannah Broadbent[1], Lucy Serpell[2,3], Lorna Richards[4], Eric Johnson-Sabine[4], Nicky Boughton[5], Linette Whitehead[5], Janet Treasure[1], Ulrike Schmidt[1*] and on behalf of the MOSAIC trial group

Abstract

Background: This study is part of a series of process evaluations within the MOSAIC Trial (Maudsley Outpatient Study of Treatments for Anorexia Nervosa and Related Conditions). This randomised controlled trial (RCT) compared two psychological treatments, the Maudsley Model for Treatment of Adults with Anorexia Nervosa (MANTRA) and Specialist Supportive Clinical Management (SSCM) for adult outpatients with Anorexia Nervosa. The present process study integrates quantitative (treatment acceptability and credibility) and qualitative (written) feedback to evaluate patients' treatment experiences.

Method: All 142 MOSAIC participants were asked to (a) rate treatment acceptability and credibility on visual analogue scales (VAS) at six and 12 months post-randomisation, and (b) provide written feedback regarding their views on their treatment at 12 months. Transcripts were first analysed thematically and then rated according to the global valence of feedback (positive, mixed/negative).

Results: 114/142 (80.3 %) MOSAIC participants provided VAS data and 82 (57.7 %) provided written feedback. At 12 months, MANTRA patients gave significantly higher acceptability and credibility ratings compared to SSCM patients. A significantly higher proportion of MANTRA patients provided written feedback. MANTRA patients also tended to write in more detail and to give globally more positive feedback when compared to individuals receiving SSCM. Qualitative themes suggest that patients experienced the two treatments differently in terms of characteristics and outcomes.

Conclusions: This study highlights the benefits of incorporating qualitative and quantitative data into RCT process evaluations. MANTRA patients were more willing to express their views on treatment and generally felt more positively about this than those receiving SSCM.

Keywords: Anorexia nervosa, MANTRA, Randomised–controlled trial, Specialist supportive clinical management, Process evaluation

* Correspondence: ulrike.schmidt@kcl.ac.uk
[†]Equal contributors
[1]Section of Eating Disorders, Department of Psychological Medicine, Institute of Psychiatry, Psychology and Neuroscience, King's College London, PO Box 59SE5 8AF London, UK
Full list of author information is available at the end of the article

Background

Anorexia nervosa (AN) is a highly debilitating mental disorder which is challenging to treat and expensive to manage, especially in adults with a more enduring form of the illness [1]. The UK National Institute for Health and Care Excellence [2] and the US National Institute of Mental Health [3] have emphasized the need for the development and evaluation of new approaches to the treatment of AN as at present, there is little high quality empirical evidence to support a preferred psychological treatment [4].

Whilst randomised controlled trials (RCTs) remain the gold standard for evaluating treatment outcomes, process evaluations integrated into trials provide crucial information regarding factors involved in treatment success, such as fidelity and quality of implementation, potential causal mechanisms, and contextual factors associated with variation in outcomes [5]. Such process evaluations are used to supplement quantitative outcomes by providing a more complete picture of the treatment approach [6]. This puts an emphasis on meanings, experiences, and views of all the participants in order to understand treatment in the natural setting [7]. Evaluations aim to identify the potential "active ingredients" of a particular treatment approach, and explore interactions between patients and therapists [6].

The present study is the second stage of a planned process evaluation conducted as part of a large multi-centre RCT, the Maudsley Outpatient Study of Treatment for Adults with Anorexia Nervosa and Related Conditions (MOSAIC). The MOSAIC trial compared two outpatient treatments. The first is a novel therapy, Maudsley Model of Treatment for Adults with Anorexia Nervosa (MANTRA) [8–10], and the second, Specialist Supportive Clinical Management (SSCM) is a more established treatment that was developed as a standardised form of treatment as usual, emphasising the importance of the non-specific curative factors of therapeutic relationships and active interest of the therapists in the progress of their patients. This treatment has been shown to be superior to cognitive behavioral therapy and interpersonal psychotherapy at end of treatment [11], but with effects lessening over time [12, 13]. Full details on the MOSAIC trial [14], MANTRA [8–10, 15, 16] and SSCM [11, 17] can be found elsewhere. Both treatments were found to be effective, with MANTRA having advantages in more severely ill patients [18].

In the first stage of our process evaluation, we explored both therapist and patient experiences of MANTRA and SSCM using in-depth qualitative interviews [19, 20]. There was a high level of agreement between therapists' and patients' views of these two treatments, their unique and overlapping features and relative strengths and weaknesses.

A limitation of the study on patients' views [19] was that because of resource constraints only a small proportion ($n = 17$) of participants from one of the study centres were included and they were interviewed at different stages of treatment, i.e. without the benefit of having experienced a full course of treatment. Oakley et al. [21] have highlighted several methodological issues to be considered in conducting process evaluations within RCTs: All participating treatment sites should be included as well as both qualitative and quantitative data, and importantly, process data should be analysed *prior* to the outcome data to minimize potential biases in interpreting results. The present study has taken into account the aforementioned criteria, in addition to approaching all available MOSAIC trial patients to obtain generalisable results and assessing their feedback after the completion of all treatment sessions, in order to supplement the earlier study by Lose et al. [19].

Accordingly, the aim of the current study was to conduct a process evaluation prior to analysis of outcome data to investigate patients' experiences of two different treatments within a large RCT of outpatient treatment of AN. The main objective was to combine participants' quantitative treatment acceptability and credibility ratings at 12 months with qualitative written feedback. It was hoped that the patients' qualitative feedback could shed more light on the factors associated with their treatment ratings.

Materials and Method

Participants

MOSAIC trial participants were 142 adults (98 % female) with a DSM-IV-TR (2000) diagnosis of AN or Eating Disorder Not Otherwise Specified AN type (EDNOS-AN), recruited between June 2010 and November 2012 from four treatment centres in the UK: South London and Maudsley NHS Foundation Trust; North East London Foundation Trust Eating Disorders Service; Barnet, Enfield & Haringey Mental Health NHS Trust; Oxford Health NHS Foundation Trust. For inclusion in the trial, participants needed a body mass index (BMI) of below 18.5 kg/m^2 and the absence of any major mental or physical co-morbidities that warranted their own treatment. There was no lower BMI limit provided patients were medically stable. After initial assessment, including a range of eating disorder (ED) and other outcome measures, participants were randomly allocated to receive either 20 once-weekly sessions of MANTRA or SSCM plus four monthly follow-up sessions. Optional additional sessions with a dietician and sessions including a family member were also offered. Patients with a BMI of $\leq$ 15 kg/m^2 at the start of treatment were offered 30 weekly sessions. Therapists were expected to see patients in both treatment conditions to control for therapist effects. Follow-up research assessments were carried out at six months (approximately at the end of weekly treatment sessions) and 12 months (end of follow-up sessions). Full details of in- and exclusion criteria and trial procedures can be found elsewhere [14].

Informed consent was obtained from all individual participants included in the study. Ethical approval for the MOSAIC trial was obtained from the Central London REC 4, National Research Ethics Service, Royal Free Hospital, London, (Reference: 10/H0714/9). The trial is registered with Current Controlled Trials: ISRCTN67720902.

Measures

Eating Disorders Examination (EDE) [22]

The EDE measures eating disordered thoughts and behaviors. The EDE is a semi-structured diagnostic interview that generates 4 subscale scores, the mean of which gives an overall global score. Higher scores indicate more serious eating disordered psychopathology. It has been shown to have good reliability and discriminant validity [23, 24]. EDE interviews were carried out by trained assessors. Inter-rater reliability was checked through second scoring every 10th interview.

Treatment acceptability and credibility

Acceptability and credibility of treatment were assessed using two 10 cm visual analogue scales (VAS). Participants were asked to place a vertical mark on each scale to indicate how they would rate themselves in relation to two questions: 1) 'How *acceptable* did you find the type of treatment you received from your therapist during this study?' and 2) 'To what extent do you feel that the treatment you received has *helped you* to reduce your eating disorder behaviors?' On the two scales, 0 cm corresponds to 'completely unacceptable' and 'not at all' and 10 cm represents 'completely acceptable' and 'very much so' respectively. As a treatment's 'credibility' may be difficult for patients to conceptualize, we operationalised it as the reduction of eating disorder behaviours to assess how the treatment has been effective. Helpfulness of treatment is a key aspect of established credibility scales [25]. Scores for treatment acceptability and treatment credibility were calculated separately and to one decimal place.

Participant written feedback form

This qualitative feedback form asked two questions: (1) 'What was your experience of therapy in the MOSAIC trial?' and (2) 'Do you have any comments or suggestions?' Participants were informed that anonymised quotes might be used in publications and a tick box was provided if participants wished to opt out from this (2/82 participants used this option). To protect anonymity, all participants who completed the written feedback were assigned a pseudonym.

Procedure

Demographic and clinical information including age, age of onset, illness duration, BMI, and EDE global score were collected at baseline (pre-randomisation) assessment. Process evaluation data were part of the planned 6- and 12 month follow-up assessments. Ratings of acceptability and credibility were obtained at both 6- and 12-month follow-up assessments in order to capture changing views over time. Written feedback was collected at 12 months only. In all cases, participants were posted the process questionnaires to complete in their own time prior to attending the planned follow-up appointment.

At the time of data collection, research assessors did not read written feedback forms in order to ensure they remained blind to patient treatment allocation. Instead a separate researcher (KAZ), who was not involved in data collection, read and transcribed the feedback for analysis.

Data analysis

Quantitative analysis

Analyses were conducted with IBM SPSS Statistics Version 20 software. Baseline demographic and clinical characteristics were compared between the two treatment groups and between patients who did or did not provide process evaluation data. Independent *t*-tests were conducted to compare the acceptability and credibility ratings given by MANTRA and SSCM patients at 6-month and12-month follow up assessments.

Qualitative analysis

Participants' written feedback forms were transcribed verbatim and imported into NVivo 10 by researcher KAZ. Data were analysed using Braun and Clarke's [26] six phase thematic analysis process from a realist epistemological standpoint. The approach used is similar to that of our first published process evaluation of the MOSAIC trial [19, 20], in which coding was driven by the information obtained from the participants' feedback.

All 82 written feedback responses were transcribed into the software package, before being read and re-read to familiarize the researcher with the data and allow for initial generation of ideas. Through repeated re-reading of the transcripts the researcher identified patterns of common issues raised and data were systematically coded (i.e. a code representing the most basic segment or element of the raw data). At this early stage, as many codes as possible were generated and collated, then grouped into overarching themes and subthemes.

Subsequently, codes and themes were constantly reviewed and refined, discarded, combined or split. Broad, higher-order themes and subthemes were labeled and organized to include all relevant codes.

KAZ, BR and US, researchers blind to treatment outcome, completed data triangulations to improve validity and reliability of the resulting themes, noting down over-arching themes and additional ideas. They came together to consolidate their findings, discussing any disagreements until a consensus was reached. The frequencies with which the codes and themes occurred were calculated and the numbers of words in the transcripts were counted, using the word count facility in Microsoft Office Word 2007. The final thematic map is presented in Fig. 1.

Global valence ratings of feedback

In a separate step, two researchers (KAZ, BR) independently rated the overall global valence of participants' responses on the feedback form as overall positive, mixed or overall negative. Feedback was rated as overall positive if the experience of therapy was described using only favorable, approving, enthusiastic descriptions (e.g. *"BRILLIANT... Really feel that I have been so lucky to be here and it has made all the difference between recovery and not"*), as mixed if there clearly were some positive and some negative descriptions (e.g. *"Mainly positive – although I don't think it was very positive or useful for the state I was in at the time so didn't make best use of the trial"*), and as overall negative if the person described their experience in dismissive, disapproving or unenthusiastic terms (e.g. *"Useless and made me worse until landed up in hospital again"*). Seven irrelevant responses were excluded (e.g. where participants had exclusively focused their feedback on the research process or were unable to give appropriate feedback on treatment due to receiving a very limited number of sessions). The ratings were finalised when a consensus was agreed upon. These ratings were subsequently used as comparisons between treatment groups in our quantitative analyses.

Results

Quantitative analyses

114 of 142 MOSAIC participants (80.3 %) provided acceptability or credibility ratings at six- or 12-month follow-up. There were no baseline differences in age, age of onset, illness duration, BMI or EDE global score between those who did (n =114) or did not (n =28) provide any feedback at 6-month or12 month follow-up. In addition, 82 of the 142 MOSAIC participants (57.7 %) also provided written feedback. Participants who did or did not provide written feedback did not significantly differ from each other on baseline demographic or clinical characteristics.

A total of 60 MANTRA and 54 SSCM patients provided either quantitative and/or qualitative views on their treatment at 6- or12-month follow-up. MANTRA and SSCM patients who provided any feedback did not differ significantly from each other on baseline demographic or clinical characteristics (see Table 1). A significantly higher proportion of MANTRA patients (48/60,

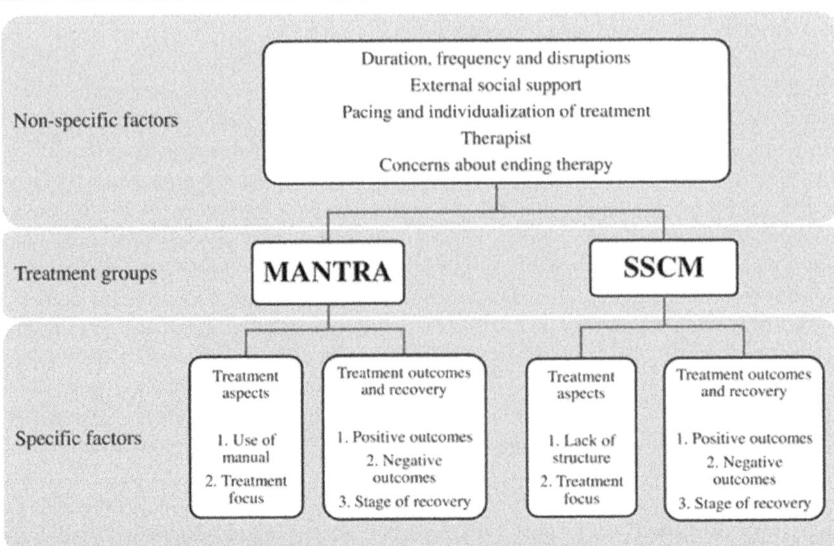

Fig. 1 Thematic map of participants' written feedback

Table 1 Baseline demographic and clinical characteristics of process evaluation participants split by treatment group

	MANTRA n = 60	SSCM n = 54	*t*	*df*	*p*
Age (years), mean (*SD*)	27.0 (8.1)	25.9 (7.6)	.779	112	.438
Age of onset (years), mean (*SD*)	17.7 (6.8)	18.6 (7.0)	-.710	106	.480
Illness duration (years), mean (*SD*)	9.3 (8.2)	7.4 (6.8)	1.351	108	.179
EDE global score, mean (*SD*)	3.2 (1.3)	3.4 (1.3)	-.674	112	.502
BMI (kg/m^2) mean (*SD*)	16.7 (1.2)	16.7 (1.3)	-.048	111	.961

Note. MANTRA: The Maudsley Model of Anorexia Nervosa Treatment for Adults, SSCM: Specialist Supportive Clinical Management, EDE: Eating Disorders Examination, BMI: Body Mass Index

80 %) provided written feedback compared to those receiving SSCM (34/54, 62.9 %) (Pearson's Chi-Square 4.028; df =1; p = 0.045).

Whilst at six months there was no significant difference on acceptability and credibility between the two treatments, at 12 months. MANTRA patients rated their treatment as significantly more acceptable and credible than SSCM patients (see Table 2).

In the written feedback, the mean number of words used was higher in the MANTRA group (M = 107.8, SD = 72.6) compared with the SSCM group (M = 90.6, SD = 47.3) although this difference was not statistically significant (t =1.296; df = 79.9; p = 0.199). After excluding participants who had given an irrelevant written feedback response [MANTRA: 4/48 (8.3 %); SSCM: 3/34 (8.9 %)], assessment of global valence showed that in the MANTRA group, 35/44 participants (79.5 %) were positive about their treatment and 9/44 (20.5 %) either had mixed views or felt negatively about treatment, whereas in the SSCM group, 19/31 (61.3 %) were positive and 12/31 (38.7 %) mixed or negative. Differences between the two treatments were not significant (Pearson's Chi-square value = 2.377; p = 0.123).

Table 2 Treatment acceptability and treatment credibility ratings across six- and 12- month follow up split by treatment group

6-month follow up	MANTRA n = 55	SSCM n = 47	*t*	*df*	*p*
Treatment acceptability, mean (*SD*)	8.5 (2.0)	8.0 (2.2)	1.331	100	.186
Treatment credibility, mean (*SD*)	6.4 (3.1)	5.8 (2.7)	1.052	100	.295
12-month follow up	**MANTRA n = 50**	**SSCM n = 43**	***t***	***df***	***p***
Treatment acceptability, mean (*SD*)	8.6 (1.8)	7.8 (2.3)	2.010	91	.047*
Treatment credibility, mean (*SD*)	6.8 (3.1)	5.5 (2.7)	2.244	91	.027*

Note. *p < .05. MANTRA: The Maudsley Model of Anorexia Nervosa Treatment for Adults, SSCM: Specialist Supportive Clinical Management, EDE: Eating Disorder Examination, BMI: Body Mass Index

In both treatment groups, those who provided positive feedback also gave significantly higher acceptability and credibility ratings at 12 months than those who gave mixed or negative feedback. In the MANTRA group, mean acceptability ratings for participants giving positive feedback were: M = 9.4, SD = 0.9 and for those giving mixed or negative feedback were: M = 5.6, SD = 1.6, ($t(41)$ = 9.725, p < .01). Respective numbers for credibility ratings were positive: M = 8.1, SD = 2.1; mixed or negative: M = 3.0, SD = 1.6, ($t(41)$ = 6.956, p < .01). In SSCM, mean acceptability ratings for people giving positive feedback were: M = 8.6, SD = 1.5 and for those giving mixed or negative feedback were: M = 5.8, SD = 3.2, ($t(26)$ = 3.160, p < .01). Respective credibility ratings were positive: M = 7.3, SD = 1.8; mixed or negative: M = 3.1, SD = 2.5, ($t(26)$ = 5.307, p < .01).

Qualitative analyses

Themes were grouped according to whether they were MANTRA-specific, SSCM-specific, or non- specific, as well as if they were positive or negative to highlight aspects of the treatment that participants liked or did not like. For MANTRA, specific treatment features were use of the manual and exercises and the focus on cognitive and emotional aspects of AN. For SSCM, treatment-specific factors included the focus on weight and eating and lack of structure. Treatment outcomes and recovery describe the positive and negative outcomes, and stage of recovery at the end of treatment. Non-specific factors describe those shared between the two treatment groups such as duration and frequency of treatment, external support and the patient-therapist relationship. Several similar themes were identified in Lose et al.'s [19] paper and the same theme names have been used here for consistency. The resulting themes and sample quotations are presented in Table 3, and the thematic map in Fig. 1.

Table 3 Themes and sample quotations based on written feedback

MANTRA	
Themes and Subthemes	Quotes
Treatment aspects	
1. Use of manual	
Positive (n = 10)	M3 "Many of the exercises that we went through in the sessions made me really think about why I felt and acted the way I did and what I really want from life."
Negative (n = 2)	M23 "I found the workbook didn't help me as I wasn't learning anything new."
2. Treatment focus	
Positive (n = 4)	M19 "Not too focused on solely the eating disorder per se, but on the many different factors/ difficulties that encourage and maintain the eating problems (and other difficulties)."
Negative (n = 2)	M43 "Did not find it that helpful. I did not feel that [the therapist] dealt with either the root of the problem, why I lack confidence, or how to deal with it."
Treatment outcomes and recovery	
1. Positive outcomes	
Effect on understanding AN symptoms and their impact on behavior (n = 8)	M16 "[The treatment] was great in helping me to see it as a disease with symptoms as opposed to something wrong with me as a person."
	M32 "I feel that the therapy has given me a much greater understanding of why I keep this illness and what the illness gives me. I strongly believe that I needed this insight to be able to work on recovery."
Effect on feelings and thought processes (n = 13)	M7 "I found it beneficial as I was able to start to question the [anorexic] voices and thoughts I had regarding food – whereas before I was unable to challenge them and simply accepted them as fact."
	M41 "By no means have I completely let go of anorexia but I've taken so many more steps than I felt capable of before. I have reappraised myself, my eating, and my illness and feel more hopeful than I have in years."
Effect on eating habits and weight (n = 7)	M3 "The food plans we made also helped me to learn how to eat normally and I now rarely worry about what I eat."
	M33 "I think strategies… help me to manage my anxiousness around food and have increased my self-management of my food intake."
Effect on communication (n = 3)	M1 "[Expressing my feelings to others] has been really beneficial as I can tell people when I am struggling, instead of letting the eating disorder do the talking."
2. Negative outcomes (n = 1)	M24 "I do not feel [the therapy] has necessarily AIDED recovery."
3. Stage of recovery (n = 9)	M25 "I still have my fears about gaining weight, weighing myself and find it very difficult to change. Maybe I was/am expecting too much and there is no magic/instant cure or solution to my problems with ED."
	M42 "I consider myself to be almost completely recovered at this point and very excited about moving forward."
SSCM	
Treatment aspects	
1. Lack of structure	
Positive (n = 1)	S34 "I was pleased to have been given the freedom and time to find a lot of answers and strength for myself, but having the security of monitoring and treatment behind me."
Negative (n = 2)	S23 "I did not feel like there was a secure plan in place for that there were set goals or targets, which I would have found helpful."
	S33 "Didn't like the unstructured approach of SSCM, would have preferred more tailored one like MANTRA to ensure lots of aspects of anorexia… were covered."
2. Focus on Nutrition	
Positive (n = 1)	S9 "We talked a lot about food and meal plans and provided me with all the material to work out what I needed to eat and open my eyes to what healthy eating and nutrients really mean."
Negative (n = 4)	S11 "The fact that I got weighed each week terrified me… [The therapist] started talking about 2500 calorie diet, this is when I said no I can't do it."
	S31 "I also found the therapy too focused on food (encouragement to eat) as opposed to exploring feeling and behaviors. I would have liked to explore why I do this to myself. I am still struggling to understand this."

Table 3 Themes and sample quotations based on written feedback *(Continued)*

Treatment outcomes and recovery	
1. Positive outcomes	
Effect on understanding AN symptoms and their impact on behavior (n = 4)	S7 "I do feel that the therapy has given me a better foundation and understanding of my behavior to work from."
	S31 "During the therapy I became aware of my issues and realized that most of my physical problems are due to the same issue."
Effect on feelings and thought processes (n = 1)	S26 "I hope it has set me up with the right mental tools to be able to analyze situations better (both related and unrelated to food)."
Effect on eating habits and weight (n = 2)	S27 "I still have a lot of negative eating disordered thoughts but I'm at a healthy weight so I suppose that is a positive."
Effect on communication (n = 2)	S30 "Felt that I could be very open and honest even when I knew what I was feeling or saying would expose my underlying desire to keep my eating disorder."
2. Negative outcomes (*n* = 2)	S1 "Anything new I have tried I have not tried more than once or made a permanent part of my diet… And sometimes I feel I say or agree to things just to please my therapist."
	S33 "Ended up being admitted as an inpatient due to low mood and then daycare treatment for [eating disorders]."
3. Stage of recovery (*n* = 4)	S17 "I felt like the therapy did not get very far… I don't know if any therapy can ever stop [the illness]."
	S26 "I hope with carrying on the therapy for a bit I will be able to return to eating healthily."
Non-specific	
1. Duration, frequency and disruptions of therapy (*n* = 11)	M12 "I do not feel that it was long enough and I have definitely regressed."
	S14 "I found it difficult to maintain changes to my diet only seeing the therapist once a week, perhaps more regular appointments would help people continue their recovery independently."
	S12 "Unfortunately, my therapist was away for quite a few weeks during my weekly sessions and this did set me back a bit, and feel I still have quite a way to go."
2. External social support (*n* = 9)	S31 "It was very useful to have my family involved in the therapy."
	S21 "I would have liked to have group sessions so I didn't feel so abnormal about thoughts I was having."
3. Pacing and individualization of treatment (*n* = 8)	M27 "I appreciated the way it was individualized and went at the pace that suited me."
	S11 "I think a slower pace, I was not at all ready mentally to increase food."
4. Therapist (*n* = 31)	M7 "My psychologist was fantastic with me. I feel I learned a lot from her and even though I have now stopped seeing her, I still remember a lot of what we covered and can use it to continue challenging my thoughts."
	S7 "After developing a therapist/patient relationship… I was able to feel as though I could trust her advice over my thoughts."
	M48 "The therapist I was given I believe failed to deliver this treatment in an acceptable and appropriate manner."
5. Concerns about ending therapy (*n* = 9)	M44 "I notice an immediate change back to some old behaviors within two weeks of ceasing weekly sessions."
	S27 "I am scared of getting ill again."

Note. MANTRA: The Maudsley Model of Anorexia Nervosa Treatment for Adults, SSCM: Specialist Supportive Clinical Management

MANTRA

Treatment aspects

Use of manual

Positive Ten participants gave positive comments about the MANTRA manual and its exercises. They remarked on its flexibility and ability to be tailored to their needs. Participants also felt that the resources were enjoyable to use, helped them gain better understanding of their illness and provided them with skills to facilitate change. They valued the focused tasks and useful analogies in aiding their reflection and recovery. Even though two participants found the exercises "repetitive" (M20) or "uncomfortable to do" (M16), they indicated that they understood the importance of the issues addressed.

Negative Two participants did not find the manual useful, as they felt that the exercises were too difficult, or that they did not learn anything new from the resources.

Treatment focus

Positive Four participants felt that MANTRA's focus on cognitive, emotional and interpersonal factors, instead of primarily nutrition, helped them better understand their illness.

Negative In contrast, one participant reported that MANTRA did not address the issue of self-confidence which she felt was key for her illness and another would have preferred more help with nutrition.

Treatment outcomes and recovery

Positive outcomes

Effect on understanding ED symptoms and their impact on behaviour Eight participants said that they had benefited from acquiring a greater understanding of AN and of themselves, including the factors contributing to AN, symptoms and their negative impact on their life. Participants were able to see AN as an illness with symptoms separate from their identity. Reflection also helped them to identify, face, and tackle issues from their past and present. Participants highlighted that these factors helped them in their recovery.

Effect on feelings and thought processes Thirteen participants also referred to ways in which the treatment contributed to altered ways of thinking, reappraising their approach to situations in a more adaptive way. This enabled them to challenge negative thoughts, reduce anxiety, accept weight gain, and gain confidence in recovery.

Effect on eating habits and weight Seven participants described positive changes in their eating and weight and linked this to other improvements in their life, such as resuming their education and boosting their self-confidence.

Effect on communication Three participants indicated greater expression of feelings towards others around them, enabling them to open up about their illness to close others.

Negative outcomes

One participant commented that the treatment did not help with her recovery but did not elaborate as to why this was the case.

Stage of recovery

Several MANTRA participants commented on their stage of recovery. Two conveyed that they still had difficulties with eating, weight gain, and relationships with others. Even though they acknowledged they had not attained full recovery, seven participants expressed hope and excitement, as well as the recognition that recovery would be a difficult but not insurmountable challenge.

SSCM

Treatment aspects

Two distinct features of SSCM were highlighted by patients: focus on weight and eating and its lack of structure.

Lack of structure

Positive One participant liked the freedom associated with the treatment, as it enabled her to express herself fully with the guidance of the therapist.

Negative Two participants disliked the lack of treatment structure, and would have preferred a more structured and comprehensive approach.

Focus on nutrition

Positive One participant found SSCM's focus on weight and eating favourable in supporting recovery.

Negative Four participants indicated that the focus on weighing and nutritional advice was distressing or unsuitable for their needs. They stated that a focus on other aspects of AN, such as body image, or its emotional and psychological aspects would have been preferable.

Treatment outcomes and recovery

Positive outcomes

Effect on understanding ED symptoms and their impact on behaviour Four SSCM patients expressed that they had gained greater understanding of AN and of themselves, which helped them identify problems that needed addressing.

Effect on feelings and thought processes One participant indicated that they experienced altered ways of thinking, in terms of an improved ability to analyse situations and to positively compare themselves to others.

Effect on eating habits and weight Two participants described achieving normal eating, weight gain, and a greater understanding and respect for their body.

Effect on communication Two participants found the therapy useful in encouraging expression of feelings towards the therapist and close others.

Negative outcomes

Two SSCM patients felt that the treatment did not benefit them as they required an additional inpatient admission.

Stage of recovery

Four participants shared their outlook regarding their own recovery. One expressed hopefulness about healthy eating, whilst the other three expressed that the therapy did not enable them to achieve long-lasting changes or that recovery was perceived to be impossible.

Non-specific factors

Duration, frequency and disruptions in treatment

Eight participants ($M = 5$, $S = 3$) commented on the duration of treatment and frequency of therapy sessions, with some ($M = 1$) being satisfied and others ($M = 4$, $S = 3$) wishing for a greater number or frequency of sessions. Three participants ($M = 1$, $S = 2$) were dissatisfied about temporary disruptions in their therapy that they felt had contributed to their condition worsening.

External social support

Participants valued the importance of social support during their therapy and recovery. Five ($M = 4$, $S = 1$) individuals felt that more involvement of family members and close others would have been beneficial. Four participants ($M = 1$, $S = 3$) suggested that the involvement of other currently ill or recovered AN patients could serve as friends who truly understood their illness and provide role models for recovery.

Pacing and individualisation of treatment

Five participants ($M = 4$, $S = 1$) commented that their treatment was flexible, individualized and relevant for their needs. This included the flexibility of treatment, meeting with a dietician for nutritional advice, and treatment moving at a comfortable pace. Three participants ($M = 1$, $S = 2$), however, felt that their treatment was not individualized enough.

Therapist

A total of 31 participants ($M = 21$, $S = 10$) mentioned their therapists in their written feedback; 27 ($M = 19$, $S = 8$) gave positive comments, including favorable qualities, such as being understanding, sympathetic, non-judgmental, kind, considerate to their needs, welcoming, intuitive, compassionate, and empathic. Furthermore, they also commented on the therapists' expertise, and the development of the therapist-patient relationship. Three participants ($M = 1$, $S = 2$), however, expressed dissatisfaction about a change of therapist and disrupted therapy, and one MANTRA patient felt that their therapist lacked training in conducting the treatment.

Concerns about ending therapy

Several participants ($M = 7$, $S = 2$) expressed concerns about ending therapy, including fear of returning to old behaviours and suggested including more follow-up support.

Discussion

This study is the second stage of a process evaluation integrated into a large scale RCT of two outpatient psychological therapies in adults with AN. This evaluation combined the use of both quantitative and qualitative measures to assess patients' treatment experiences.

Findings show that at 12 months post-randomisation i.e. at the end of both weekly and follow up treatment sessions, MANTRA patients rate their treatment as significantly more acceptable and credible than patients receiving SSCM. This result is strengthened by the clear agreement between the global valence of the qualitative written feedback and quantitative VAS ratings at 12-month follow-up, in that participants who provided overall positive written feedback also rated their treatment as significantly more acceptable and credible than participants who gave mixed or negative written feedback.

It is also of note that, although overall proportions of MANTRA and SSCM patients who provided some process feedback did not differ, significantly more MANTRA patients gave written feedback when compared to SSCM. Those MANTRA patients who did respond also tended to give a more detailed account of their experiences (as assessed by number of words used). This difference might be explained by the fact that MANTRA aims to reduce AN patients' emotion avoidance and suppression, and to increase emotional clarity and adaptive emotion regulation, such as emotional expressivity [27]. Arguably willingness to express views about one's treatment experience is a facet of this. Alternatively, it may be that MANTRA patients are simply more practiced in using writing as a form of expression compared to SSCM patients, given that therapeutic writing exercises are incorporated into this treatment, but not into SSCM.

Overall, themes that arose from the thematic analysis replicate those found in our earlier paper which used qualitative interviews in a subset of patients from one participating centre [19]. Participants highlighted both treatment specific (e.g. MANTRA: manual, exercises, comprehensive focus; SSCM: focus on nutrition, lack of structure) and non-specific factors (e.g. relationship with therapist, treatment pacing, duration, frequency and disruption, external social support and concerns about ending therapy) as important aspects of their treatment.

Thus MANTRA and SSCM were experienced somewhat differently in terms of their focus, strengths and challenges, but there were also some overlapping features.

The perceived differences between treatments, both positive and negative, were to an extent, in line with the specific focus and targets of each treatment. MANTRA targets motivational, cognitive, emotional and interpersonal maintaining factors of AN with the aim of effecting nutritional changes via broader cognitive and emotional changes. In contrast, SSCM centrally focuses on improving eating and weight and other topics for discussion arise as chosen by patients, session by session. Thus, in MANTRA many participants valued the flexible, individually tailored manual-based approach and the focus on thoughts and feelings. A small number of patients however, experienced certain therapeutic exercises as unhelpful or even as patronising, and felt the manual-based approach did not address their unique problems or teach them anything new. Whilst these more critical views may be legitimate and appropriate there is a possibility that they may at least in part be linked to AN patients' detail-focused perfectionist cognitive style, that makes some individuals dismissive of anything that is not a perfect fit. It is important for therapist to be aware of this possibility.

In SSCM, patients who gave positive feedback commended the clear focus on nutrition and freedom offered, whereas others saw the focus on nutrition as negative, generating anxiety and distress. SSCM's lack of structure was also seen as unhelpful by some, in facilitating exploration of certain aspects of their illness.

In addition, across treatment groups disappointment regarding failure to reach desired improvements or a continuation of significant ED symptoms associated with more negative feedback. Thus mixed or negative feedback about treatment appeared to be due to a range of reasons, some to do with the therapeutic focus, content, delivery or structure, others with patients' mixed feelings about change or disappointment about limited progress.

As expected, due to feedback being collected at the end of treatment the theme of recovery and life beyond therapy was more prominent in the present evaluation than in our earlier interview study [19]. More MANTRA patients addressed this issue than those receiving SSCM. In general, MANTRA patients expressed greater satisfaction with their progress and excitement about working towards their future, despite the recognition that achieving recovery would remain challenging. Of the few SSCM patients mentioning this theme one individual expressed pessimism about recovery whilst the other remained hopeful.

Several non-specific factors were mentioned by a substantial number of patients. This suggests the importance of basic factors such as structure, duration and timing for the success of a treatment and the difficulties that arise from disruptions through therapist illness or departure. The single most commonly mentioned theme by a long way, unsurprisingly was that of the therapeutic relationship A previous study on therapist characteristics preferred by AN patients identified factors (acceptance, vitality, challenge and expertise) associated with a good therapeutic relationship and also unhelpful therapist characteristics (disregard, prejudice, passivity, pampering) [28]. The views of patients in the present study largely confirm these findings. Overall, our findings support the implications highlighted in the earlier process evaluations of the MOSAIC Trial [19, 20]. More specifically, the importance of non- specific factors, such as therapist characteristics, individualisation of treatment and social support are emphasized.

Since the completion of the process study, the study's main outcomes have been published [18]. Findings show that MANTRA patients attended significantly more treatment sessions and a higher proportion of MANTRA patients were treatment completers. Whilst overall there were no significant differences at 12 months between MANTRA and SSCM on BMI, eating disorders psychopathology, distress levels and other outcomes, MANTRA appeared to be advantageous in more underweight patients in terms of facilitating greater weight gain at both 6 and 12 months. This suggests that MANTRA patients' view of this treatment as more acceptable, credible and all round positive is at least in part rooted in better clinical outcomes.

The 'three-legged stool' principle of evidence-based medicine [29, 30] suggests that in choosing one intervention over another, best available research evidence about efficacy, clinical expertise and patient preference all need to be considered. With this in mind MANTRA can be recommended over SSCM.

Finally, due to the more positive initial treatment experience, individuals' receiving MANTRA may be more willing to have further treatment should this become necessary. This is particularly important for the many individuals with AN who have a chronic and/or relapsing course of the illness.

This study has several strengths and limitations. Firstly, over 80 % of MOSAIC trial participants provided some process feedback and there were no baseline differences between those who did and did not provide these data. Thus, our findings are likely to be representative of the views shared by the whole MOSAIC trial sample. Secondly, treatment acceptability and credibility ratings were supported by the written feedback provided. Thirdly, participants were recruited from all treatment sites involved in the MOSAIC trial and data were obtained and analysed before trial outcomes are known.

Finally, bias in the interpretation of qualitative data was reduced through performing data triangulations.

The study also has a number of limitations. First, a significantly higher proportion of MANTRA patients compared to SSCM patients provided written feedback. The fact that the SSCM group were more selected may have biased the results. Second, although the use of written feedback, enabled participants to express their opinions freely and independently (i.e. away from their therapists'), the questions asked were broad and the written nature of the feedback did not allow for probing and exploration of key issues as a qualitative interview would. It might have been helpful to include detailed questions in order to obtain more in-depth feedback regarding different treatment components and outcomes. Third, the feedback represents participants' retrospective recollections of treatment at the time point of assessment, and there may have been some recall bias. However, this would have operated similarly in both treatments. Fourth, some of the qualitative themes were only reported by one or two participants. Thus caution is required in interpretation of these findings. Nonetheless, current results replicate those obtained from semi-structured interviews carried out as part of the previous evaluation [19].

Fifth, our assessment of credibility was limited to helpfulness of treatment and thus rather narrow. Established expectancy/credibility scales [25] also include other aspects, such as how logical a particular therapy rationale seems to the patient and whether they would recommend a treatment to a friend or another person in their situation. It is possible that use of a broader credibility scale would have yielded different responses.

A final limitation is the lack of a treatment expectancy measure taken at the start of therapy. However, in the previous pilot trial comparing MANTRA with SSCM a treatment expectancy measure was included and both treatments were viewed as equally credible and positive [15].

Conclusions

Together with our earlier interview paper [19] on patients' views of their treatment this study is very much a first attempt to capture some of the qualitative views of patients receiving the two study treatments and is somewhat exploratory in its nature. MANTRA patients viewed their treatment as more acceptable, credible and generally more positive in comparison to patients receiving SSCM at 12 months. Participants also highlighted the useful components of and outcomes associated with their treatment. MANTRA patients valued the use of the manual and the focus on cognitive, emotional and interpersonal factors, while SSCM patients mentioned its less structured nature and focus on nutrition. This study, together with the previous process evaluation [19], suggests that many individuals with AN perceive MANTRA as a viable treatment option. Further studies should include more sophisticated methods of evaluating treatment process to address the dearth of research in this area.

Competing interests

US and JT are the developers of MANTRA.

Author contributions

US and BR conceived and designed the study. LR, EJS, NB, NW, JT, US contributed to the coordination, supervision and treatment delivery of the study. BR, AK, AL, MK, HD and HB made substantial contributions to acquisition of data. KAZ, BR and US analysed and interpreted the data and drafted the manuscript. All authors contributed to revising it critically for important intellectual content; and all authors read and approved the final manuscript.

Acknowledgement

This article presents independent research commissioned by the National Institute for Health Research (NIHR) under its Programme Grants for Applied Research scheme (RP-PG-0606-1043). The views expressed in this publication are those of the author(s) and not necessarily those of the NHS, the NIHR or the Department of Health. US and JT receive salary report from the NIHR Biomedical Research Centre for Mental Health, South London and Maudsley NHS Foundation Trust and Institute of Psychiatry, King's College London.

Author details

[1]Section of Eating Disorders, Department of Psychological Medicine, Institute of Psychiatry, Psychology and Neuroscience, King's College London, PO Box 59SE5 8AF London, UK. [2]Hope Wing, Porters Avenue Health Centre, North East London Foundation Trust, Dagenham, Essex, UK. [3]Eating Disorders Research Group, Research Dept. of Clinical, Educational & Health Psychology, University College London, London, UK. [4]The Phoenix Wing, St Ann's Hospital, Barnett, Enfield and Haringey Mental Health Trust, Tottenham, London, UK. [5]Oxford Adult Eating Disorder Service, Cotswold House, Warneford Hospital, Oxford NHS Foundation Trust, Oxford, UK.

References

1. Zipfel S, Giel KE, Bulik CM, Hay P. Schmidt U. Anorexia nervosa, aetiology, assessment and treatment. Lancet Psychiatry 2015; In press.
2. National Institute for Clinical and Health Care Excellence . Eating disorders: core interventions in the treatment and management of anorexia nervosa, bulimia nervosa and related eating disorders. British Psychological Society (UK). NICE Clinical Guideline No.9; 2004.
3. Agras WS, Brandt HA, Bulik CM, Dolan-Sewell R, Fairburn CG, Halmi KA, et al. Report of the National Institutes of Health workshop on overcoming barriers to treatment research in anorexia nervosa. Int J Eat Disord. 2004;35:509–21.
4. Hay PJ, Claudino AM, Touyz S, Abd Elbaky G. Individual psychological therapy in the outpatient treatment of adults with anorexia nervosa. Cochrane Database Syst Rev. 2015;7:CD003909.
5. Craig P, Dieppe P, Macintyre S, Michie S, Nazareth I, Petticrew M. Developing and evaluating complex interventions: the new Medical Research Council guidance. BMJ. 2008;337:a1655.
6. Crawford MJ, Weaver T, Rutter D, Sensky T, Tyrer P. Evaluating new treatments in psychiatry: the potential value of combining qualitative and quantitative research methods. Int Rev Psychiatry. 2002;14:6–11.
7. Pope C, Mays N. Qualitative research in health care. Chichester: John Wiley & Sons; 2008.
8. Schmidt U, Treasure J. Anorexia nervosa: Valued and visible. A cognitive-interpersonal maintenance model and its implications for research and practice. Br J Clin Psychol. 2006;45:343–66.
9. Schmidt U, Wade TD, Treasure J. The Maudsley Model of Anorexia Nervosa Treatment for Adults (MANTRA): Development, Key Features, and Preliminary Evidence. J Cog Psychotherapy. 2014;28:48–71.

10. Treasure J, Schmidt U. The Cognitive-Interpersonal Maintenance Model of Anorexia Nervosa Revisited: A summary of the evidence for cognitive, socio-emotional and interpersonal predisposing and perpetuating factors. J Eat Disord. 2013;1:13.
11. McIntosh VV, Jordan J, Carter FA, Luty SE, McKenzie JM, Bulik CM, et al. Three psychotherapies for anorexia nervosa: a randomized, controlled trial. Am J Psychiatry. 2005;162:741–7.
12. Carter FA, Jordan J, McIntosh VV, Luty SE, McKenzie JM, Frampton C, et al. The long-term efficacy of three psychotherapies for anorexia nervosa: A randomized, controlled trial. Int J Eat Disord. 2011;44:647–54.
13. Touyz S, Le Grange D, Lacey H, Hay P, Smith R, Maguire S, et al. Treating severe and enduring anorexia nervosa: a randomized controlled trial. Psychol Med. 2013;43:2501–11.
14. Schmidt U, Renwick B, Lose A, Kenyon M, Dejong H, Broadbent H, et al. The MOSAIC study-comparison of the Maudsley Model of Treatment for Adults with Anorexia Nervosa (MANTRA) with Specialist Supportive Clinical Management (SSCM) in outpatients with anorexia nervosa or eating disorder not otherwise specified, anorexia nervosa type: study protocol for a randomized controlled trial. Trials. 2013;14:160.
15. Schmidt U, Oldershaw A, Jichi F, Sternheim L, Startup H, McIntosh V, et al. Out-patient psychological therapies for adults with anorexia nervosa: randomised controlled trial. Br J Psychiatry. 2012;201:392–9.
16. Wade TD, Treasure J, Schmidt U. A case series evaluation of the Maudsley Model for treatment of adults with anorexia nervosa. Eur Eat Disord Rev. 2011;19:382–9.
17. McIntosh VV, Jordan J, Luty SE, Carter FA, McKenzie JM, Bulik CM, et al. Specialist supportive clinical management for anorexia nervosa. Int J Eat Disord. 2006;39:625–32.
18. Schmidt U, Magill N, Renwick B, Keyes A, Kenyon M, Dejong H, et al. The Maudsley Outpatient Study of Treatments for Anorexia Nervosa and Related Conditions (MOSAIC): Comparison of the Maudsley Model of Anorexia Nervosa Treatment for Adults (MANTRA) with specialist supportive clinical management (SSCM) in outpatients with broadly defined anorexia nervosa: A randomized controlled trial. J Consult Clin Psychol. 2015;83:796–807.
19. Lose A, Davies C, Renwick B, Kenyon M, Treasure J, Schmidt U. Process Evaluation of the Maudsley Model for Treatment of Adults with Anorexia Nervosa Trial. Part II: Patient Experiences of Two Psychological Therapies for Treatment of Anorexia Nervosa. Eu Eat Disord Rev. 2014;22:131–9.
20. Waterman-Collins D, Renwick B, Lose A, Kenyon M, Serpell L, Richards L, et al. Process Evaluation of the MOSAIC Trial, Part I: Therapist Experiences of Delivering Two Psychological Therapies for Treatment of Anorexia Nervosa. Eur Eat Disord Rev. 2014;22:122–30.
21. Oakley A, Strange V, Bonell C, Allen E, Stephenson J. Process evaluation in randomised controlled trials of complex interventions. BMJ. 2006;332:413–6.
22. Fairburn CG. Cognitive behavior therapy and eating disorders. New York: Guilford Press; 2008.
23. Cooper Z, Cooper PJ, Fairburn CG. The validity of the eating disorder examination and its subscales. Br J Psychiatry. 1989;154:807–12.
24. Rizvi SL, Peterson CB, Crow SJ, Agras WS. Test-retest reliability of the eating disorder examination. Int J Eating Disord. 2000;28:311–6.
25. Devilly GJ, Borkovec TD. Psychometric properties of the credibility/ expectancy questionnaire. J Behav Ther Exp Psychiatry. 2000;31:73–86.
26. Braun V, Clarke V. Using thematic analysis in psychology. Qual Res Psychol. 2006;3:77–101.
27. Oldershaw A, Lavender T, Sallis H, Stahl D, Schmidt U. Emotion generation and regulation in anorexia nervosa: A systematic review and meta-analysis of self-report data. Clin Psychol Rev. 2015;39:83–95.
28. Gulliksen KS, Espeset EM, Nordbø RH, Skårderud F, Geller J, Holte A. Preferred therapist characteristics in treatment of anorexia nervosa: the patient's perspective. Int J Eat Disord. 2012;45:932–41.
29. Lilenfeld S. Evidence-Based Practice: The Misunderstandings Continue. Published on January 27, 2014. http://www.psychologytoday.com/blog/the-skeptical-psychologist/201401/evidence-based-practice-the-misunderstandings-continue
30. Sackett DL, Rosenberg WM, Gray JA, Haynes RB, Richardson WS. Evidence based medicine: what it is and what it isn't. BMJ. 1996;312:71–2.

'Feelings stronger than reason': conflicting experiences of exercise in women with anorexia nervosa

Liv-Jorunn Kolnes

Abstract

Background: Individuals with anorexia nervosa frequently feel ambivalent about treatment and weight restoration, and drop out and relapse rates in treatment are high. Increased insight into the function of the eating disorder is considered essential for achieving long-lasting, meaningful change. However, research investigating the functions of anorexia nervosa tends to focus on the role of the disease *per se*. Distinctions are rarely made across features. In particular, the subjective experience, understanding and sense making of the engagement in compulsive exercise in individuals with anorexia nervosa has received little attention. By using a qualitative methodological approach, this paper aims to expand on prior findings by examining how patients with anorexia nervosa understand and make sense of the experience of exercise in the context of their lives and treatment programme.

Methods: Semi-structured interviews were conducted with six females, four of whom were former athletes. Transcripts were subjected to interpretative phenomenological analysis (IPA).

Results: Two overarching themes emerged in the analysis of the larger study of which this paper is a part; 'paradoxical functions of exercise' and 'diverging experiences of exercise'. Diverging experiences of exercise is the focus of this paper. Firstly, in spite of being severely underweight and suffering from exhaustion, as well as having a clear awareness of the associated negative health effects, participants were engaged in a continuous cycle of rigorous and excessive exercise, which consumed extensive amounts of time and energy. Secondly, the results demonstrate how exercise routines negatively control and interfere with the participants' involvement in the social world. Thirdly, the manner in which participants speak about their exercise reveals their wording to be characterized by efforts to downplay the extent of their actual immersion in exercise. Issues of control and ambivalence about treatment and recovery can be considered potential triggers for the participants' engagement with exercise. Implicit meanings are elaborated upon and discussed in relation to existing literature.

Conclusions: The material provides increased insight into the multi-layered meanings of exercise for individuals with anorexia nervosa. It also suggests alternatives to current ways of understanding and approaching exercise that may enable this issue to be addressed in a more meaningful way in therapy. Qualitative approaches can make a valuable contribution to furthering such understanding.

Keywords: Anorexia nervosa, Compulsive exercise, Ambivalence and control, IPA

Correspondence: l.j.kolnes@nih.no
Norwegian School of Sport Sciences, PB 4014 Ullevål Stadion, 0806 Oslo, Norway

Background

While anorexia nervosa is a serious illness commonly associated with high levels of medical and psychological complications [1, 2], it is also recognised that individuals with anorexia nervosa may have positive feelings about their illness [3–5]. It is therefore not surprising that such individuals frequently feel ambivalent about treatment and weight restoration, and that drop-out and relapse rates in treatment are high [6, 7]. Attempts to produce long-lasting, meaningful change during the treatment of eating disorders focus on reducing psychiatric distress, producing changes in self-concept, and providing increased insight into the function of the eating disorder for the individual [8]. However, research into the functions of anorexia nervosa tends to focus on sense making or the role of the disease *per se* (e.g., [9–11]). Distinctions are rarely made across features, such as between explicit functions of restrictive eating and intense exercise routines, all of which are considered core parts of anorexia nervosa (restrictive subtype). In particular, little attention has been paid to the subjective experience, understanding and sense making of compulsive exercise in individuals with this disorder. Accordingly, existing work may not fully capture the means by which individuals make sense of the diverse practices and features that are part of their illness, or how these relate to one another.

Compulsive exercise is associated with increased levels of disordered eating attitudes and behaviours and considered an important component in the development and maintenance of anorexia nervosa (e.g., [12, 13]), particularly the restrictive subtype [14–16]. Preoccupation with exercise in the eating disorders has long been associated with weight- and body shape concerns [17–19]. In view of the assumption that individuals with anorexia nervosa have difficulties in identifying and regulating their emotions [20–23], it is assumed that the regulation and neutralizing of negative emotions also makes an important contribution to compulsive exercise [24–28]. There are, however, concerns that compulsive exercise may become the usual method by which emotions are regulated and that this may prevent the individual from exploring alternative ways of managing difficult feelings [8, 29]. Currently, there is no agreement among researchers and clinicians regarding what constitutes excessive versus compulsive exercise in this context. The most consistent support for a term that captures adherence to strict and recurring exercise routines maintained in spite of negative consequences, appear to be for the term *compulsive exercise* [30]. Excessive exercise may also be comprehended as a continuum characterized by increased prioritizing of exercise routines over other activities in parallel with increased exercise tolerance, which may gradually become more noticeable and progress into compulsive exercise [31].

While physical activity is commonly associated with health benefits, in the context of anorexia nervosa, exercising is a complex, multi-layered dimension that needs further understanding. It has been shown that heavy exercising in individuals with anorexia nervosa is accompanied by an increased risk of medical complications [2, 18], longer length of hospitalization [19], moderate clinical results [32], and an increased prospect of relapse after recovery [7, 33]. Studies of exercise in people with anorexia nervosa have in the main used standardized measures or fixed self-report surveys. These may not entirely capture the meaning of exercise for people who exercise compulsively. With few exceptions [34–37], qualitative investigations of the experience of exercise in individuals with anorexia nervosa are sparse. In an auto ethnographic paper, Axelsen [35] describes challenging experiences connected with the shift from being an anorectic to becoming a devoted triathlete. She gives an account of how her engagement with exercise developed from walking the dog as a 'time out' from difficult feelings to gradually becoming more compulsive and interfering negatively with her societal life. Having received psychological and medical care for her illness, she regained some weight, although her exercising became increasingly excessive after she quit treatment. Eventually, Axelsen reached a turning point and began training for a triathlon. This new training gradually helped Axelsen regain weight and reconnect with her body in what was perceived to be a more healthful manner than her previous exercising [35]. It also entailed engagement in social interactions with training peers. Successively, she identifyed her self more with being an athlete, than with being an anorectic. Given that the core beliefs and feelings that maintained the exercise routines did not seem to have been sufficiently challenged, it could, however, be suggested that she had mainly replaced one compulsion with another in the process of becoming a devoted triathlete. Yet, she maintains that the engagement in triathlon became a journey into some sense of recovery, and that the new compulsion was more balanced and healthy than the former, whilst also representing a sense of belonging and a positive lifestyle [35]. Employing a thematic analytic approach, Moola et al. [36] explore experiences of physical activity in Canadian women previously hospitalized for their anorexia nervosa. Despite expressing serious health issues due to exercise routines, the women engaged in compulsive exercising motivated by weight concerns and anxiety reduction. The authors describe confusion among patients and staff about what is considered physical activity and what represents eating disorder psychopathology and how this gave rise to challenging situations [36]. Furthermore, the women's engagement in any physical activity was frequently considered to compromise treatment goals, and attempts to deal with problematic exercise in hospital treatment were characterized by exercise restriction [36]. In a narrative inquiry study, Young et al. [34] examine the role of exercise across the lifespan in a mostly Australian sample of women with anorexia nervosa. This study illustrates the transformation of exercise from being balanced and enjoyable during childhood into compulsive and rule-driven exercising during their illness [34]. Whilst providing emotion regulation and a sense of being in control in the participants, concomitant to previous research, exercise contributed to prolonged progress and relapse and was considered a prominent feature in sustaining the illness [34]. The findings of a qualitative report focusing on the meaning women with anorexia nervosa make of their experience with exercise are complemental to these studies. In addition to taking part in high levels of exercising to escape and regulate feelings, the results illuminate how feelings deriving from past and present challenging life experiences resonate as bodily sensations, and how participants turn to exercise to ease off embodied distress stemming from such feelings [37]. This study further demonstrate the significant meaning of exercise to the women's sense of self and identity, and how their sense of self entangle with an anorectic and an athletic identity, a complementary identification giving increased connotation to the reluctance and ambivalence towards change apparent in some of the participants [37].[1]

Given the challenges and confusions connected with the understanding and management of exercise during treatment [36] and the assumption that compulsive exercise is a major emotion-regulation strategy that contributes to maintaining the illness [29], an understanding of how individuals with anorexia nervosa make sense of their engagement in such exercise is now needed. Indeed, it is imperative to challenge the view that exercise is a more acceptable behaviour than disturbed eating or dieting in this context [38]. By using a qualitative methodological approach, the current paper aims to expand the aforementioned findings by examining how individuals with anorexia nervosa restrictive subtype understand and make sense of the experience of exercise in the context of their lives and treatment programme.

Methods

To address the issue central to this study, interpretative phenomenological analysis (IPA) has been employed. IPA is concerned with understanding the person-in-context, and exploring individuals' relatedness to the world. IPA is a phenomenological and hermeneutical research approach [39, 40]. Phenomenological philosophy is valuable as it offers a rich source of beliefs about how to examine and understand lived experience, which is unique to the person's embodied and situated relationship to the world [40, 41]. IPA is inspired by *phenomenology* as it is concerned with trying to understand the individuals's personal perception or account of an experience, as opposed to attempting to produce an objective record of the experience itself [40]. IPA connects with *hermeneutics* in that phenomenological examination is an interpretative process. In the examination of how a phenomenon appears, the analyst offers an interpretative account of what it means for the participant to have such concerns [42]. IPA also links up with an *ideographic* commitment, situating participants in their particular contexts, exploring their personal perspectives, starting with a detailed examination of each case before moving to more general claims [40]. As the aim is to reveal something of the experience of each given person, IPA studies usually involve a small number of participants. The rationale of sampling in IPA is based on producing a clearly situated, circumscribed and transparent account of what has been found within contexts, and within homogenous populations [42]. It is not assumed that there will be a place to stop where one can claim that this is enough data, or that 'saturation' has been achieved. IPA is concerned with keeping the numbers low, in order to look for rich detail, similarity and difference, shade and nuance, such that 'saturation' is reached in terms of what has been taken from the individual case or these cases. IPA has increasingly been used among health and social care professionals as it allows for an in-depth exploration and a nuanced account of individuals with a health condition, at the same time as it pays attention to explicit content and implied meanings.

It may be noted that a unique part of the broader study of which this paper is a part, involves a body examination frequently applied in Norwegian psychomotor physiotherapy with the aim of providing insight about bodily tension and constriction in the participants. Due to its separate character and focus on how clients' functional impairments may guide exercise and physical therapy interventions in a beneficial way, the results of the body assessment and a discussion of relevant implications for treatment will be detailed in a separate paper.

Participants

Six women who were undergoing intensive in- or outpatient treatment for anorexia nervosa participated in this study. All of these women were attending residential or day treatment at eating disorder services in Norway. Intensive treatment is commonly recommended for patients with anorexia nervosa who have a low BMI, and weight restoration is often the primary goal. The inpatient treatment programmes impose non-negotiable weight gain expectations and restricted engagement in exercise (usually restricted to walking 15 – 30 min, two to three times per day). To achieve depth and richness of data, it was essential that the sample of interviewees was homogenous and shared particular criteria related to the research question [43]. Participants selected were over the age of 18, they had a clinical diagnosis of anorexia nervosa restricting subtype and were considered compulsive exercisers. The diagnosis was provided by their consultant psychiatrist or psychologist using ICD 10 [44]. For inclusion in this study, compulsive exercise was defined as 'moderate to vigorous exercise for more than six hours per week for a minimum of 1 month before hospitalisation' [45]. This definition does not capture qualitative aspects of exercise, yet it is utilized in relevant literature [46]. It takes into consideration that exercise for more than six hours weekly may have harmful effects (e.g., overuse injuries, decreased bone density, stress fractures) for individuals with anorexia nervosa who are severely underweight [2, 47]. Four participants were involved in competitive sports in their teens, prior to the onset of the illness. The sample only includes women, as there were no men admitted to the units during the recruitment phase meeting the inclusion criteria. The participants' ages, duration of illness and length of treatment are listed in Appendix 1. Their body mass index (BMI) was between 15.2 and 19.2 at the time of the interview, while lowest BMI had been between 12.6 and 14.5. The participants were asked to take part in the study by their physician or psychotherapist. One woman, still fulfilling the inclusion criteria, but who recently had resigned from the service, was asked to take part by the author. To protect participants' anonymity and safeguard confidentiality, names and identifying features were altered. The study was given ethical approval by the Regional Ethics Committee of Southern Norway and administrative consent was granted by the hospital units involved. Participants were given written information regarding the research and were informed of the possibility of withdrawing from the interview at any time. Informed consent was gathered from all women.

The interview schedule

The interview schedule consisted of open-ended questions. Participants were initially encouraged to recount the history and status of their eating disorder and experiences with exercise, including their interest in sport prior to the onset of anorexia nervosa. Next, they were asked to elaborate on their thoughts and feelings related to exercising, the functions and meanings it has for them, and how their training may influence other aspects of their lives (e.g., Can you describe your exercise and activities during a day and week? What are your thoughts/feelings about exercise, and about why you exercise? Does your exercise influence other aspects of your life? If so, in what way?). The interview procedure was flexible in order to allow interesting points emerging during the interview to be followed up. For instance, in the course of the interview, prompting by asking particular questions (e.g., How long are your walks? Do you do any strength training? If so, what do you do specifically? What about activity when in your room? What do you do when on leave?) was used in order to obtain balanced responses about the scope of the participants' experience with exercise. The author conducted the interviews during second half of 2013 in a private room at the units or at the author's workplace. The interviews lasted for 50–90 min, they were audiotaped and subsequently transcribed verbatim by the author.

Data analysis

The analysis closely adhered to the four-stage process described by Smith et al. [40]. In the first step, the author read the primary transcript a number of times in order to become familiar with the data. Any significant or interesting initial comments were recorded during this reading. Secondly, initial notes were transformed into emerging themes while paying attention not to overstate relations between the participants' own words and the researchers' interpretations. During the third stage, the emergent themes were examined for patterns and connections, and clustered according to conceptual similarities. These clusters were subsequently labelled according to the conceptual nature of the themes in each cluster. Next, a table of themes was produced and sub-themes were nested with supporting quotes from the participant. Quotes were coded (e.g., A: Agnes/3: page number/C: quote 3 on page) to safeguard the possibility of revisiting the transcript to check the context of the extract. Transcripts for the next five participants were then read and subjected to the same analytic process. When considering individual cases during data analysis in an IPA study, we are inevitably influenced by what has been found in previous cases. To allow new themes to emerge, it is crucial to maintain the rigour of systematically following the steps outlined by IPA for each case [40]. Thus, individual cases were considered on their own terms, allowing new themes to emerge within each case. After conducting the analysis for each case, cross-case patterns were established and documented in a table of themes for the group. This information was transformed into a narrative account supported by verbatim extracts from the participants. An experienced IPA researcher reviewed and audited the analytic journey to ensure firm grounding in the transcripts. Two overarching themes emerged during the analysis, 'paradoxical functions of exercise' and 'diverging experiences of exercise', of which the second is the focus of this present paper.

Issues of quality and validity

To demonstrate scientific rigour and trustworthiness, the criteria outlined by Yardley [48] for assessing validity and quality in qualitative psychology are considered useful for ensuring high quality of research with IPA [40]. These criteria include sensitivity to context, commitment and rigour, coherence and transparency, and impact and importance. Smith [49] has made suggestions to guide IPA research output, by recommending that sufficient quotations from the data are used to illustrate the points made and to show density for each theme (e.g., for N = 1–3, quotations are needed from every participant per theme; for N = 4–8, quotations are needed for at least three participants per theme). The present study adheres to Yardley and Smith's guidelines concerning scientific rigour.

Reflexivity

The author of this paper has a doctoral degree in sport sciences. She is a physiotherapist specialist in Norwegian psychomotor physiotherapy (NPMP[2]), and has a number of years of experience of working with individuals with anorexia nervosa. Reflexivity involves the need for the researcher to recognise that she always brings her own horizons of experience and fore-conceptions to the encounter and that phenomena are continuously interpreted in the light of these. While presumptions may hinder the process of allowing the new (e.g., person, text) to speak in its own voice, they might also represent a way in to the new. The author recognises that her past experiences and understandings inevitably colour her perceptions. Nevertheless, these may also be helpful in the interpretation process, by allowing her to empathise and understand the participants' voices and to help her explore in depth the meaning of significant events and processes [40].

Results

Two superordinate themes were identified in the analysis of the larger study of which this paper is a part: *'Paradoxical functions of exercise'* and *'diverging experiences of exercise'*. To ensure richness of the phenomenological description and the exploratory interpretative account of the participants concerns within each overarching theme, the two themes are examined in two separate papers. This present article reports on *diverging experiences of exercise*, due to its rich examination of participants' challenging relationship with exercise. The analysis of *paradoxical functions of exercise* reporting on exercise as a means of regulating feelings and easing off embodied emotional distress, as well as the experience and meaning of exercise for the participants' self and identity, are published in a separate paper [37]. Subthemes in all participants are illustrated in Appendix 2.

Diverging experiences of exercise

Key features of this superordinate theme are experiences of exercise as a rigorous and comprehensive entity limiting the participants' social and relational worlds. Accounts of how the participants experience and relate to compulsive exercise and what it is like to be engaged in such exercise are examined first. Secondly, the manner in which exercise is prioritized over and limits involvement in the social world is explored. Thirdly, the paradoxical wording that characterizes the participants' descriptions of their engagement in exercise is presented, along with their tendency to minimize and redefine their engagement with physical activity.

'I feel like I am being compelled to exercise': Ambivalence and control

This theme illustrates participants' diverging experiences with exercise and how compulsions, rules, routines and conflicting feelings accompany this engagement. The analysis is introduced by extracts from Agnes and Hedda illustrating some of the main features of the participants' accounts[3]:

> Agnes: When it first started, I was very thin. (..) In the end, I found myself eating and training, eating and training. It became a constant vicious circle (..). Every time I was full, I exercised or threw up. (..) I have been doing several things on top of the training sessions, such as working out compulsively in the midst of other activities and doing push-ups wherever possible. This has increased more and more, (..) there were around 200 before breakfast (..) in between taking a shower, preparing breakfast, and then in the afternoon and before going to bed. (..) I had to do push-ups while visiting friends, or at the university. (..) Ultimately, it was like being on autopilot, as I constantly had to do more than the day before and exercise longer or harder or run further, even though I was exhausted and desperate since I was short of energy. Once I fainted on the spinning bike. Still, I could not take a step back and see that something was wrong. I could not take a break and breathe and look at what was actually going on, and why I needed this. I just remained with this obsession.

> Hedda: If I go to the gym (..) I cannot only strength train (..), I must run first, even if I have run in the morning. I also cycle, to and from work, which is probably 20 or 30 km (..). I do not run less than 10 km, preferably 20 km on weekdays. If I have the chance, I run closer to 30 km at weekends. (..) It has to be a whole number of kilometres, it cannot be 9.7 km or 10.5 it has to be 10 or 11. (..) I also used to have several rules in the gym, but since it was so demanding to have so many schemes about which equipment to use and for how long and stuff, I cut it out. (..) It was like 45 min on the treadmill, 30 min on

the step machine and 10 min on the rowing machine, then back to the treadmill for 20 min, a little weight-training (..), and three times this and that. I was very stressed out by it. (..) I felt that it was only exercise characterized by hatred. It was just tiring. I did not enjoy it at all.

In these extracts, Agnes and Hedda describe very powerfully how exercise has become increasingly compulsive, controlling and structured around particular rules and routines. They engage in a perpetuating cycle of exercise and food restraint, consuming extensive amounts of time and energy in their lives. Hedda experiences part of her training at a fitness centre as exhaustive and aversive, but managed to cut this part of her training out. Agnes describes her engagement in training as an automatic entity that is beyond her control and persists in exercising despite being physically exhausted or nearly collapsing. This experience gives rise to a sense of lacking control and feelings of powerlessness. Agnes clearly expresses an understanding of her training routines as out of place. She also reflects on why she needs to train and why she cannot let go of it, apparently unable to connect with the underlying thoughts and feelings triggering the obsession to exercise. In contextualizing this account within Agnes' narrative as a whole, it becomes evident that Agnes struggles with loneliness and feelings of not being good enough when comparing herself to family and friends.

Those participants who were athletes before the onset of the eating disorder (e.g., Hedwig and Rebecca) were engaged in healthy exercise when they first entered the sport and training arena in their childhood or early teens, though their training successively escalated into a more intense endeavour. Here, Hedwig and Rebecca illuminate how they have pushed themselves to extreme fatigue during training and competitions:

Hedwig: I remember I took part in a couple of long-distance competitions and I was nervous about how it would work out. People thought I was crazy, but it went really well... I only used to eat one meal per day, so it is difficult to understand how I managed... I do not really get it, since I had not eaten. I must have been exercising in a kind of adrenaline intoxication. (..) At times, when I was training at the gym, I could get so exhausted that I nearly fainted, sort of. Because when I do not eat anything during the day and exercise hard, I gets totally worn-out. (..) More or less, I have been doing the same type of training, no matter how exhausted I have been.

Rebecca: I used to exercise a lot when I was an athlete. It was like several hundred hours per year when in high school. Though, after a while I was not allowed to train. (..) I remember being constantly unwell. They thought it was a virus, kind of. But I had that drive to exercise and continued to train, so I did not get any better... I lost more and more weight that year.

These extracts further emphasize the intensity of the drive or compulsion to exercise. Bodily signs of fatigue and exhaustion are ignored, as the women persist in training and competing regardless of being physically ill and lacking energy. Despite a clear awareness of exercise being at odds with their current health condition and nutritional status, they exercise intensively.

In the following extract, Nora describes similar experiences whilst comparing aspects of her training with 'torture' and with a 'vicious circle' of exhaustion:

Nora: It is simply so tiring and boring (..). They are all the same movements and over such a long time, it is almost like torture. Yet, I must exercise. (..) I feel that if I have not trained one day, then I cannot eat. But then I must eat. I would like to refrain from exercise and get out of this cycle, but I do not know if I can. It is hopeless. (..) It is such a vicious circle wherein I need to exercise to be able to eat and rest, and then it is gone. Then along comes the next cycle and the next cycle. There is no end to the tormenting of myself. (..) I try to be more moderate or not exercise at all, I do not know which is the easiest. Every day I decide this has to end, but when I wake up it is the same roundabout again. (..) It really surprises me how it is possible to see that training is not the right thing for me now, yet, I still choose to exercise. When I think rationally, my body should rest, that would be best for me... But then again I have other feelings that are stronger than reason, which force me to exercise. Indeed, it is compulsory.

Here, Nora feels caught up in a never-ending 'roundabout' of exercising and eating that bears resemblance to feelings of being tortured or tormented. Indeed, an internal battle is taking place within Nora, in which she struggles with conflicting feelings and thoughts about her body needing rest and the simultaneous obligation to exercise. At the same time, she recognises that the 'outcome' of exercising is short-lived (i.e., 'then it is gone'). Clearly, ambivalence seems to be of relevance to Nora's engagement with exercise. She too recognises that her exercise regime influences her health negatively, nevertheless, she feels forced to exercise, as the urge to exercise is 'stronger than reason'. Moreover, and analogous to Agnes' experience in the first extract, Nora appears to experience powerlessness as she feels unable to moderate or stop the training. This feeling of lacking control over exercise signifies her belief that giving up exercising is impossible in her current situation. Importantly, she seems unable to explain why she needs to train or why she has such intense feelings that feed the compulsion to train excessively. In the next extract, Hilde exemplifies how exercise generates feelings of powerlessness, while at the same time also provides feelings of being in control:

> Hilde: I actually never sit down. If I watch TV, I either walk on a step machine, or cycle on a spinning cycle, or I walk back and forth while trying to see what is going on. I cannot sit still. Before I attended treatment, I only sat down during meal times, or else I felt I did not deserve to sit still. I was incredibly restless, so it was difficult to relax. (..) No matter where I was heading, I walked or I cycled, also back and forth from work. In addition, I did a lot of walking while working. (..) I feel like I am being compelled to exercise, as if someone has decided that now you must exercise or everything will be chaos. Since I can be really short-tempered, I feel I will be awful to be with if I do not exercise. (..) It is like a remote control (..). The main challenge right now is to be in treatment five days per week... I feel that the threat is enormous, because there are five days each week that I cannot decide... Thus, I exercise a lot during leave to compensate for the time at the unit.

Hilde's engagement in exercise is extreme. She feels she is not worthy of sitting still and is continually active in one way or another. In addition to replacing public transportation with physical activity (e.g., walking or cycling), she has a work situation that allows for extensive walking during the day. Her need to be physically active seems to have a regulatory function in terms of escaping and controlling difficult feelings, or as a means of expressing problematic feelings. It may be hypothesized that the role of exercise in consolidating herself and escaping difficult feelings relates to problematic experiences in her past. During the interview, she conveyed having been sexually assaulted in her early teens, and that she only recently had begun acknowledging and articulating these experiences in therapy.[4]

Based on the phenomenological perspective that the body offers us the means to interact with and understand the world [41], it may be suggested that Hilde's personal story and the associated unsolved feelings are imprinted in her body, her earlier life experiences are embodied [50]. Accordingly, the use of extensive exercise in particular when on leave from the hospital, to relieve and escape bodily distress and embodied feelings, gives her a sense of disruption and a feeling of control. Thus, her exercising appears to have multi-layered meanings, as she not only trains to compensate for exercise restrictions and meal plans when in hospital, but also to consolidate herself in order to endure the awakening of embodied feelings taking place in current psychotherapy. In view of this, the prospect of losing the means (here: exercise) by which she controls some of her feelings appears overwhelming. It is interesting how she uses the metaphor 'remote control' to describe her drivenness towards exercise. References to feelings of being externally controlled suggest that her obligation to exercise seems beyond her control. It may be assumed that the battle around lacking control versus taking control relates to her body and to a process where the body is brought back from being an object from which she has separated herself in the years following the assaults (objective body) into a body that currently engages with her lived world (subjective body) (see e.g. [51] for details on this distinction).

In this last quote, Agnes expands on the experience of feeling controlled by exercise and at the same time retaining control through exercising when on leave:

> Agnes: It has been very difficult to follow the treatment plan and not being allowed to go out. (..) Thus, I have been over-active when home on leave, as I need to compensate for all those hours that I am not entitled to exercise at the unit. Though this is not something I want to carry on with. It has been extremely difficult to resist the need to do small errands, walk back and forth in the halls, and do anything that represents some sort of physical activity. I can see the control this has had over me, such as when on leave, I have been running up and down the stairs, or I have written applications for leave in order to meet friends in town and instead walked around the city for hours. (..) Even though I say yes to treatment, on the other hand, I insist on having the control that I feel I have.

Although treatment guidelines for anorexia nervosa commonly require individuals to refrain from compulsive exercising and to commit themselves to a meal plan, Agnes retains control by exercising heavily during leave. While the engaging in such exercise regimes prevents her from exploring alternative ways of dealing with problematic feelings, the prospect of exercising on leave seems to facilitate her commitment to the treatment process. In explicitly disclosing that while accepting treatment, she insists on retaining control, Agnes illustrates very powerfully how control and ambivalence are key to the participants' engagement in exercise. Such ambivalence may indicate that the individuals are perhaps not ready for recovery.

'I should rather have trained': Limiting the societal and relational world

This theme examines how exercise negatively interferes with the participants' relationships with the social world in a variety of ways. In the following extract, Agnes illustrates how adhering to strict exercise schemas impedes and obstructs her engagement in the societal world:

> Agnes: It has controlled me a lot, so that I have been unable to accept invitations. I have scheduled when to exercise, when to eat and go to bed, it has turned into routines that I have not been able to change. Therefore, it has affected me such that I cannot take part in many societal things. I have spent a lot of time by myself, since training is more important. (..) Also, I have made many weird and stupid excuses to family and friends about why I could not take part in events. As a result, I have been lying a lot... to those around me... Today I find it problematic to say that I have lied, or that they will realise that I have been lying, or why I have lied. Thus, it has been problematic to let anyone get close to me.

Agnes communicates very powerfully how daily routines around training and meals limit involvement in the societal world and how this produces a feeling of being socially isolated from family and peers. Moreover, Agnes illuminates challenging experiences connected with being in close relationships. Since the masking of intense training has been going on for years, it is extremely difficult for her to engage in close relations with family and friends, as this cover up invokes feelings of embarrassment and shame. Accordingly, in order to avoid disclosing the various practices that form a part of her anorexia, she chooses to avoid relating to people emotionally. Yet, this withdrawal from social situations can result in a loss of social connectedness and of the prospect of acquiring close friends, leading to further social isolation and distress. The following extracts from Hedwig and Hedda further demonstrate how, when tailoring their daily lives to fit their training regimes, exercise is preferred to taking part in the social and relational sphere:

> Hedwig: It destroys everything. (..) Because, if I come home from work and a friend all of a sudden calls and asks if we can go out and eat sushi, if I did that, it would definitely have clashed with a planned training session, and that would be a disaster. I have very strict routines around exercise. The training is always more important, it is utterly rigid.

> Hedda: If something social comes up (..), then I must think through the day in detail... If I say yes to be social, and if I cannot squeeze in at least a five-kilometre run or something like that, I must do some planning and make sure I can do some additional running the day after. That way, I manage to let go of a training session. But as a rule, if it is a weekday, I usually just say that I have to work and there will not be any socialising.

Hedwig is deeply concerned about the prospect of social events getting in the way of her training activities, which are considered more crucial. The phrasing emphasizes how her training habits are categorically fixed and not up for negotiation. Hedda seems to experience slightly more flexibility regarding her exercise routines. Even though she commonly chooses training instead of engaging in social events, she sometimes manages to postpone some of her exercise activities if something social comes up.

In the next extract, Hilde further describes dilemmas associated with excessive training, food restraint and taking part in the social world:

> Hilde: If I have the opportunity to train, I easily choose not to attend weddings and such things. (..) Yet, it is not only about exercise, it is also about the fact that, basically, food is always included in social settings. When I was truly ill, I was so withdrawn that I shut myself in and avoided everything that included food. (..) Even though spending time with friends can help me refrain from exercise, this may also cause an irritation to build up, because during the whole visit I would only be concerned about that I should rather have been training. (..) I have tried to spend time with friends, but then I only train later. Thus, it does not really work as a long-term distraction.

Here, Hilde describes difficulties connected to engaging in situations that include food, as these make it more challenging to take part in the social world. Moreover, while spending time with friends and family has the potential to be a positive force in her life, helping to reduce the obligation to exercise, spending time with others may also trigger the compulsion to exercise even more. As such, the societal appears ambiguous, as it merely becomes a short interruption that causes further negative feelings to build up. This experience emphasizes the intensity of the compulsion to exercise and the difficulties that may evolve from social participation. Compared to Agnes and Hilde, Hedda seems able to engage somewhat more with the relational world, as she lives with her long-term partner whom she describes as being understanding about her illness, and who takes on an active role in the recovery process. However, living in a close relationship is also challenging in terms of potential disagreements about exercise:

> Hedda: If I am going out for a run, he tries to negotiate a bit. So before I run, I have to eat or drink some of those energy products, or something like that. When we are at the gym he comes over and tells me that 'now you have run enough, now you should do some strength training'... Before, I could push him away, in a way. Now, I know he is right, so there is no point in getting into an argument with him. (..) Still, if he says 'no, I do not think you should exercise today', I get really angry. In the end, he gives in. He does not manage to resist my anger, sort of.

While exercise is to some extent a subject open to negotiation, it is also clearly a matter producing tension and conflict in Hedda's relationship with her partner. A clear sense of ambivalence is taking place, such as when Hedda first admits that her partner is right that she should reduce her training, but in the very next sentence insists on having her own way if they disagree. While her partner attempts to support her in the recovery process, she is not interested in him having too much impact upon her level of exercise. This need to have full control over the amount and intensity of training may reflect a typical position of ambivalence in individuals going through the treatment and recovery process of anorexia nervosa. As described by a number of participants in this study, they choose treatment, whilst at the same time insisting on retaining the sense of control provided by their exercise routines.

The participants' accounts illuminate how exercise in general is prioritized over taking part in the social world and over involvement in close relationships, and how social relations produce feelings of ambivalence. While spending time with friends may provide some distraction, being social may also increase the intensity of negative feelings, leading to further exercising. It may be that these experiences not only relate to avoidance of internal discomfort and difficult feelings, but also to avoidance of 'taking up space' and of connecting with others, since this involves emotional commitment.

'I only went for long walks': Minimizing and rephrasing

This theme illustrates the participants' paradoxical wording with respect to their engagement in exercise. In speaking about their various exercise routines, their speech is habitually flavoured with phrases that minimize the scale and intensity of the training activity, or which imply that their activity is not 'real' exercise. Hedwig vividly illustrates this point:

> Hedwig: Earlier (..), I did not exercise as such, I only went for long walks, maybe two to three hours per day. (..) When I am at the unit, I just do some stretching. I try to stretch every day, but it is not exercising. I only stretch the body, stretch the arm like that, once on each side. I also stretch in order to do the splits, since it is important for me to continue to do them (..). I do not know if that counts as exercise. (..) Then I do sit-ups every night, maybe five or ten sit-ups (..) Besides, when brushing my teeth, I now and then do knee bends, say I do ten knee bends. But I do not consider this to count as exercise. At times, I do a few push-ups. It is not much really, maybe I do around sixty push-ups, other days I do not do any.

Here, Hedwig gives a detailed account of her engagement in comprehensive physical activities during her day at the unit. It is noteworthy that in spite of reporting an extensive amount of push-ups, she instantly refers to these as 'a few push-ups' and 'it is not much really', emphasizing that what she does is not regarded as real exercising. Nora and Rebecca equally talk down their training, as illustrated in the next quotes:

> Nora: Since I was admitted to the hospital, I have been doing some training similar to aerobics... I lift my arms and legs, and do a few steps. (..) I only exercise for about one hour or so. Then I do some strength training for the stomach and the back. In one day, we are talking about two hours altogether. The strength training is very easy, I get no increase in pulse, but it gives me a feeling of having done something.

> Rebecca: Since I am not entitled to exercise, I walk a great deal instead. I walk everywhere. In a day, maybe I walk for three hours. That is how I manage to keep my activity levels down, sort of, such that I do not exercise or run, or other such things.

While describing her activity as 'I lift my arms and legs', 'I do a few steps' and 'the strength training is very easy', Nora concurrently admits to undertaking two hours of aerobic and strength training each day. Rebecca conveys how despite being aware that exercise is not acceptable due to her low body weight, she still walks extensively to compensate for 'real' training, from which she manages to abstain when in treatment. As such, she substitutes one energetic physical activity (i.e., running) with a seemingly more moderate activity (walking for hours), proposing that such 'moderate' activity is not actual training. Similarly, Hilde makes a distinction between her own level of exercise and the training she thinks other individuals with anorexia are undertaking:

> Hilde: Compared to those that you have to deal with, it is not much. Generally, I run between 10 or 15 km four times a week. Mostly, I run 10 km three times a week and one long distance run. (..) For the moment, I am not supposed to train at all, but I probably exercise, yes, it must be as much as three times per week.

In comparing herself to what she assumes to be the level of exercise in other study participants, Hilde assumes that she trains less than they do. Yet, while at once admitting that she should not be training when receiving treatment, she describes an activity level apparently at odds with her current treatment programme. Eventually, she recognizes that her level of activity can be considered exercising. Relatedly, Nora uses daily routines to justify parts of her activity when on leave. By referring to imaginary errands, she conceals the actual level of activity to her family:

> Nora: It was really difficult. I made up excuses, for instance, if I went for a walk, I said I would go for a walk and that I would go via the grocery shop, or something like that. The truth was, however, that I was walking the whole time, and that I did not go via the shop. (..) I said this every so often to hide how much it really was.

The accounts of this theme capture the manner in which the women articulate their training, and how this may blur, minimize, conceal or redefine the real level of exercising. Once again, ambivalence is of relevance as the participants display a clear understanding of the need to be cautious about exercising due to their present health situation, but at the same time engage in prolonged exercising. Given a treatment programme obliging the individuals to refrain from exercise, the participants' tendency to minimize their level of physical activity may be a way of expressing a seeming loyalty to the treatment plan. By talking down their engagement in exercise, they avoid disclosing their real activity levels, as well as potential discussions with staff about increased nutrition following the elevated energy expenditure. More importantly, such minimizing may prevent the theme of exercise commitment from being adressed in therapy and participants from exploring the diverse functions that exercise may have for them.

Discussion

The purpose of this study is to explore how participants with anorexia nervosa restricting subtype experience and understand their engagement with exercise in the context of their lives. The analysis presents a range of conflicting experiences expanding on previous findings on the experience of exercise in this area. Firstly, in spite of being severely underweight and suffering from exhaustion and feelings of hopelessness, as well as having a clear awareness of the associated negative health effects, participants are engaged in a continuous cycle of rigorous and excessive exercise (e.g., aerobics, strength training, stretching, running or walking multiple hours per day) consuming extensive amounts of time and energy in their lives. They habitually replace transportation with exercise and convert work situations into physical efforts. Some participants even compare their drive towards exercise with torture and hatred. These findings are consistent with recent qualitative work showing how individuals with anorexia nervosa persist in exercising despite pain and injuries in muscles and joints and frequently describe their partaking in such exercise regimes as 'gruelling' and 'demon-like' [35, 36].

While some participants do not seem to connect with the underlying thoughts and feelings triggering the compulsion to exercise, others experience exercise as a moderator for difficult feelings and bodily distress connected with negative events of the past (e.g., sexual assaults). This resonates with former studies (e.g., [24, 25]) and is exemplified by Hilde, who exercises to self-regulate in order to endure the emotional distress arising from ongoing psychotherapy. The idea that problematic past experiences are reflected in the body adheres to phenomenological literature, proposing that we interact with and understand the world through our bodies [41]. In line with phenomenological perspectives, as well as theoretical underpinnings of Norwegian psychomotor physiotherapy [50], the material calls attention to the salient value of a person's life experiences (i.e., physical, psychological and social strain) and how these are embedded in the body and may invoke bodily tension and distress. If such feelings are continuously controlled and suppressed by rigorous exercise and restrictive eating patterns and underlying conflicts and meanings are not addressed, this may prevent the individual from engaging fully in the treatment process.

As has been shown in previous work [5, 34, 52, 53], the material demonstrates diverging experiences of being in control and losing control in individuals with anorexia nervosa. While these findings may be illustrative of the power of the obligation towards exercise, they also reflect accompanying feelings of powerlessness regarding the ability to moderate or change such activities. Though exercise appears functional in terms of emotion distraction, bolstering of self and identity, and in retaining a sense of structure and control, rigorous exercising also generates feelings of lacking control. For instance, the material illustrates the experience of an external power (i.e., 'remote-control') struggling against and controlling the participants more reasonable self, similar to notions of an 'anorectic voice' discussed in foregoing literature (e.g., [54]). Also, a number of the participants recount sensations of their exercising being imposed by an 'autopilot' or compulsions 'stronger than reason', similar to the notion of an 'internal voice' driving the anorexic behaviour put forward in previous work [36, 55]. Yet, while accepting treatment, the women insist on having a sense of autonomy and control, and retain such control through exercising extensively when on leave from the units. Paradoxically, exercise seems to facilitate coping with enhanced internal stress and conflicting feelings associated with gaining weight when in the recovery process. These observations indicate strong feelings of ambivalence towards altering exercise routines and foster doubts to whether the participants are ready to fully submit themselves to the requirements of the treatment programme.

Secondly, the findings demonstrate how exercise routines negatively control and interfere with the participants' involvement in the social and relational world. In contrast to a beneficial approach to exercise, in which exercise is organized to fit into life in general, for the women in this study, life in general is organized around exercise. As found in prior studies [4, 9, 10, 35, 53], extensive engagement in exercise instead of taking part in the societal world causes difficulties in maintaining close relationships. For instance, instead of disclosing the concealed and unduly taxing exercise routines to family and friends, some participants rather choose lonesomeness. While struggling with associated feelings of shame and guilt, close relationships that might involve intimacy and emotional connection are avoided. For those remaining in close relationships, exercise may be an issue open to negotiation, whilst also producing disagreements and conflicts, as shown in Hedda's account. Furthermore, while socialising may represent a distraction from the obligation to exercise, this interruption is merely temporary and may intensify problematic feelings still further, resulting in further exercising.

Such restricted participation in the social world is problematic for these individuals as it may produce social isolation and a loss of social and interpersonal connectedness, elements considered critical for young adults in their becoming a self and in the shaping of social support [56, 57]. A restricted social life may lead to a lack of relational skills and of confidence in making and maintaining relationships in general [10]. Limited social connectedness may further reinforce negative attributions of the self and others, resulting in a sense of aloneness that connects the participant even more strongly to the anorectic identity. Whereas involvement in the social world represents a challenge causing conflicting feelings and ambivalence in the participants, previous research has established that maintaining connections with social supports and involvement in social activities outside treatment may also have positive impacts in terms of preventing social isolation, developing interpersonal skills, and promoting recovery in individuals with an eating disorder [58–61].

Thirdly, this study illuminates the manner in which participants speak about their experience of exercise, and how their wording is characterized by a reduction and rephrasing of their actual immersion in exercise. Diverse training regimes are commonly described as not being 'real exercise'. The verbalizing of training appears to be rather paradoxical and works to blur and conceal what is actually going on. Given the participants' health status following enduring underweight status and the accompanying medical vulnerabilities [2], the high activity level reported by the participants clearly represents a threat to their physical health. These findings concur with a few other papers showing how language may serve to minimize the level of exercise [62, 63]. In support of such curtailing of the level of physical activity in the eating disorders is a paper examining self-reported (by the writing of a diary) versus objectively assessed (by using an accelerometer) moderate to vigorous physical activity. This study reveal a higher objectively measured than subjectively reported physical activity level in individuals with an eating disorder compared to healthy controls [62].[5] Such reductive phrasing of the engagement in training is of clinical importance as it may prevent experiences of exercise from coming to the fore, thus limiting the opportunity to explore the meaning and function of exercise, and to investigate alternative ways of thinking and interacting with problematic feelings and the social world.

In sum, the analysis shows that conflicting feelings and emotional distress build up when taking part in a treatment process where weight gain is required and exercise strictly regulated. Thus, participants engage in a perpetuating cycle of extensive exercising which interferes with their health, social and interpersonal life, as well as the process of recovery. Accordingly, issues of control and ambivalence about treatment and recovery can be considered potential triggers for the women's' engagement with exercise when undergoing treatment. Such ambivalence and the associated lack of readiness to relinquish the problematic behaviour maintaining the eating disorder are considered key dimensions in the symptom presentation of individuals with anorexia nervosa [4, 5, 8, 64]. Notably, this ambivalence has been shown to persist throughout treatment in individuals with anorexia nervosa, who will gain weight in treatment [64]. Being caught up in ambivalence is, however, problematic as it may prevent the women from engaging themselves fully in the recovery process.

Concerning implications of this study for treatment, it is essential that core beliefs about self and behaviour that maintain such ambivalence need to be challenged. To offer a more meaningful treatment for those who engage in compulsive exercising, it is imperative to increase the understanding of beliefs and feelings perpetuating exercising for the particular individual in her situated context. It has been suggested that the foundation for achieving such an understanding, is a functional therapeutic relationship and an acknowledging of the significance of exercising for the individual [8]. One therapeutic approach leading to long-lasting change in a female former athlete ('Deborah') who exercised almost continuously in combination with restrictive dietary routines, has been illustrated by Geller [8]. Drawing on cognitive-behavioural and motivational approaches, a reformulation of maladaptive beliefs was achieved, along with a reprioritization and strengthening of values associated with relationships and personal development. As provided in Geller [8], the strengthening of patients' self-confidence and relational skills may help them make autonomous decisions about their lives so that the need for maladaptive coping strategies, such as exercising compulsively, is reduced [8]. Thus, instead of focusing heavily on food and weight gain issues in the therapeutic programme, there is a need to target wider life-related and psychological issues which are important to the individual client and which could enable her/him to challenge the basis of her/his emotional distress [5, 59, 65, 66].

Along with increased understanding of the function and meaning of exercise for the individual client, the manner in which exercise and physical activity are comprehended and approached in treatment programmes may also need some reconsideration. Restricting activity entirely in patients with anorexia nervosa while they are in a treatment situation involving increased emotional distress may cause further difficulties, and has been shown to be counterproductive due to its potential to weaken 'the already fragile grasp of perceived control' ([67], p. 60) in these individuals. Restricting a problematic, but nevertheless reachable, coping strategy for managing the self and the emotions may hamper the capacity and motivation of these individuals to manage the treatment situation, particularly since their repertoire for articulating difficult feelings and thoughts is otherwise limited. The difficulty for persons with anorexia nervosa to fully anticipate the experiences they will have upon reducing exercise and gaining weight may explain some of their ambivalence towards change. The clients may possibly benefit from increased knowledge about bodily functioning, qualities of physical activities and how these relate to nutritional requirements. To increase treatment compliance, one option may be to carefully implement, in a manner complementary to cognitive-behavioural and motivational work (e.g., [8, 68]), a nutritionally supported exercise programme to accompany the process of medical stabilization. Some foregoing studies suggest that exercise interventions of moderate intensity may engender positive aspects for medically stable patients, such as increased psychological well-being, reduced anxiety and increased compliance to treatment [13, 69–71]. A tailored exercise programme combined with an opportunity to reflect on the experience before, during or after the session, has shown a reduction in obligatory attitudes towards exercise [72]. Thus, a diversity of supervised and individually tailored activities with the aim of increasing body awareness, muscular strength, bodily stability and balance could be introduced to medical stable patients. Such interventions could, however, appear more meaningful and health beneficial for the client if they were founded on bodily assessments accomplished by physiotherapists having explicit expertise regarding the examining of the body and identifying bodily impairments and resources. It could be noted that improved awareness of the body may be favourable for multiple reasons, as it may perhaps help integrating the body as one's own, and improve emotional awareness and the ability to attune oneself to problematic feelings and the social world [73, 74].

The methodological approach and limited sample of this research may connect with both the strengths and limitations of the study. The use of a qualitative methodology, such as IPA, is particularly suitable for exploring and situating the means by which participants make sense of their experiences. In applying this approach, rich detail, nuance and difference to the examination of the experience of exercise in women with anorexia nervosa and how they make sense of these experiences from their personal and contextualized perspectives are provided. An in-depth exploration of personal experiences and meanings in this area seems suitable as it may engender detailed and renewed insight into the participant's relatedness to and engagement with exercise. In order to produce a clearly situated and transparent account, the findings are from a small homogenous sample of participants. Yet, it is hoped that this idiographic illumination of the understanding and sensemaking of the experience of exercise in individuals with anorexia nervosa can provide increased insight into the intricacy surrounding exercise that can inform and benefit clinical and therapeutic interventions. It is assumed that the visibility of the context of the participants and the research process offer readers to estimate transferability to other similar contexts [40]. Overall, qualitative approaches, such as IPA, can make valuable contributions to furthering the understanding of participants personal concerns, and what these concerns means for the individual in a given context.

Conclusion

In conclusion, the present study adds detail to our knowledge of exercise in women with anorexia nervosa, and to how they make sense of these in the context of their lives. It seems that, despite the functional aspects of regulating feelings and bodily distress, as well as the fuelling of the self through exercising [37], the women's engagement in a continuing cycle of exercise are accompanied by challenging experiences affecting their health, social lives and recovery process negatively. It appear that a sense of being in control and strong feelings of ambivalence towards change are essential triggering factors regarding the women's preoccupation with exercise. However, such immersion in exercise may keep the women trapped in their ambivalence, subsequently preventing them from exploring other ways of dealing with problematic feelings and strengthening the self. These findings illuminate the necessity of comprehending and addressing the phenomenon of exercise in patients with anorexia nervosa on multiple levels. In addition to adapting exercise interventions in accordance with the medical situation and level of weight gain (e.g., [13, 34, 72]), these interventions could be grounded on individual body assessments in order to become more health beneficial and motivating for the client. Moreover, personal beliefs and feelings that are preservative to the ambivalence triggering the problematic exercise behaviour needs to be acknowledged and investigated in more detail during treatment.

Endnotes

[1]The findings presented in this article is part of the larger study of which the present article is also a part.

[2]Norwegian psychomotor physiotherapy (NPMP) acknowledges the body as the centre of experiences and knowledge through which we take in information and interact with the surroundings. As such, personal experiences and stories are imprinted in and reflected in our bodies, they become embodied. The method is based on the understanding that posture, respiration, muscle tension and body awareness are closely related to emotional and psychological strain [50].

[3]... Illustrates a pause in speech. (..) Illustrates that words not adding meaning are omitted.

[4]Hilde's experience of exercise in terms of emotion regulation and escape has been explored in more detail in the paper dealing with the first superordinate theme [37].

[5]It may be noted that only 8 out of 59 participants in the eating disorder sample had anorexia nervosa [62].

Appendices

Appendix 1

Table 1 Participants

Pseudonym	Age	Duration of eating disorder, years	Time in treatment
Agnes	26	13	1 year
Hedda	30	15	2 years
Hedwig	27	12	6 months
Hilde	39	23	2 years
Rebecca	23	6	5 years
Nora	50	4	3 years

Appendix 2

Table 2 Superordinate theme: Diverging experiences of exercise

	Agnes	Hedda	Hedwig	Hilde	Rebecca	Nora
Subtheme 1: 'I feel like I am being compelled to exercise': Ambivalence and control	x	x	x	x	x	x
Subtheme 2: 'I should rather have trained': Limiting the societal and relational world	x	x	x	x	x	x
Subtheme 3: 'I only went for long walks': Minimizing and rephrasing	-	-	x	x	x	x

Competing interests
The author declares that he has no competing interests.

Acknowledgements
The author is indebted to the women who shared their experiences and insight through interviews.
The author is grateful for financial support provided by the Norwegian ExtraFoundation for Health and Rehabilitation and the Norwegian Council for Mental Health.
The research was conducted at the Norwegian School of Sport Sciences, Oslo, Norway.

References

1. Beumont PJV, Touyz SW. What kind of illness is anorexia nervosa? Eur Child Adolesc Psychiatry. 2003;12(1):i20–4. doi:10.1007/s00787-003-1103-y.
2. Mehler PS, Brown C. Anorexia nervosa - medical complications. J Eat Disord. 2015;3:11. doi:10.1186/s40337-015-0040-8.
3. Nordbo RH, Espeset EM, Gulliksen KS, Skarderud F, Geller J, Holte A. Reluctance to recover in anorexia nervosa. Eur Eat Disord Rev. 2012;20(1):60–7. doi:10.1002/erv.1097.
4. Serpell L, Treasure J, Teasdale J, Sullivan V. Anorexia nervosa: friend or foe? Int J Eat Disord. 1999;25(2):177–86. http://www.ncbi.nlm.nih.gov/pubmed/10065395.
5. Williams S, Reid M. Understanding the experience of ambivalence in anorexia nervosa: the maintainer's perspective. Psychol Health. 2010;25(5):551–67. http://www.ncbi.nlm.nih.gov/pubmed/20204933.

6. Zeeck A, Hartmann A, Buchholz C, Herzog T. Drop outs from in-patient treatment of anorexia nervosa. Acta Psychiatr Scand. 2005;111(1):29–37. http://www.ncbi.nlm.nih.gov/pubmed/15636591.
7. Carter JC, Blackmore E, Sutandar-Pinnock K, Woodside DB. Relapse in anorexia nervosa: a survival analysis. Psychol Med. 2004;34(4):671–9. doi:10.1017/S0033291703001168.
8. Geller J. Mechanisms of action in the process of change: helping eating disorder clients make meaningful shifts in their lives. Clin Child Psychol Psychiatry. 2006;11(2):225–37.
9. Espindola CR, Blay SL. Anorexia nervosa's meaning to patients: a qualitative synthesis. Psychopathology. 2009;42(2):69–80. http://www.ncbi.nlm.nih.gov/pubmed/19225241.
10. Fox JR, Diab P. An exploration of the perceptions and experiences of living with chronic anorexia nervosa while an inpatient on an eating disorders unit: an Interpretative Phenomenological Analysis (IPA) study. J Health Psychol. 2015;20(1):27–36. doi:10.1177/1359105313497526.
11. Fox AP, Larkin M, Leung N. The personal meaning of eating disorder symptoms: an interpretative phenomenological analysis. J Health Psychol. 2011;16(1):116–25. doi:10.1177/1359105310368449.
12. Davis C. Eating disorders and hyperactivity: a psychobiological perspective. Can J Psychiatry. 1997;42(2):168–75.
13. Thien V, Thomas A, Markin D, Birmingham CL. Pilot study of a graded exercise program for the treatment of anorexia nervosa. Int J Eat Disord. 2000;28(1):101–6.
14. Davis C, Katzman DK, Kirsh C. Compulsive physical activity in adolescents with anorexia nervosa: a psychobehavioral spiral of pathology. J Nerv Ment Dis. 1999;187(6):336–42. http://www.ncbi.nlm.nih.gov/pubmed/10379720.
15. Dalle Grave R, Calugi S, Marchesini G. Compulsive exercise to control shape or weight in eating disorders: prevalence, associated features, and treatment outcome. Compr Psychiatry. 2008;49(4):346–52. http://www.ncbi.nlm.nih.gov/pubmed/18555054.
16. Bewell-Weiss CV, Carter JC. Predictors of excessive exercise in anorexia nervosa. Compr Psychiatry. 2010;51(6):566–71. http://www.ncbi.nlm.nih.gov/pubmed/20965301.
17. Brewerton TD, Stellefson EJ, Hibbs N, Hodges EL, Cochrane CE. Comparison of eating disorder patients with and without compulsive exercising. Int J Eat Disord. 1995;17(4):413–6.
18. Shroff H, Reba L, Thornton LM, Tozzi F, Klump KL, Berrettini WH, et al. Features associated with excessive exercise in women with eating disorders. Int J Eat Disord. 2006;39(6):454–61. doi:10.1002/eat.20247.
19. Solenberger SE. Exercise and eating disorders: a 3-year inpatient hospital record analysis. Eat Behav. 2001;2(2):151–68.
20. Gilboa-Schechtman E, Avnon L, Zubery E, Jeczmien P. Emotional processing in eating disorders: specific impairment or general distress related deficiency? Depress Anxiety. 2006;23(6):331–9. doi:10.1002/da.20163.
21. Oldershaw A, Hambrook D, Stahl D, Tchanturia K, Treasure J, Schmidt U. The socio-emotional processing stream in Anorexia Nervosa. Neurosci Biobehav Rev. 2011;35(3):970–88. http://www.ncbi.nlm.nih.gov/pubmed/21070808.
22. Fox JRE. A qualitative exploration of the perception of emotions in anorexia nervosa: a basic emotion and developmental perspective. Clin Psychol Psychother. 2009;16(4):276–302. http://www.ncbi.nlm.nih.gov/pubmed/19639644.
23. Pemberton K, Fox JR. The experience and management of emotions on an inpatient setting for people with anorexia nervosa: a qualitative study. Clin Psychol Psychother. 2013;20(3):226–38. doi:10.1002/cpp.794.
24. Boyd C, Abraham S, Luscombe G. Exercise behaviours and feelings in eating disorder and non-eating disorder groups. Eur Eat Disord Rev. 2007;15(2):112–8. doi:10.1002/erv.769.
25. Bratland-Sanda S, Martinsen EW, Rosenvinge JH, Ro O, Hoffart A, Sundgot-Borgen J. Exercise dependence score in patients with longstanding eating disorders and controls: the importance of affect regulation and physical activity intensity. Eur Eat Disord Rev. 2011;19(3):249–55. doi:10.1002/erv.971.
26. Lawson R, Waller G, Lockwood R. Cognitive content and process in eating-disordered patients with obsessive-compulsive features. Eat Behav. 2007;8(3):305–10. doi:10.1016/j.eatbeh.2006.11.006.
27. Meyer C, Taranis L. Exercise in the eating disorders: terms and definitions. Eur Eat Disord Rev. 2011;19(3):169–73. http://www.ncbi.nlm.nih.gov/pubmed/21584910.
28. Fairburn CG, Cooper Z, Shafran R. Cognitive behaviour therapy for eating disorders: a "transdiagnostic" theory and treatment. Behav Res Ther. 2003;41(5):509–28. http://www.ncbi.nlm.nih.gov/pubmed/12711261.
29. Geller J, Cockell SJ, Hewitt PL, Goldner EM, Flett GL. Inhibited expression of negative emotions and interpersonal orientation in anorexia nervosa. Int J Eat Disord. 2000;28(1):8–19.
30. Taranis L, Touyz S, Meyer C. Disordered eating and exercise: development and preliminary validation of the compulsive exercise test (CET). Eur Eat Disord Rev. 2011;19(3):256–68. http://www.ncbi.nlm.nih.gov/pubmed/21584918.
31. Le Grange D, Eisler I. The link beween anorexia nervosa and excessive exercise: a review. Eat Disord Rev. 1993;1(2):100–19.
32. Casper RC, Jabine LN. An eight-year follow-up: outcome from adolescent compared to adult onset anorexia nervosa. J Youth Adolesc. 1996;25(4):499–517. http://apps.webofknowledge.com/InboundService.do?SID=N2CUGuD9wog3mj8DCss&product=WOS&UT=WOS%3AA1996VJ20900008&SrcApp=EndNote&DestFail=http%3A%2F%2Fwww.webofknowledge.com&Init=Yes&action=retrieve&SrcAuth=ResearchSoft&customersID=ResearchSoft&Func=Frame&IsProductCode=Yes&mode=FullRecord.
33. Strober M, Freeman R, Morrell W. The long-term course of severe anorexia nervosa in adolescents: survival analysis of recovery, relapse, and outcome predictors over 10–15 years in a prospective study. Int J Eat Disord. 1997;22(4):339–60. http://www.ncbi.nlm.nih.gov/pubmed/9356884.
34. Young S, Rhodes P, Touyz S, Hay P. The role of exercise across the lifespan in patients with anorexia nervosa: a narrative inquiry. Adv Eat Disord. 2015;3(3):237–50. doi:10.1080/21662630.2015.1027947.
35. Axelsen M. The power of leisure: "I Was an Anorexic; I'm Now a Healthy Triathlete". Leis Sci. 2009;31(4):330–46.
36. Moola FJ, Gairdner S, Amara C. Speaking on behalf of the body and activity: investigating the activity experiences of Canadian women living with anorexia nervosa. Ment Health Phys Act. 2015;8:44–55. doi:10.1016/j.mhpa.2015.02.002.
37. Kolnes L-J, Rodriguez-Morales L. The meaning of compulsive exercise in women with anorexia nervosa: An interpretative phenomenological analysis. Mental Health and Physical Activity. http://www.sciencedirect.com/science/article/pii/S1755296615000356.
38. Johnston O, Reilly J, Kremer J. Excessive exercise: from quantitative categorisation to a qualitative continuum approach. Eur Eat Disord Rev. 2011;19(3):237–48. doi:10.1002/erv.970.
39. Smith JA. Beyond the divide between cognition and discourse: using interpretative phenomenological analysis in health psychology. Psychol Health. 1996;11(2):261–71. http://apps.webofknowledge.com/InboundService.do?SID=N2CUGuD9wog3mj8DCss&product=WOS&UT=WOS%3AA1996UB66300006&SrcApp=EndNote&DestFail=http%3A%2F%2Fwww.webofknowledge.com&Init=Yes&action=retrieve&SrcAuth=ResearchSoft&customersID=ResearchSoft&Func=Frame&IsProductCode=Yes&mode=FullRecord.
40. Smith JA, Larkin M, Flowers P. Interpretative phenomenological analysis: theory, method and research. Los Angeles: Sage; 2009.
41. Merleau-Ponty M. Phenomenology of perception. Phénoménologie de la perception. London: Routledge; 2012.
42. Larkin M, Watts S, Clifton E. Giving voice and making sense in interpretative phenomenological analysis. Qual Res Psychol. 2006;3(2):102–20. http://ovidsp.uk.ovid.com/sp-3.18.0b/ovidweb.cgi?QS2=434f4e1a73d37e8cac529f721181381a03cc0d87e43bdb0bf8504a7fd95d05f5ee1d246eac532c2968680ec8b82ac25480b9eda085f6ea26ba3ed2f63c12e6ab9940532131432ee244727e01c95ec3a0db68f8a4e5cfe39a7da346e3afbb539b4353f099ddbdcc5f2b23bf8afc201727f402733aef82d48bad1aa9c35adb1e8895cbfe44a4b21e892e33996128a1f5a31bcfe33c800a7ceed923ce77ed731277c06583ce3e11b81e25e8bcf43dca31327c1894f00a688eb9dda5f2e35122e1cb73f96d600c3a2eb4c38f26b9b4956baae02bd27e0e5b7281.
43. Smith JA, Osborn M. Interpretative phenomenological analysis. Qualitative psychology: A practical guide to research methods. Thousand Oaks, CA: Sage Publications, Inc; US; 2003. p. 51–80.
44. World Health O. ICD-10: International statistical classification of diseases and related health problems : tenth revision. 2nd ed. Geneva: World Health Organization; 2004.
45. Davis C, Katzman DK, Kaptein S, Kirsh C, Brewer H, Kalmbach K, et al. The prevalence of high-level exercise in the eating disorders: etiological implications. Compr Psychiatry. 1997;38(6):321–6. http://www.ncbi.nlm.nih.gov/pubmed/9406737.
46. Bratland-Sanda S, Sundgot-Borgen J, Ro O, Rosenvinge JH, Hoffart A, Martinsen EW. Physical activity and exercise dependence during inpatient treatment of longstanding eating disorders: an exploratory study of

excessive and non-excessive exercisers. Int J Eat Disord. 2010;43(3):266–73. doi:10.1002/eat.20769.
47. Grinspoon S, Thomas E, Pitts S, Gross E, Mickley D, Miller K, et al. Prevalence and predictive factors for regional osteopenia in women with anorexia nervosa. Ann Intern Med. 2000;133(10):790–4.
48. Yardley L. Dilemmas in qualitative health research. Psychol Health. 2000; 15(2):215–28. http://apps.webofknowledge.com/InboundService.do?SID=N2CUGuD9wog3mj8DCss&product=WOS&UT=WOS%3A000087200300007&SrcApp=EndNote&DestFail=http%3A%2F%2Fwww.webofknowledge.com&Init=Yes&action=retrieve&SrcAuth=ResearchSoft&customersID=ResearchSoft&Func=Frame&IsProductCode=Yes&mode=FullRecord.
49. Smith JA. Evaluating the contribution of interpretative phenomenological analysis. Health Psychol Rev. 2011;5(1):9–27. doi:10.1080/17437199.2010.510659.
50. Bunkan BH, Thornquist E. Psychomotor therapy: an approach to the evaluation and treatment of psychosomatic disorders. Int Perspect Phys Ther. 1990;5:45–74. Psychological and Psychosomatic Problems.
51. Finlay L. The body's disclosure in phenomenological research. Qual Res Psychol. 2006;3(1):19–30. http://ovidsp.uk.ovid.com/sp-3.18.0b/ovidweb.cgi?QS2=434f4e1a73d37e8cac529f721181381a599031bd6da183259834ff959aca35128d93a7e252f80e88a8069d080e4e3ad3b42c33224abf20a3d82e1a624a4aaeb292da819375c2d7aee43628b0116737ff66ac6fc910a2d8268e815fdc3778049ddb6b297ca92b04bd7a4e3ac3418def9ba0153ab01d911b411e357132176294b1679b0f3a5cfed3fba5fb376bec6808da8e10d0873511637eab98103dd8fbc5ef0fec0dfb8af9bd0d60250c758f01749940a4a763d9531e07fc0d80401f6df6000dfb9d2dbfd2165d1bfbc1e490494e141ee49ee62767f525.
52. Dignon A, Beardsmore A, Spain S, Kuan A. 'Why i won't eat': patient testimony from 15 anorexics concerning the causes of their disorder. J Health Psychol. 2006;11(6):942–56. http://www.ncbi.nlm.nih.gov/pubmed/17035265.
53. Williams S, Reid M. 'It's like there are two people in my head': a phenomenological exploration of anorexia nervosa and its relationship to the self. Psychol Health. 2012;27(7):798–815. http://www.ncbi.nlm.nih.gov/pubmed/21736500.
54. Jenkins J, Ogden J. Becoming 'whole' again: a qualitative study of women's views of recovering from anorexia nervosa. Eur Eat Disord Rev. 2012;20(1):e23–31.
55. Tierney S, Fox JR. Living with the anorexic voice: a thematic analysis. Psychol Psychother. 2010;83(Pt 3):243–54. doi:10.1348/147608309X480172.
56. Smith JA, Osborn M. Pain as an assault on the self: an interpretative phenomenological analysis of the psychological impact of chronic benign low back pain. Psychol Health. 2007;22(5):517–34. http://apps.webofknowledge.com/InboundService.do?SID=N2CUGuD9wog3mj8DCss&product=WOS&UT=WOS%3A000248222500002&SrcApp=EndNote&DestFail=http%3A%2F%2Fwww.webofknowledge.com&Init=Yes&action=retrieve&SrcAuth=ResearchSoft&customersID=ResearchSoft&Func=Frame&IsProductCode=Yes&mode=FullRecord.
57. House JS, Umberson D, Landis KR. Structures and processes of social support. Annu Rev Sociol. 1988;14:293–318. http://www.annualreviews.org/doi/abs/10.1146/annurev.so.14.080188.001453.
58. Bell L. What can we learn from consumer studies and qualitative research in the treatment of eating disorders? Eat Weight Disord. 2003;8(3):181–7.
59. Cockell SJ, Zaitsoff SL, Geller J. Maintaining change following eating disorder treatment. Prof Psychol Res Pract. 2004;35(5):527–34.
60. Federici A, Kaplan AS. The patient's account of relapse and recovery in anorexia nervosa: a qualitative study. Eur Eat Disord Rev. 2008;16(1):1–10. http://www.ncbi.nlm.nih.gov/pubmed/18074326.
61. Weaver K, Wuest J, Ciliska D. Understanding women's journey of recovering from anorexia nervosa. Qual Health Res. 2005;15(2):188–206. http://www.ncbi.nlm.nih.gov/pubmed/15611203.
62. Bratland-Sanda S, Sundgot-Borgen J, Ro O, Rosenvinge JH, Hoffart A, Martinsen EW. "I'm not physically active - I only go for walks": physical activity in patients with longstanding eating disorders. Int J Eat Disord. 2010;43(1):88–92. http://www.ncbi.nlm.nih.gov/pubmed/19728373.
63. Bamber D, Cockerill IM, Rodgers S, Carroll D. "It's exercise or nothing": a qualitative analysis of exercise dependence. Br J Sports Med. 2000;34(6):423–30.
64. Geller J, Zaitsoff SL, Srikameswaran S. Tracking readiness and motivation for change in individuals with eating disorders over the course of treatment. Cogn Ther Res. 2005;29(5):611–25. http://apps.webofknowledge.com/InboundService.do?SID=N2CUGuD9wog3mj8DCss&product=WOS&UT=WOS%3A000232858000008&SrcApp=EndNote&DestFail=http%3A%2F%2Fwww.webofknowledge.com&Init=Yes&action=retrieve&SrcAuth=ResearchSoft&customersID=ResearchSoft&Func=Frame&IsProductCode=Yes&mode=FullRecord.
65. Reid M, Burr J, Williams S, Hammersley R. Eating disorders patients' views on their disorders and on an outpatient service: a qualitative study. J Health Psychol. 2008;13(7):956–60. http://www.ncbi.nlm.nih.gov/pubmed/18809647.
66. Corstorphine E. Cognitive - emotional - behavioural therapy for the eating disorders: working with beliefs about emotions. Eur Eat Disord Rev. 2006; 14(6):448–61. http://apps.webofknowledge.com/InboundService.do?SID=N2CUGuD9wog3mj8DCss&product=WOS&UT=WOS%3A000242774400013&SrcApp=EndNote&DestFail=http%3A%2F%2Fwww.webofknowledge.com&Init=Yes&action=retrieve&SrcAuth=ResearchSoft&customersID=ResearchSoft&Func=Frame&IsProductCode=Yes&mode=FullRecord.
67. Moola FJ, Gairdner SE, Amara CE. Exercise in the care of patients with anorexia nervosa: a systematic review of the literature. Men Health Phys Act. 2013;6(2):59–68. http://apps.webofknowledge.com/InboundService.do?SID=N2CUGuD9wog3mj8DCss&product=WOS&UT=WOS%3A000209230500001&SrcApp=EndNote&DestFail=http%3A%2F%2Fwww.webofknowledge.com&Init=Yes&action=retrieve&SrcAuth=ResearchSoft&customersID=ResearchSoft&Func=Frame&IsProductCode=Yes&mode=FullRecord.
68. Geller J, Dunn EC. Integrating motivational interviewing and cognitive behavioral therapy in the treatment of eating disorders: tailoring interventions to patient readiness for change. Cogn Behav Pract. 2011;18(1):5–15. http://apps.webofknowledge.com/InboundService.do?SID=N2CUGuD9wog3mj8DCss&product=WOS&UT=WOS%3A000286648400002&SrcApp=EndNote&DestFail=http%3A%2F%2Fwww.webofknowledge.com&Init=Yes&action=retrieve&SrcAuth=ResearchSoft&customersID=ResearchSoft&Func=Frame&IsProductCode=Yes&mode=FullRecord.
69. Beumont PJ, Arthur B, Russell JD, Touyz SW. Excessive physical activity in dieting disorder patients: proposals for a supervised exercise program. Int J Eat Disord. 1994;15(1):21–36.
70. Szabo CP, Green K. Hospitalized anorexics and resistance training: impact on body composition and psychological well-being. A preliminary study. Eat Weight Disord. 2002;7(4):293–7.
71. Chantler I, Szabo CP, Green K. Muscular strength changes in hospitalized anorexic patients after an eight week resistance training program. Int J Sports Med. 2006;27(8):660–5. http://www.ncbi.nlm.nih.gov/pubmed/16874594.
72. Calogero RM, Pedrotty KN. The practice and process of healthy exercise: an investigation of the treatment of exercise abuse in women with eating disorders. Eat Disord. 2004;12(4):273–91. http://www.ncbi.nlm.nih.gov/pubmed/16864521.
73. Kolnes L-J. Embodying the body in anorexia nervosa–a physiotherapeutic approach. J Bodywork Mov Ther. 2012;16(3):281–8. http://www.ncbi.nlm.nih.gov/pubmed/22703737.
74. Øien AM, Iversen S, Stensland P. Narratives of embodied experiences - therapy processes in Norwegian psychomotor physiotherapy. Adv Physiother. 2007;9(1):31–9.

Overvaluation of shape and weight in adolescents with anorexia nervosa: does shape concern or weight concern matter more for treatment outcome?

Catherine E. Byrne[1*], Andrea E. Kass[2], Erin C. Accurso[3], Sarah Fischer[1], Setareh O'Brien[4], Alexandria Goodyear[4], James Lock[5] and Daniel Le Grange[6]

Abstract

Background: Overvaluation of shape and weight is a key diagnostic feature of anorexia nervosa (AN); however, limited research has evaluated the clinical utility of differentiating between weight versus shape concerns. Understanding differences in these constructs may have important implications for AN treatment given the focus on weight regain. This study examined differences in treatment outcome between individuals whose primary concern was weight versus those whose primary concern was shape in a randomized controlled trial of treatment for adolescent AN.

Methods: Data were drawn from a two-site randomized controlled trial that compared family-based treatment and adolescent focused therapy for AN. Chi-square tests and logistic regression analyses were conducted.

Results: Thirty percent of participants presented with primary weight concern ($n = 36$; defined as endorsing higher Eating Disorder Examination (EDE) Weight Concern than Shape Concern subscale scores); 60 % presented with primary shape concern ($n = 72$; defined as endorsing higher EDE Shape Concern than Weight Concern scores). There were no significant differences between the two groups in remission status at the end of treatment. Treatment did not moderate the effect of group status on achieving remission.

Conclusions: Results suggest that treatment outcomes are comparable between adolescents who enter treatment for AN with greater weight concerns and those who enter treatment with greater shape concerns. Therefore, treatment need not be adjusted based on primary weight or primary shape concerns.

Keywords: Overvaluation, Weight, Shape, Anorexia nervosa

Background

A key diagnostic feature of anorexia nervosa (AN) is an overvaluation of shape and weight [1, 2], with patients tending to evaluate their self-worth in terms of their shape and weight. The Diagnostic and Statistical Manual for Mental Disorders (DSM-5) includes the third diagnostic criterion for AN as "disturbance in the way in which one's body weight or shape is experienced, undue influence of body weight or shape on self-evaluation, or denial of the seriousness of the current low body weight" [2]. The gold-standard interview assessment of eating disorder pathology, the Eating Disorder Examination (EDE), includes 'shape concern' and 'weight concern' as two separate subscales [3]. With the exception of one overlapping question, the weight concern subscale and the shape concern subscale on the EDE are comprised of different questions, suggesting the assessment conceptualizes shape and weight concerns as different constructs with distinct latent psychopathology and of separate clinical importance.

Despite the hypothesized clinical importance of distinguishing weight from shape, many factor analytic studies have demonstrated that weight and shape concerns may not represent separate constructs. In fact, two comprehensive literature reviews have demonstrated that factor

* Correspondence: cbyrne7@masonlive.gmu.edu
[1]Department of Psychology, George Mason University, Fairfax, VA, USA
Full list of author information is available at the end of the article

analyses have generally failed to discriminate between a shape concern factor and weight concern factor on the EDE and EDE-Questionnaire (EDE-Q; the self-report questionnaire of the EDE), suggesting that separating shape and weight concerns may not be a meaningful distinction for many people [4, 5]. However, the research to-date has focused primarily on the validity of the EDE and the EDE-Q as an assessment tool, but the clinical utility of separating these constructs remains a gap in the literature. Additionally, although the psychometric properties of these assessment tools indicate that concerns about weight and shape may overlap, neuroimaging studies indicate that individuals with AN have a neurobiologically distinct response to the estimation of their own body shape [6]. Individuals with AN appear to misperceive their own body shape as larger than the body shape of healthy controls, and also perceive certain body shapes as more desirable than others. These perceptions are associated with unique regions of neural activation, indicating that concerns about 'shape' itself are important to patients with AN, and that these misperceptions occur regardless of the actual body weight of the individual [7, 8].

It is necessary for eating disorder treatment research to not only determine the overall efficacy of a particular treatment, but to also identify factors that influence treatment response [9]. Distinguishing predictors that may be modifiable over the course of treatment is of significant importance in successful treatment outcome and the precise delivery of treatment services. Weight (i.e., the number on the scale) is highly relevant to the treatment of both adolescents and adults with AN. Family-based treatment (FBT), which is efficacious for treating adolescents with AN [10], considers weight restoration and re-feeding primary treatment targets, with little discussion topics outside of weight progress in the beginning sessions [11]. Additionally, cognitive-behavioral therapy for AN also prioritizes weight regain during treatment, including "weekly weighing" at every therapy session [12].

Given the focus of weight as a treatment target for patients with AN, it is possible that individuals who endorse heightened valuation of their weight compared to their shape may experience greater difficulty tolerating weight gain, resulting in poorer treatment outcomes. Moreover, given that early weight gain in treatment predicts better outcomes for adolescents with AN [13, 14], understanding factors that may impact treatment engagement and response may inform subpopulations for whom treatment tailoring may be indicated. A better understanding of the clinical importance of shape and weight concerns in this population may help to improve treatment efficacy.

Using data from a two-site randomized controlled trial (RCT) of treatment for adolescents with AN, the purpose of this study was to examine differences in treatment outcome between individuals whose primary concern was weight compared to those whose primary concern was shape. Though reviews of the psychometric properties of the EDE and EDE-Q show that data do not support a distinction between the weight concern and shape concern subscales, the prognostic clinical value of evaluating these as separate concepts has yet to be explored. To our knowledge, this is the first evaluation of weight concern and shape concerns as separate constructs predicting treatment outcome for individuals with AN. Additionally, to our knowledge, this is the first evaluation examining the predictive clinical utility of separating weight concern items and shape concern items during the eating disorder symptom assessment process. We hypothesized that adolescents who endorsed heightened valuation of their weight compared to their shape would experience greater difficulty tolerating weight gain, resulting in poorer treatment outcome.

Method

Participants & procedure

Data were drawn from a two-site RCT (Chicago and Stanford) that compared family-based treatment (FBT) and adolescent-focused therapy (AFT) [10]. Adolescents ($N = 121$) meeting DSM-IV criteria for AN, excluding the criterion requiring the absence of at least three menstrual cycles, were randomly assigned to one of the two treatments. Each treatment was delivered for a total of 24 h (twenty-four 1-h sessions for adolescents receiving FBT, thirty-two 45-min sessions for adolescents receiving AFT) over 12 months. In-person study assessments were conducted at baseline and end of treatment (EOT).

For the purposes of the current analyses, participants considered having 'primary weight concern' (PWC; $n = 36$, 30 %) endorsed higher baseline EDE Weight Concern subscale scores than Shape Concern subscale scores; participants considered having 'primary shape concern' (PSC; $n = 72$, 60 %) endorsed higher baseline EDE Shape Concern subscale scores than Weight Concern subscale scores. Additionally, for the purposes of this study, participants with equal weight and shape concern subscale scores ($n = 13$, 10 %) were excluded from the analyses.

At end of treatment, normal weight was defined as ≥ 95 % of expected body weight for sex, age, and height. Treatment remission was defined as achieving both normal weight and a global EDE score within 1 standard deviation (SD) of published norms (1.59) [15, 16]. Full disclosure of the purpose of the study, the benefits and risks to patients' participation, and the confidential nature of information obtained during the study is explained to participants per ethics board requirements. The Institutional Review Boards at both sites approved this study, and all adolescents and at least one parent gave informed assent and consent, respectively. Further details of this the study design and main outcome findings are reported elsewhere [10].

Measures

Weight

Weight in pounds was objectively measured by trained assessors at baseline, at every treatment session, and at EOT. At each study assessment, participants were weighed wearing a hospital gown on a balance-beam scale that was regularly recalibrated.

Eating Disorder Examination (EDE)

The EDE is a semi-structured interview used to assess eating disorder pathology [17]. The EDE (version 12.0) was administered at baseline and EOT. The EDE was used to assess psychological and behavioral symptoms of an eating disorder, yielding four subscales (Restraint, Eating Concern, Shape Concern, Weight Concern) and a global score, which indicates level of overall eating disorder pathology. Scores range from 0 to 6, with higher scores indicating greater severity of eating disorder pathology. The EDE has demonstrated good reliability and validity and has been utilized in many studies of youth with eating disorders [5].

Analysis plan

Analyses were conducted using SPSS Version 22.0. Chi-square tests were used to evaluate between-group differences at baseline between PWC and PSC groups on demographic variables and on treatment condition. Treatment outcome at the end of treatment (i.e., achieving remission or achieving normal weight) was compared by PWC or PSC group using chi-square tests. Logistic regression was used to evaluate the interaction between PWC versus PSC and treatment condition on the proportion of participants achieving remission or achieving normal weight at end of treatment. *P*-values less than 0.05 were considered statistically significant.

Results

Participants were mostly females (89.8 %) with a mean age of 14.47 years ($SD = 1.6$). Participants identified as 75 % non-Hispanic Whites ($n = 81$), 8.3 % Hispanic White ($n = 9$), 11.1 % Asian ($n = 12$), and 5.6 % as Other ($n = 6$). Mean percent expected body weight was 80.6 % ($SD = 3.58$) using Centers for Disease Control and Prevention growth charts. The average duration of illness was 11.9 months ($SD = 12.0$). Mean difference in 'shape concern' scores and 'weight concern' scores on the EDE among participants was 0.89 ($SD = 0.31$). Adolescents with PWC did not differ significantly from those with PSC on age, gender, racial/ethnic minority status, duration of illness (months), baseline percent expected body weight, baseline EDE global score, treatment dropout status, or prior hospitalization ($ps > .165$) (See Table 1).

No significant differences were found at baseline between the PWC and PSC groups by treatment condition ($\chi^2 = 0.464$, $p = .496$). There were no significant differences between the two groups across treatments in the proportion of participants achieving remission ($\chi^2 = 0.702$, $p = .482$; PWC achieving remission $n = 12$, 33.3 %, PSC achieving remission $n = 18$, 30 %) or normal weight ($\chi^2 = 0.204$, $p = .659$; PWC achieving normal weight $n = 13$, 42 %, PSC achieving normal weight $n = 23$, 31.1 %). The interaction between the effect of PWC/PSC group status and treatment condition was not associated with achieving remission (Exp(B) = 0.495, $p = .457$) or normal weight (Exp(B) = 1.300, $p = .775$) post treatment.

A secondary analysis was conducted among participants with clinically-significant baseline weight and shape pathology. Specifically, analyses were conducted among the subset of participants ($N = 26$) with an EDE score greater than or equal to 4 on either the weight concern subscale ($n = 5$) or the shape concern subscale ($n = 21$), given that a score of 4 on a subscale is considered clinically significant [18, 19]. Mean difference in EDE 'shape concern' and 'weight concern' scores among this subset was 1.14. There were no significant differences

Table 1 Baseline and demographic variables

	Primary Weight Concern ($n = 36$)	Primary Shape Concern ($n = 72$)	Statistic	*p*-value
	Mean (SD)	Mean (SD)		
Age (in years)	14.17 (1.483)	14.62 (1.626)	$t(106) = 1.39$	.165
Duration Ill (mo)	11.64 (9.04)	12.09 (13.28)	$t(106) = .184$	.855
Percent EBW	80.91 (3.90)	80.43 (3.43)	$t(106) = -.646$	.520
	n (%)	*n* (%)		
Female	32 (90.2 %)	65 (88.9 %)	$\chi^2(1) = 0.051$	.532
White	26 (72.2 %)	55 (76.4 %)	$\chi^2(1) = 0.431$	.934
Prior Hospitalization	17 (47.2 %)	32 (44.4 %)	$\chi^2(1) = 0.075$	.472
Treatment Dropout	9 (25 %)	18 (25 %)	$\chi^2(1) = 0.589$	.745

Key: *mo* months, *EBW* Expected Body Weight

between these two groups across treatments in the proportion of participants achieving remission ($\chi^2 = 1.250$, $p = .264$) or normal weight ($\chi^2 = 1.544$, $p = .214$).

Discussion

The current study was an exploratory analysis, examining weight concern and shape concern as separate constructs predicting remission from eating disorder treatment among adolescents with AN. Given the importance of overvaluation of shape and weight as a key clinical characteristic of AN, it is of clinical significance to understand the ways in which these concerns may separately influence the outcome of treatment. Results of this study revealed there were no differences in demographics, weight, or eating disorder pathology between adolescents who presented to treatment with primary weight concern versus with primary shape concern, nor was there a significant difference in clinical outcomes (i.e., remission, normal weight) at the end of treatment. Further, the interaction between treatment group did not moderate the effect of primary weight versus shape concerns on achieving remission or normal weight at end of treatment. Thus, results of this study suggest no significant differences between the two constructs on predicting treatment results among adolescents with AN and indicate that individuals with higher weight concerns are as likely as those with higher shape concerns to have good treatment outcome.

Results of the study were contrary to the hypothesis that, given the focus on weight regain as a treatment target for AN, individuals who place a higher value on weight than shape may have less successful treatment outcomes. Although weight (i.e., the specific number on the scale) restoration is often a primary treatment target for adolescents with AN, it is possible that changes in weight are quickly associated with changes in shape, reducing the prognostic utility of these two constructs to differentiate clinical outcomes by the end of treatment. Further research to understand changes over the course of treatment in weight concerns and shape concerns may be beneficial for informing whether temporal differences impact treatment outcome.

Study results also contribute to the assessment literature on weight versus shape concerns regarding the prognostic value of assessing these features as separate constructs. Although the original validation study of the EDE showed that the weight concern and shape concern subscales could not be combined despite being closely associated with one another [20], several factor analytic studies have failed to differentiate between a shape concern factor and weight concern factor on the EDE and EDE-Q [5], which is consistent with our study findings. Thus, results from the present study further inform assessment issues by calling into question whether it is clinically meaningful to assess shape concern and weight concern as separate constructs in terms of its prognostic value for AN treatment outcomes.

There are several limitations of the current study that should be noted. First, this study defined primary weight concern and primary shape concern as any difference between these two subscales, regardless of the magnitude of this distinction, as the limited sample size of adolescents in the study precluded setting a more conservative distinction between the groups. Accordingly, the mean difference of 0.89 (SD = 0.31) was small, which may have limited the capacity to observe differences in outcome between these groups. However, this also suggests that the mean difference between weight and shape concern tends to be low, which is in keeping with a unified weight and shape concern construct. Additionally, the current study examined a treatment-seeking sample of adolescents with AN, and thus study results may not generalize to other eating disorder samples.

Conclusions

Despite these limitations, this study represents the first to examine whether weight concern and shape concern differentially impact treatment outcome for adolescents with AN. This study makes a clinical contribution in understanding the influence that weight concern and shape concern have as two separate components of AN, and suggests that treatment outcomes are comparable between adolescents who overvalue one or the other. Further, it challenges the clinical relevance of assessing weight concern and shape concern as separate constructs.

Abbreviations

AFT: adolescent-focused therapy; AN: anorexia nervosa; DSM-5: Diagnostic and Statistical Manual for Mental Disorders; EDE: Eating Disorder Examination; EOT: end of treatment; PSC: primary shape concern; PWC: primary weight concern; RCT: Randomized control trial; SD: standard deviation.

Competing interests

Dr. Daniel Le Grange and Dr. James Lock receive consultant fees from the Training Institute for Child and Adolescent Eating Disorders, LLC. Dr. Le Grange and Dr. Lock also receive royalties from Guilford Press and Routledge.

Authors' contributions

CEB conceived of the study and helped draft the manuscript. AEK, SF, SO, and AG helped draft the manuscript. ECA, AEK, and SF provided statistical support. JL and DLG served as primary investigators of the RCT and helped draft the manuscript. All authors read and approved the final manuscript.

Funding

Funding for this work was supported by: T32 MH082761, T32 HS000078, R01-MH-070621, and R01-MH-070620.

Author details

[1]Department of Psychology, George Mason University, Fairfax, VA, USA. [2]Department of Medicine, The University of Chicago, Chicago, IL, USA. [3]Department of Psychiatry, University of California, San Francisco, CA, USA. [4]Department of Psychiatry and Behavioral Neuroscience, The University of Chicago Medicine, Chicago, IL, USA. [5]Department of Psychiatry and Behavioral Sciences, Stanford University, Palo Alto, CA, USA. [6]Department of Psychiatry and Department of Pediatrics, University of California, San Francisco, CA, USA.

References

1. Attia E. Anorexia nervosa: Current status and future directions. Annu Rev Med. 2010;61:425–35.
2. American Psychiatric Association. Diagnostic and statistical manual of mental disorders (5th ed.). Washington, DC: American Psychiatric Association. 2013.
3. Cooper Z, Fairburn CG. The Eating Disorder Examination: a semi-structured interview for the assessment of the specific psychopathology of eating disorders. Int J Eat Disorder. 1987;6:1–8.
4. Carrad I, Rebetez M, Mobbs O, Van der Linden M. Factor structure of a French version of the eating disorder examination-questionnaire among women with and without binge eating disorder symptoms. Eat Weight Disorder. 2015;20:137–44.
5. Berg KC, Peterson CB, Frazier P, Crow SJ. Psychometric evaluation of the eating disorder examination and eating disorder examination-questionnaire: a systematic review of the literature. Int J Eat Disorder. 2012;45:428–38.
6. Gaudio S, Quattrocchi CC. Neural basis of a multidimensional model of body image distortion in anorexia nervosa. Neurosci Biobehav Rev. 2012; 36(8):1839–47.
7. Sachdev P, Mondraty N, Wen W, Gulliford K. Brains of anorexia nervosa patients process self-images differently from non-self images: an fMRI study. Neuropsychologia. 2008;46(8):2161–8.
8. Mohr HM, Zimmermann J, Roder C, Lenz C, Overbeck G, Grabhorn R. Separating two components of body image in anorexia nervosa using fMRI. Psychol Med. 2010;40(9):1519-29.
9. Kraemer HC, Wilson GT, Fairburn CG, Agras WS. Mediators and moderators of treatment effects in randomized clinical trials. Arch Gen Psychiatry. 2002; 59(10):877–83.
10. Lock J, Le Grange D, Agras S, Moye A, Bryson S, Jo B. Randomized clinical trial comparing family-based treatment to adolescent focused therapy for adolescents with anorexia nervosa. Arch Gen Psychiatry. 2010;67:1025–32.
11. Lock J, Le Grange D. Treatment Manual for Anorexia Nervosa, Second Edition A Family-Based Approach. New York, New York: Guilford Press; 2013.
12. Murphy R, Straebler S, Cooper Z, Fairburn C. Cognitive Behavioral Therapy for Eating Disorders. Psychiatr Clin North Am. 2010. 33(3): 611–27
13. Accurso EC, Ciao AC, Fitzsimmons-Craft EE, Lock JD, Le Grange D. Is weight gain really a catalyst for broader recovery?: The impact of weight gain on psychological symptoms in the treatment of adolescent anorexia nervosa. Behav Res Ther. 2014;56:1.
14. Le Grange D, Lock J, Accurso EC, Agras SW, Darcy A, Forsberg S, et al. Relapse from remission at two-to four-year follow-up in two treatments for adolescent anorexia nerovsa. J Am Acad Child Adolesc Psychiatry. 2014;53(11):1162–7.
15. Couturier J, Lock J. (2006) What is remission in adolescent anorexia nervosa? A review of various conceptualizations and quantitative analysis. Int J Eat Disord. 2006;39(3):175–83.
16. Couturier J, Lock J. What is recovery in adolescent anorexia nervosa? Int J Eat Disord. 2006;39(7):550–5.
17. Fairburn CG, Cooper Z. The Eating Disorder Examination. In: Fairburn CG, Wilson GT, editors. Binge Eating: Nature, Assessment and Treatment. New York: Guilford; 1993. p. 317–60.
18. Mond JM, Hay PJ, Rodgers B, Owen C. Eating disorder examination questionnaire (EDE-Q): Norms for young adult women. Behav Res Ther. 2006;44:53–62.
19. Carter JC, Stewart DA, Fairburn CG. Eating Disorder Examination Quesetionnaire: Norms for young adolescent girls. Behav Res Ther. 2001;39:625–32.
20. Cooper Z, Cooper PJ, Fairburn CG. The validity of the eating disorders examination and its subscales. Br J Psychiatry. 1989;154:807–12.

Permissions

All chapters in this book were first published in JED, by BioMed Central; hereby published with permission under the Creative Commons Attribution License or equivalent. Every chapter published in this book has been scrutinized by our experts. Their significance has been extensively debated. The topics covered herein carry significant findings which will fuel the growth of the discipline. They may even be implemented as practical applications or may be referred to as a beginning point for another development.

The contributors of this book come from diverse backgrounds, making this book a truly international effort. This book will bring forth new frontiers with its revolutionizing research information and detailed analysis of the nascent developments around the world.

We would like to thank all the contributing authors for lending their expertise to make the book truly unique. They have played a crucial role in the development of this book. Without their invaluable contributions this book wouldn't have been possible. They have made vital efforts to compile up to date information on the varied aspects of this subject to make this book a valuable addition to the collection of many professionals and students.

This book was conceptualized with the vision of imparting up-to-date information and advanced data in this field. To ensure the same, a matchless editorial board was set up. Every individual on the board went through rigorous rounds of assessment to prove their worth. After which they invested a large part of their time researching and compiling the most relevant data for our readers.

The editorial board has been involved in producing this book since its inception. They have spent rigorous hours researching and exploring the diverse topics which have resulted in the successful publishing of this book. They have passed on their knowledge of decades through this book. To expedite this challenging task, the publisher supported the team at every step. A small team of assistant editors was also appointed to further simplify the editing procedure and attain best results for the readers.

Apart from the editorial board, the designing team has also invested a significant amount of their time in understanding the subject and creating the most relevant covers. They scrutinized every image to scout for the most suitable representation of the subject and create an appropriate cover for the book.

The publishing team has been an ardent support to the editorial, designing and production team. Their endless efforts to recruit the best for this project, has resulted in the accomplishment of this book. They are a veteran in the field of academics and their pool of knowledge is as vast as their experience in printing. Their expertise and guidance has proved useful at every step. Their uncompromising quality standards have made this book an exceptional effort. Their encouragement from time to time has been an inspiration for everyone.

The publisher and the editorial board hope that this book will prove to be a valuable piece of knowledge for researchers, students, practitioners and scholars across the globe.

List of Contributors

Kristy Zwickert and Elizabeth Rieger
Research School of Psychology (Building 39), Australian National University, Canberra, ACT 0200, Australia

Marisol Perez and Ashley Kroon Van Diest
Department of Psychology, Texas A&M University, 4235 TAMU, College Station, TX 77843-4235, USA

Shannon Cutts
Mentor CONNECT, Houston, Texas, USA

Julia K Moore
Princess Margaret Hospital for Children, Perth, Australia
The School of Paediatrics and Child Health, University of Western Australia, Perth, Australia

Hunna J Watson
Princess Margaret Hospital for Children, Perth, Australia
Centre for Clinical Interventions, Perth, Australia
The School of Paediatrics and Child Health, University of Western Australia, Perth, Australia
The School of Psychology and Speech Pathology, Curtin University, Perth, Australia

Emily Harper and Julie McCormack
Princess Margaret Hospital for Children, Perth, Australia

Thinh Nguyen
The School of Psychiatry and Clinical Neurosciences, University of Western Australia, Perth, Australia

Alina Coman
Regional Eating Disorders Service (RASP), Division of Mental Health and Addiction, Oslo University Hospital-Ullevål, P.O. Box 4956 Nydalen, Oslo N-0424, Norway
Centre for Medical Ethics, University of Oslo, P.O. Box 1130, Blindern, Oslo N-0318, Norway

Finn Skårderud
Regional Eating Disorders Service (RASP), Division of Mental Health and Addiction, Oslo University Hospital-Ullevål, P.O. Box 4956 Nydalen, Oslo N-0424, Norway
Institute of Special Needs Education, University of Oslo, Sognsveien 250, Oslo N-0863, Norway

Deborah L Reas
Regional Eating Disorders Service (RASP), Division of Mental Health and Addiction, Oslo University Hospital-Ullevål, P.O. Box 4956 Nydalen, Oslo N-0424, Norway

Bjørn M Hofmann
Centre for Medical Ethics, University of Oslo, P.O. Box 1130, Blindern, Oslo N-0318, Norway

Katrina Kostro
Columbia University Medical Center, New York, NY, USA
Weill Cornell Medical College, New York, NY, USA

Jessica B Lerman
Weill Cornell Medical College, New York, NY, USA

Evelyn Attia
Columbia University Medical Center, New York, NY, USA
Weill Cornell Medical College, New York, NY, USA

Janet Treasure and Ulrike Schmidt
Department of Psychological Medicine, King's College London, Institute of Psychiatry, The Basement, P059, 103 Denmark Hill, London SE5 8AF, UK

Camilla Lindvall Dahlgren
Regional Department for Eating Disorders, Division of Mental Health and Addiction, Oslo University Hospital, Ullevål HF, Oslo, Norway
Department of Psychiatry, Centre for Research on Eating Disorders at Oxford (CREDO), University of Oxford, Warneford Hospital, Oxford, UK

Øyvind Rø
Regional Department for Eating Disorders, Division of Mental Health and Addiction, Oslo University Hospital, Ullevål HF, Oslo, Norway
Division of Mental Health and Addiction, Institute of Clinical Medicine, University of Oslo, Oslo, Norway

Karina L Allen
1Telethon Institute for Child Health Research, Centre for Child Health Research, The University of Western Australia, PO Box 855, West Perth, WA, Western Australia
2School of Psychology, The University of Western Australia, Crawley, Western Australia

Ross D Crosby
Department of Clinical Neuroscience, University of North Dakota School of Medicine and Health Sciences, Fargo, North Dakota, USA
Department of Biostatistics, Neuropsychiatric Research Institute, Fargo, North Dakota, USA

Wendy H Oddy
Telethon Institute for Child Health Research, Centre for Child Health Research, The University of Western Australia, PO Box 855, West Perth, WA, Western Australia

Susan M Byrne
School of Psychology, The University of Western Australia, Crawley, Western Australia

Sau F Leung
School of Nursing, The Hong Kong Polytechnic University, Hung Hom, Kowloon, Hong Kong, China

Joyce LC Ma
Department of Social Work, The Chinese University of Hong Kong, Shatin, New Territories, Hong Kong, China

Janice Russell
Discipline of Psychiatry, Faculty of Medicine, Sydney Medical School, University of Sydney, Sydney, NSW 2006, Australia

Caroline Bentley and Kassandra Gratwick-Sarll
Research School of Psychology, Australian National University, Canberra, ACT 0200, Australia

Jonathan Mond
Research School of Psychology, Australian National University, Canberra, ACT 0200, Australia
Department of Psychology, Macquarie University, Sydney, Australia

Liv Sand, Mari Hysing and Kjell Morten Stormar
Regional Centre for Child and Youth Mental Health and Welfare, Uni Health, PO Box 7810, N-5020 Bergen, Norway

Bryan Lask
Gt Ormond St Hospital for Children NHS Foundation Trust, Great Ormond Street, London WC1N 3JH, UK

Sarah Young, Paul Rhodes and Stephen Touyz
Clinical Psychology Unit, Mackie Building K01, School of Psychology, University of Sydney, Sydney, NSW 2006, Australia

Phillipa Hay
School of Medicine, University of Western Sydney, Locked Bag 1797, Penrith, NSW 2751, Australia
School of Medicine, James Cook University, Townsville, North Queensland, Australia

Michael Wm MacGregor and Paige Lamborn
University of Saskatchewan, Saskatoon, Saskatchewan, Canada

Matilda E Nowakowski and Stephanie Cassin
Department of Psychology, Ryerson University, 350 Victoria Street, Toronto, Ontario M5B 2K3, Canada

Traci McFarlane
Department of Psychology, Ryerson University, 350 Victoria Street, Toronto, Ontario M5B 2K3, Canada
Eating Disorder Program, The Toronto General Hospital, 200 Elizabeth Street, Toronto, Ontario M5G 2C4, Canada

Karina L Allen
Telethon Institute for Child Health Research, Centre for Child Health Research, The University of Western Australia, PO Box 855, West Perth, WA, Australia
School of Psychology, The University of Western Australia, Crawley, WA, Australia

Lisa Y Gibson
Telethon Institute for Child Health Research, Centre for Child Health Research, The University of Western Australia, PO Box 855, West Perth, WA, Australia

Elizabeth A Davis
Telethon Institute for Child Health Research, Centre for Child Health Research, The University of Western Australia, PO Box 855, West Perth, WA, Australia
Department of Endocrinology and Diabetes, Princess Margaret Hospital for Children, Subiaco, Australia

Neil J McLean and Susan M Byrne
School of Psychology, The University of Western Australia, Crawley, WA, Australia

Sarah Fogarty
School of Medicine, Western Sydney University, Richmond, Australia
National Institute of Complementary Medicine, Western Sydney University, PO Box 2002, Homebush West, NSW 2140, Australia

Lucie M. Ramjan
School of Nursing and Midwifery, Western Sydney University, Richmond, Australia
Centre for Applied Nursing Research, Ingham Institute of Applied Medical Research, Richmond, Australia

Jennifer Bibb
Mental Health CSU, Austin Health, 145 Studley Road, Heidelberg 3084, Victoria, Australia
National Music Therapy Research Unit, Melbourne Conservatorium of Music, University of Melbourne, 151 Barry Street, Parkville 3010, Victoria, Australia

David Castle
The Body Image & Eating Disorders Treatment & Recovery Service (BETRS), St Vincent's Hospital, 104 Studley Park Rd, Kew 3101Victoria, Australia
Department of Psychiatry, University of Melbourne, Parkville 3010, Victoria, Australia

Richard Newton
Mental Health CSU, Austin Health, 145 Studley Road, Heidelberg 3084, Victoria, Australia
The Body Image & Eating Disorders Treatment & Recovery Service (BETRS), St Vincent's Hospital, 104 Studley Park Rd, Kew 3101Victoria, Australia
Department of Psychiatry, University of Melbourne, Parkville 3010, Victoria, Australia

Kelly Ann Zainal, Beth Renwick, Alexandra Keyes, Anna Lose, Martha Kenyon, Hannah DeJong, Hannah Broadbent, Janet Treasure and Ulrike Schmidt
Section of Eating Disorders, Department of Psychological Medicine, Institute of Psychiatry, Psychology and Neuroscience, King's College London, PO Box 59SE5 8AF London, UK

Lucy Serpell
Hope Wing, Porters Avenue Health Centre, North East London Foundation Trust, Dagenham, Essex, UK

Eating Disorders Research Group, Research Dept. of Clinical, Educational & Health Psychology, University College London, London, UK

Lorna Richards and Eric Johnson-Sabine
The Phoenix Wing, St Ann's Hospital, Barnett, Enfield and Haringey Mental Health Trust, Tottenham, London, UK

Nicky Boughton and Linette Whitehead
Oxford Adult Eating Disorder Service, Cotswold House, Warneford Hospital, Oxford NHS Foundation Trust, Oxford, UK

Liv-Jorunn Kolnes
Norwegian School of Sport Sciences, PB 4014 Ullevål Stadion, 0806 Oslo, Norway

Catherine E. Byrne and Sarah Fischer
Department of Psychology, George Mason University, Fairfax, VA, USA

Andrea E. Kass
Department of Medicine, The University of Chicago, Chicago, IL, USA

Erin C. Accurso
Department of Psychiatry, University of California, San Francisco, CA, USA

Setareh O'Brien and Alexandria Goodyear
Department of Psychiatry and Behavioral Neuroscience, The University of Chicago Medicine, Chicago, IL, USA

James Lock
Department of Psychiatry and Behavioral Sciences, Stanford University, Palo Alto, CA, USA

Daniel Le Grange
Department of Psychiatry and Department of Pediatrics, University of California, San Francisco, CA, USA

Index